Wrist Arthroscopy

William B. Geissler, MD

Professor and Chief, Arthroscopy and Sports Medicine
Professor, Division of Hand and Upper Extremity Surgery
Director, Hand/Upper Extremity Fellowship Program
Department of Orthopaedic Surgery and Rehabilitation
University of Mississippi Medical Center
Jackson, Mississippi

Editor

Wrist Arthroscopy

Foreword by Terry L. Whipple, MD, FACS

With 217 Illustrations in 321 Parts, 44 in Full Color

DVD
INCLUDED

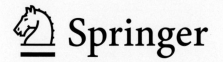

Springer

William B. Geissler, MD
Professor and Chief, Arthroscopy and Sports Medicine
Professor, Division of Hand and Upper Extremity Surgery
Director, Hand/Upper Extremity Fellowship Program
Department of Orthopaedic Surgery and Rehabilitation
University of Mississippi Medical Center
Jackson, MS 39216
USA

Library of Congress Cataloging-in-Publication Data
Wrist arthroscopy / [edited by] William Geissler.
    p. ; cm.
    Includes bibliographical references and index.
    ISBN 0-387-20897-6 (h/c : alk. paper)
    1. Wrist—Endoscopic surgery. 2. Wrist—Surgery. 3. Arthroscopy. I. Geissler, William.
    [DNLM: 1. Wrist—surgery. 2. Arthroscopy—methods. WE 830 W95512 2004]
    RD559.W7514 2004
    617.5'74—dc22   2004041828

ISBN 0-387-20897-6   Printed on acid-free paper.

Printed in China.   (MP/EVB)

9 8 7 6 5 4 3 2 1   SPIN 10941881

springeronline.com

Foreword

It is a great pleasure to introduce this techniques book and accompanying DVD on arthroscopic surgery of the wrist. Dr. William B. Geissler, uniquely qualified to address the diagnosis and treatment of wrist disorders, has devoted himself to teaching others the advantages and techniques of applying minimally invasive surgical approaches to this complex joint. He has assembled an impressive team of accomplished contributors; thus the reader will find it enjoyable, informative and particularly thorough as a reference for hand surgery.

Dr. Geissler has organized the text and DVD to the practitioner's advantage. Arthroscopic anatomy is discussed in detail. Specific diagnoses are addressed separately throughout. Newer technologies such as laser energy and electrothermal devices are addressed to illuminate their potential application in the wrist.

Arthroscopy has provided new, minimally invasive access to smaller joints as well. The distal radioulnar joint of the wrist and even the carpometacarpal joint of the thumb can now be evaluated and surgically treated in many cases by arthroscopy.

For those who are looking to master the newer surgical approaches to the hand and wrist, or for those seeking guidance for a specific surgical procedure for the wrist, this book, with an accompanying DVD, constitutes an excellent source. It surely represents the current state of the art for arthroscopic surgery of the wrist.

Terry L. Whipple, MD, FACS

Preface

Arthroscopy has revolutionized the practice of orthopedics by providing the technical capability to examine and treat intra-articular abnormalities directly. The development of wrist arthroscopy was a natural evolutionary progression from the successful application of arthroscopy to other, larger joints. The wrist is a labyrinth of eight carpal bones and multiple articular surfaces, with both intrinsic and extrinsic ligaments and a triangular fibrocartilage complex—all within a 5-cm interval. This perplexing joint continues to challenge clinicians with an array of potential diagnoses and treatments. Wrist arthroscopy has significantly advanced our knowledge and understanding of this complex joint. This is an exciting time in the field; there has been considerable growth since pioneers, such as Terry L. Whipple, MD, Gary Poehling, MD, and A. Lee Osterman, MD, reported their original descriptions of the techniques they developed from reviewing the anatomy of the wrist.

The indications and techniques for wrist arthroscopy have continued to expand since Terry L. Whipple wrote his original textbook on arthroscopic surgery of the wrist approximately 12 years ago. Much has changed as more surgeons have been exposed to wrist arthroscopy and have contributed to the field, and as arthroscopy has been applied to the thumb and smaller joint areas of the hand.

This is truly an international text. Recognized experts from around the world have contributed their latest techniques and advances in wrist arthroscopy. These authors describe their arthroscopic techniques in detail and include tips and tricks to make the procedure easier for all of us to perform. This book and DVD contain updates on commonly performed wrist arthroscopy procedures, such as debridement of tears of the triangular fibrocartilage complex (TFCC) and management of carpal instability and distal radius fractures. It also includes the very latest descriptions of arthroscopic management of acute scaphoid fractures and selected nonunions, including arthroscopic bone grafting, arthroscopic excision of both volar and dorsal wrist ganglia, new techniques in arthroscopic repair of peripheral TFCC tears, and the application of arthroscopy and debridement to arthrofibrosis of the wrist.

This book, with an accompanying DVD is intended for the surgeon who is just beginning to develop an interest in wrist arthroscopy, as well as for the experienced arthroscopist who wants to refresh his memory before performing a specific arthroscopic procedure. Subjects for the beginner include how to evaluate the painful wrist; when to order imaging studies and which studies are appropriate; understanding the complexities and mechanics of carpal instability; and general arthroscopic anatomy and setup. Complex topics such as arthroscopic proximal carpectomy, electrothermal shrinkage, and arthroscopy of the thumb carpometacarpal joints and the small joints of the hand are discussed in detail for the wrist arthroscopy expert.

ACKNOWLEDGMENTS

I would like to acknowledge a number of those who have contributed to this textbook. First, I would like to thank Terry L. Whipple, MD, who initially exposed me to the techniques of wrist arthroscopy. He demonstrated to me how precise and delicate arthroscopic surgery of the wrist is expertly performed. Next, thanks to Alan E. Freeland, MD, my mentor, friend, and colleague, who continues to instruct me in hand surgery and guide my career. Thanks also to Janis Freeland, RN, my nurse, and Tammy Chamblee, her assistant, who really run the show; Susan Fleming, who tirelessly works to keep things organized for me; Patti Corder, RN, Margie Ross, RN, Tracy Wall, RN, and Macy Gunter, ORT, and the other surgical nurses at the Methodist Rehabilitation Center and University Medical Center, who work long hours in the operating room. I also very much want to thank Merry Post for her excellent command of the English language and her constant, gentle reminders to finish the textbook—onward and upward. Thank you to Susan and Rachel Leigh, who have taught me strength and courage and every once in a while to take time to stop and smell the roses. Special thanks go to Stryker Endoscopy and Acumed Corporation for their generous support for the DVD. Most of all, I want to thank my national and international experts for sharing their latest techniques with us so that we all may continue to advance in the field of wrist arthroscopy.

William B. Geissler, MD

Contents

Contributors

Edward Akelman, MD
Professor and Vice-Chairman, Department of Orthopaedics, Brown Medical School; Chief, Division of Hand/Upper Extremity and Microvascular Surgery, Rhode Island Hospital, Providence, RI, 02905, USA

Scott Allen, MD
Clinical Instructor, Department of Orthopaedics, Brown Medical School, Providence, RI 02905, USA

Andrea Atzei, MD
Associate Professor of Hand Surgery and Reconstructive Microsurgery, Clinical Coordinator, Hand Surgery Unit, Department of Orthopaedic Surgery, University of Verona, 37100 Verona, Italy

Ryan A. Beekman, MD
Fellow, Hand and Microvascular Surgery, Department of Orthopaedic Surgery, Columbia University College of Physicians and Surgeons, New York Presbyterian Hospital, New York, NY 10032, USA

Richard A. Berger, MD, PhD
Professor, Department of Orthopaedic Surgery and Anatomy, Mayo Graduate College of Medicine; Consultant in Hand and Orthopaedic Surgery, Mayo Clinic, Rochester, MN 55905, USA

Matthew A. Bernstein, MD
Berrington Orthopaedic Specialists, Hoffman Estates, IL 60195, USA

James Chow, MD
Director, Orthopaedic Center of Southern Illinois, Clinical Assistant Professor, Southern Illinois University School of Medicine, Mt. Vernon, IL 62864, USA

Mark S. Cohen, MD
Associate Professor of Hand, Wrist, and Elbow Surgery, Department of Orthopaedics, Rush Medical Center, Midwest Orthopaedics, Chicago, IL 60612, USA

Randall W. Culp, MD
Associate Professor of Orthopaedic, Hand, and Microsurgery, Thomas Jefferson University, King of Prussia, PA 19078, USA

Scott G. Edwards, MD
Associate Professor, Orthopaedic Surgery, Georgetown University, Alexandria, VA 22310, USA

Tracy Fairplay, PT
Private Professional Hand Therapy Practice, Bologna, Italy; Hand Therapy Consultant, Department of Functional Rehabilitation and Hand Surgery, Policlinico di Moderna, 40137 Bologna, Italy

Alan E. Freeland, MD
Professor of Hand and Wrist Surgery, Department of Orthopaedic Surgery and
Rehabilitation, University of Mississippi Medical Center, Jackson, MS 39216,
USA

William B. Geissler, MD
Professor and Chief, Arthroscopy and Sports Medicine, Professor, Division
of Hand and Upper Extremity Surgery, Director, Hand/Upper Extremity
Fellowship Program, Department of Orthopaedic Surgery and Rehabilitation,
University of Mississippi Medical Center, Jackson, MS 39216, USA

Gregory J. Hanker, MD
Assistant Clinical Professor of Plastic and Reconstructive Surgery, University
of Southern California, Southern California Orthopaedic Institute, Van Nuys,
CA 91405, USA

Thomas B. Hughes, Jr., MD
Clinical Instructor, Orthopaedic Surgery, Drexel University School of
Medicine, Allegheny General Hospital, Pittsburgh, PA 15212, USA

David M. Kalainov, MD
Assistant Director, Clinical Orthopaedic Surgery, Northwestern University,
Feinberg School of Medicine, Northwestern Center for Orthopaedics, Chicago,
IL 60611, USA

Gary R. Kuzma, MD
Clinical Associate Professor, Hand Center of Greensboro, Bowman Gray
School of Medicine, Greensboro, NC 27405, USA

Jonathan H. Lee, MD
Research Fellow, Trauma Training Center, Department of Orthopaedic
Surgery, Columbia University College of Physicians and Surgeons, New York
Presbyterian Hospital, New York, NY 10032, USA

Tommy Lindau, MD, PhD
Assistant Professor of Orthopaedic Surgery, Hand Unit, Department of
Orthopedics, Lund University Hospital, 22185 Lund, Sweden

Riccardo Luchetti, MD
Associate Professor, Clinic of Plastic, Reconstructive and Hand Surgery,
Ancona University, Torrette Hospital; Department of Orthopaedics, Trauma-
tology and Surgery of the Hand, State Hospital, Republic of San Marino, 47900
Rimini, Italy

Christophe Mathoulin, MD
Head, Hand and Microsurgery Department, Hospital Tenon, Institut de la
Main, 75016 Paris, France

Greg A. Merrell, MD
Chief Resident, Department of Orthopaedic Surgery, Yale University School of
Medicine, New Haven, CT 06519, USA

Karl Michalko, MD
Assistant Professor, Department of Microsurgery, Plastic Surgery Division,
University of Rochester, Rochester, NY 14627, USA

Michael J. Moskal, MD
Clinical Instructor, Department of Orthopaedic Surgery, University of Washington, New Albany, IN 47150, USA

Daniel J. Nagle, MD
Professor, Clinical Orthopaedic Surgery, Northwestern University Medical School, Chicago, IL 60611, USA

Susan Nasser-Sharif, MD
Resident, Orthopaedic Surgery, Institut de la Main, 75016 Paris, France

A. Lee Osterman, MD
Professor of Orthopaedic and Hand Surgery, Chairman, Division of Hand Surgery, Thomas Jefferson University, King of Prussia, PA 19078, USA

Melvin P. Rosenwasser, MD
Robert E. Carroll Professor of Orthopaedic Surgery, Director of Hand and Orthopaedic Trauma Service, Columbia University College of Physicians and Surgeons, New York Presbyterian Hospital, New York, NY 10032, USA

David S. Ruch, MD
Associate Professor, Department of Orthopaedic Surgery, Co-Director, Hand Surgery Fellowship, Wake Forest University, Winston-Salem, NC 27157, USA

Felix H. Savoie III, MD
Clinical Associate Professor, Department of Orthopaedic Surgery, University of Mississippi Medical Center; Co-director, Upper Extremity Service, Mississippi Sports Medicine Orthopaedic Center, Jackson, MS 39202, USA

Sanjay K. Sharma, MD
Hand Fellow, Department of Orthopaedic Surgery, University of Washington School of Medicine, Seattle, WA 98195, USA

Walter H. Short, MD
Clinical Research Professor, Orthopedics, State University of New York Upstate Medical Institute for Human Performance, Syracuse, NY 13202, USA

Joseph F. Slade III, MD
Associate Professor of Orthopaedics and Rehabilitation, Director, Yale Hand and Upper Extremity Center, Yale University School of Medicine, New Haven, CT 06519, USA

Stephanie Sweet, MD
Clinical Assistant Professor, Department of Orthopaedic Surgery, Thomas Jefferson University, King of Prussia, PA 19078; Philadelphia Hand Center, Philadelphia, PA 19107, USA

Nathan L. Taylor, MD
Fellow, Hand and Microsurgery, Department of Orthopaedic Surgery, Columbia University College of Physicians and Surgeons, New York Presbyterian Hospital, New York, NY 10032, USA

Matthew M. Tomaino, MD
Chief of Microsurgery, Department of Orthopaedic Surgery, University of Pittsburgh Medical Center, Pittsburgh, PA 15213, USA

Thomas E. Trumble, MD
Professor, Orthopaedic Surgery, Chief, Hand and Microvascular Surgery
Service, University of Washington, Seattle, WA 98195, USA

Arnold-Peter C. Weiss, MD
Professor, Hand/Elbow Surgery and Microvascular Surgery, Department of
Orthopaedic Surgery, Brown Medical School, Providence, RI 02905, USA

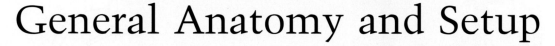

1

General Anatomy and Setup

Thomas B. Hughes, Jr., and Arnold-Peter C. Weiss

Though wrist arthroscopy was first introduced in 1979, it did not become an accepted method of diagnosis until the mid-1980s. As our technical abilities and technologies improved, wrist arthroscopy became a therapeutic modality as well as a diagnostic one.[1] It is useful in the diagnosis and treatment of triangular fibrocartilage complex (TFCC) pathology, ligamentous injuries, carpal instability, chondral defects, arthritis, carpal and radial fractures, ganglia, synovitis, and loose bodies. There is little doubt that arthroscopy will continue to play a larger role in the diagnosis and treatment of wrist pathology.

A complete understanding of the anatomy as well as appropriately sized instrumentation facilitates visualization. Precise placement of portals and adequate traction are required in wrist arthroscopy due to the small space available within the wrist joint. Once these techniques have been learned, arthroscopy can be used to treat a tremendous array of wrist pathology.

SURGICAL TECHNIQUE

Although arthroscopy without traction has been described, traction is usually recommended.[2] Several methods of traction are available. A traction tower allows precise modulation of the traction through a gearing mechanism (Figures 1.1 and 1.2). The forearm is stabilized while the traction is applied vertically through finger-traps, which permits 360-degree access to the wrist. If a traction tower is not available, a shoulder holder can be used to hold the arm vertically with a countertraction band around the arm proximal to the elbow. Weights can be added to the countertraction to adjust the tension. Finally, the wrist can be positioned horizontally on a hand table (Figure 1.3). Finger traps are placed on the index, long, and ring fingers, with 10 pounds of weight suspended over the end of the table. A bar or pulley is used to provide countertraction. The advantage of this last method is its simplicity and ease of setup.

The development of diagnostic and therapeutic indications for wrist arthroscopy would not have been possible without the development of smaller arthroscopy equipment in the 1980s. Small-bore arthroscopes and shavers are either 2.7 or 2.9 mm in diameter.[3] Arthroscopes are available with either a 30-degree or 70-degree viewing angle. An appropriately sized wrist probe is essential to fully examine the contents of the joint. A variety of hand-held graspers and punches have been developed that have expanded our ability to treat TFCC and ligament tears. A video printer is also helpful to document identified pathology and demonstrate treatments performed.

Thorough understanding of wrist anatomy is the most crucial aspect of wrist arthroscopy. Proper portal placement, identification of pathology, and successful treatment all rely on a complete understanding of the structures at risk and the ability to recognize the abnormalities present.[1,2,4–7] Placement of the portals either too proximal or too distal can cause articular cartilage injury. It is important to mark the portal sites *after* traction is applied, so that the relationships of surface landmarks are not altered. Palpation and marking of the index, middle, and ring metacarpal bases provide good landmarks for the distal edge of the carpus. The surgeon's fingertip can be rolled over the distal edge of the radius to identify the "soft spot" of the radiocarpal joint. Additionally the extensor digitorum communis, extensor pollicis longus, and extensor carpi ulnaris are all palpable if the wrist is not markedly swollen.

The portal locations are identified relative to the extensor compartments between which they pass (Figure 1.4A,B). The 3-4 portal is between the third and fourth compartment, and the cannula passes radial to the extensor digitorum communis tendon to the index finger and ulnar to the extensor pollicis longus tendon. Bony landmarks for this portal include Lister's tubercle, which is approximately 1 cm proximal to the wrist joint; and the radial aspect of the long finger, which is in line with the 3-4 portal. The surgeon should place a fingertip on Lister's tubercle and then roll the finger over the distal edge of the radius into the soft spot of the 3-4 portal. The surgeon who uses the fingernail for part of this last step can feel the extensor tendons on either side of the 3-4 portal (Figure 1.5).

The 4-5 portal passes ulnar to the extensor digitorum communis tendon to the ring finger and radial to the extensor digiti minimi tendon. The fourth compartment is palpated, and the finger is rolled over ulnarly over the tendons until it falls into the soft spot

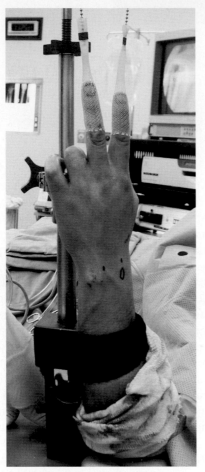

FIGURE 1.1. A specialized tower providing traction significantly aids in instrument placement.

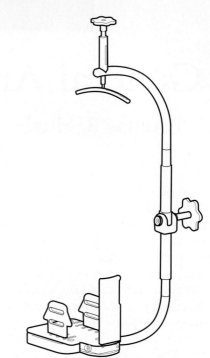

FIGURE 1.2. Diagram of a new traction tower designed by Geissler and Slade (Acumed, Beavertown, OR). The traction bar is off to the side which allows simultaneous arthroscopic and fluoroscopic evaluation of the wrist without having to move the wrist around the traction bar to obtain radiologic evaluation. Also, the traction tower can be set up so the surgeon may arthroscope or perform open surgery to the hand or wrist in either the vertical or horizontal position.

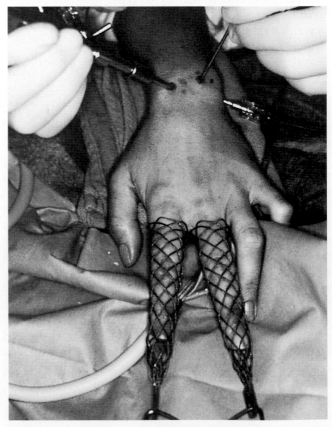

FIGURE 1.3. Alternatively, horizontal traction through finger traps and a pulley system can provide joint distraction. This type of set-up is especially useful for arthroscopic treatment of distal radius fractures.

on the ulnar side of the fourth compartment (Figure 1.6). Because of the radial inclination of the distal radius, the 4-5 portal is usually slightly proximal to the 3-4 portal (and *never* distal to the 3-4 portal). The 6-R portal lies radial to the extensor carpi ulnaris tendon and ulnar to the extensor digiti minimi tendon and can be found by moving the finger over the palpable fifth compartment. Alternatively, the surgeon can locate the prominent extensor carpi ulnaris (ECU) tendon of the sixth dorsal compartment and palpate the soft spot just radial to it and distal to the edge of the radius.

The 6-U portal is just ulnar to the extensor carpi ulnaris tendon, dorsal to the flexor carpi ulnaris, and just distal to the ulnar styloid. Any instruments placed in the 6-U portal should be introduced by "hugging" the underside of the ECU, thereby avoiding any potential injury to the ulnar neurovascular structures. Midcarpal portals can be placed on the radial and ulnar sides of the capitate approximately 1 cm distal to the 3-4 and 4-5 portals, respectively.[8]

The wrist joint is distended by the introduction of 3 to 5 mL of saline prior to trocar insertion. A separate inflow cannula can be placed throughout the procedure to keep a constant pressure or flow of the irri-

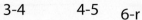

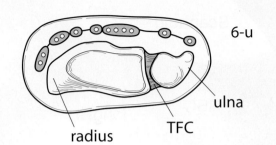

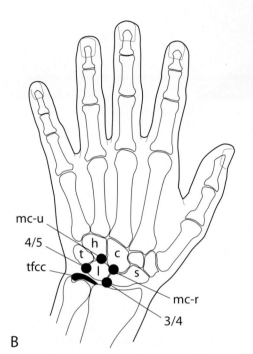

FIGURE 1.4. An illustration in cross-section (**A**) and frontal view (**B**) of the main working portals.

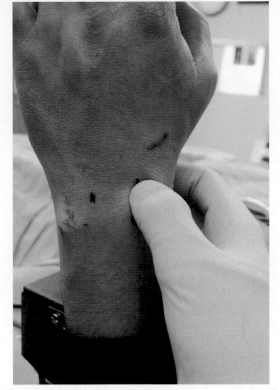

FIGURE 1.5. From Lister's tubercle, the 3-4 portal is found 1 cm distally as a soft spot when palpated by the thumb or finger.

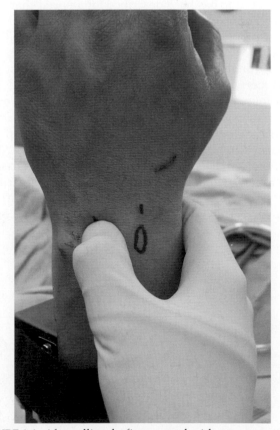

FIGURE 1.6. After rolling the finger over the 4th compartment tendons, the 4–5 portal soft spot is identified.

gant (Figure 1.7) Irrigation pumps are now available that regulate fluid volumes and pressure to avoid extravasation and decrease intraoperative bleeding. In the midcarpal joint, care should be taken to maintain the cannulas in the joint once they are placed, because extravasation of fluid makes reintroduction of the cannulas into this tight joint difficult.

A needle should be placed into the joint at the prospective portal sites prior to skin incision to confirm their location. Longitudinal portal incisions are made to avoid tendon transection by an inadvertently deep incision. Prior to making the incisions, the skin should be pulled taut against the tip of a number 11 blade so that only the skin is cut. This prevents inadvertent injury to branches of the radial sensory nerve, which run in the immediate subcutaneous tissue.

The 3-4 portal is usually established first, as this is the main viewing portal. A blunt trocar with a cannula is directed volar and proximal at a 30-degree an-

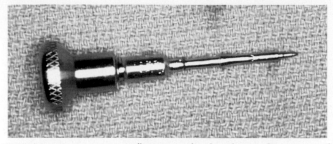

FIGURE 1.7. A custom inflow cannula placed into the 6U portal provides excellent joint irrigation.

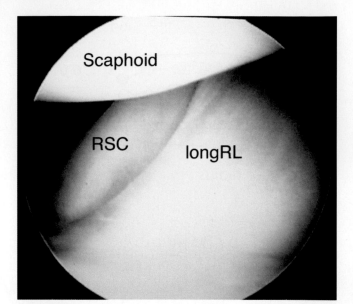

FIGURE 1.9. The radioscaphocapitate and long radiolunate ligaments run side-by-side in a proximal-radial to distal-ulnar orientation.

gle. This technique aligns the cannula with the articular surface of the radiocarpal joint. If one attempts to place the cannula into the joint perpendicular to the wrist, injury to the dorsal articular surface will occur (Figure 1.8). Once the camera is introduced, more precise placement of the remaining portals is possible. The 4-5 or 6-R portals are commonly used to insert instruments if a therapeutic arthroscopy is planned. The 6-U portal is used as the inflow portal, while the port on the camera cannula is left open to allow fluid to drain.

Other portals described include the 1-2 portal and anterior portals. The 1-2 portal passes ulnar to the extensor pollicis brevis tendon and radial to the extensor carpi radialis longus tendon. Various anterior portals have been described, but most recently a safe inside-out technique has been described for a portal that is ulnar to the flexor carpi radialis tendon and radial to the median nerve. Though these portals are not used routinely, they may be helpful in certain circumstances.

Examination of the wrist should be systematic to make certain that all areas are inspected and that pathology identified early does not distract from a thorough exam. Frequently the exam is performed beginning radially and moving ulnarly. The radial styloid and scaphoid articular surfaces are examined for degeneration as well as for surrounding synovitis. As the camera is moved ulnarly, the extrinsic volar ligaments are visible beyond the scaphoid articular surface. First the radioscaphocapitate ligament comes into view, then the long radiolunate ligament, which is about three times wider (Figure 1.9). Next, the radioscapholunate ligament (ligament of Testut) is seen, which is small and identified by the blood vessels that frequently run upon it (Figure 1.10). This usually marks the scapholunate joint and the intrinsic scapholunate ligament. Complete injury to this ligament allows the arthroscope to pass between the scaphoid and lunate, visualizing the capitate head (known as a "drive-through" sign).[1,9,10] Next, the lunate fossa of the radius and the proximal lunate articular surfaces are examined.

Attention is then turned to the triangular fibrocartilage complex (TFCC) and its attachment to the ulnar portion of the distal radius. A probe is used to perform the trampoline test, which involves ballottement of the disk of the TFCC to test the disk's integrity (Figure 1.11). When the disk is without tension or a break in the smooth contour is noted, a tear must be suspected (Figure 1.12). Both the central and pe-

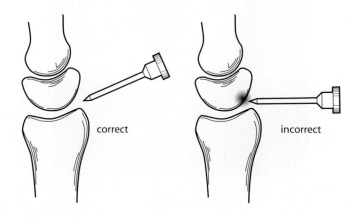

FIGURE 1.8. To avoid injury, the normal inclination of the distal radius must always be taken into consideration when entering the joint with a trocar. The usual alignment is with the trocar angled 20 to 30 degrees proximally to match the distal radius articular curve.

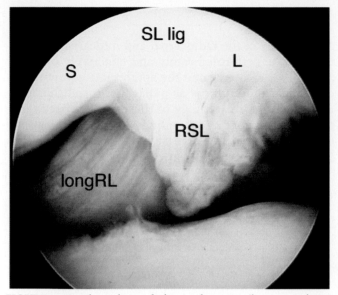

FIGURE 1.10. The radioscapholunate ligament (ligament of Testut) is a vascular structure; the distal end marks the scapholunate ligament.

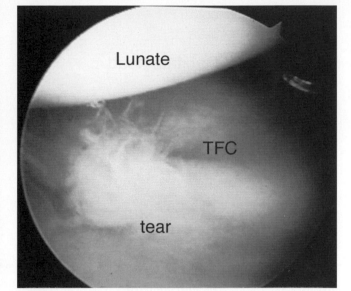

FIGURE 1.12. Loss of the trampoline effect or an obvious disruption (as in this case) indicates a TFC disk tear.

ripheral portions of the disk must be inspected, as either can lead to a loss of the tension of the TFCC. In the distal ulnar portion of the TFCC, the ulnar styloid recess can be mistaken for a tear, though it is a normal anatomic finding. The trampoline test can be helpful to confirm that this is not a tear, as the TFCC will remain taut.

Arthroscopy should continue with examination of the lunotriquetral articulation and the ulnocarpal ligaments. The lunotriquetral interosseous ligament has a concave appearance between the 2 bones (Figure 1.13). The ulnocarpal can be best visualized by switching the scope to the 4–5 or 6-R intervals. Capsular

thickenings can be identified volarly that represent the ulnolunate and the ulnotriquetral ligaments.

Following complete examination and treatment of the radiocarpal joint, the arthroscopy should continue with insertion of the arthroscope into the midcarpal joint as described earlier (Figure 1.14). Midcarpal arthroscopy has been shown to contribute to the diagnosis of pathology in 82% to 84% of cases and can significantly impact the treatment protocol.[8] The first landmark identified is usually the convexity of the proximal capitate. The scope is then turned proximally to view the scapholunate joint radially and the lunotriquetral joint ulnarly, and these joints are

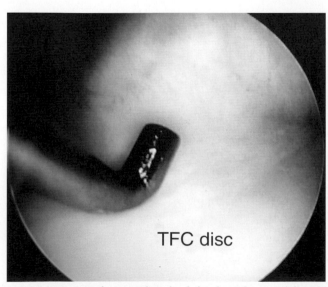

FIGURE 1.11. A probe is used to check for the tightness of the TFC articular disk by the trampoline test.

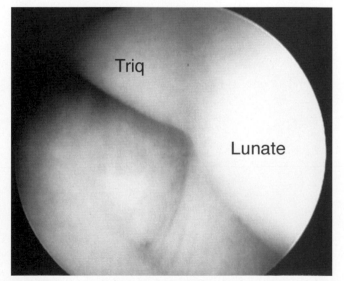

FIGURE 1.13. A slight concavity marks the lunotriquetral ligament.

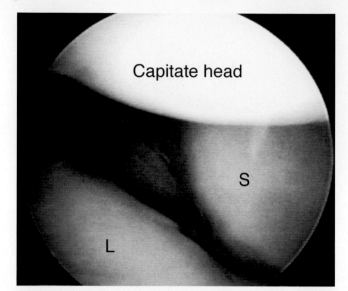

FIGURE 1.14. During midcarpal arthroscopy, excellent visualization of both the scapholunate (shown here) and the lunotriquetral articulations is accomplished.

probed to detect signs of instability. The scaphotrapeziotrapezoid (STT) joint can be visualized by moving the scope radially and distally around the capitate head, while the capitohamate joint can be viewed by moving the scope distally and ulnarly around the capitate. The articular surfaces should be examined for early arthritic changes. Visualization of a significant amount of the volar capsule between the hamate and the triquetrum is a sign of midcarpal instability.

CONCLUSION

Arthroscopy of the radiocarpal and midcarpal articulation can be performed safely and effectively once the anatomy is mastered and the appropriate equipment is obtained. Its usefulness as a diagnostic and therapeutic modality for pathology of the wrist has been demonstrated. As our understanding of wrist pathology and our technical ability increase, arthroscopy will play a larger role in the treatment of disorders of the wrist.

References

1. Geissler WB, Freeland AE, Weiss APC, et al. Techniques of wrist arthroscopy. *J Bone Joint Surg* 1999;81-A:1184–1197.
2. Ekman EF, Poehling GG. Principles of arthroscopy and wrist arthroscopy equipment. *Hand Clin* 1994;10:557–566.
3. Roth JH, Poehling GG, Whipple TL. Hand instrumentation for small joint arthroscopy. *Arthroscopy* 1988;4:126–128.
4. Bettinger PC, Cooney WP 3rd, Berger RA. Arthroscopic anatomy of the wrist. *Orthop Clin North Am* 1995;26:707–719.
5. Botte MJ, Cooney WP, Linscheid RL. Arthroscopy of the wrist: anatomy and technique. *J Hand Surg* 1989;14-A:313–316.
6. North ER, Thomas S. An anatomic guide for arthroscopic visualization of the wrist capsular ligaments. *J Hand Surg* 1988;13A:815–822.
7. Buterbaugh GA. Radiocarpal arthroscopy portals and normal anatomy. *Hand Clin* 1994;10:567–576.
8. Viegas SF. Midcarpal arthroscopy: anatomy and portals. *Hand Clin* 1994;10:577–587.
9. Weiss APC, Akelman E, Lambiase R. Comparison of the findings of triple-injection cinearthrography of the wrist with those of arthroscopy. *J Bone Joint Surg* 1996;78-A:348–356.
10. Weiss AP, Sachar K, Glowacki KA. Arthroscopic debridement alone for intercarpal ligament tears. *J Hand Surg* 1997;22A:344–349.

2

Arthroscopic Wrist Anatomy

Jonathan H. Lee, Nathan L. Taylor, Ryan A. Beekman, and Melvin P. Rosenwasser

Wrist arthroscopy allows excellent visualization of the articular surfaces of the carpal bones and ligaments that is not possible via an open arthrotomy.[1] Arthroscopy of the wrist is now a primary method of evaluating and treating many intra-articular wrist conditions, including triangular fibrocartilage complex tears, chondral injuries, distal radius fractures, carpal fractures, wrist ligament injuries, loose bodies, and ganglia (Table 2.1).[2] A thorough knowledge of overall wrist anatomy, including topographic landmarks, extracapsular tendon and neurovascular structures, and intracapsular ligamentous and osseus structures is essential to proper diagnosis and treatment.[3] Chapter 1 outlined the basic setup and surface topography of the wrist joint, as well as the creation of the standard radiocarpal and midcarpal portals. This chapter will focus on the internal anatomy of the radiocarpal, midcarpal, distal radioulnar joint, and thumb carpometacarpal joint.

A thorough understanding of the topographic anatomy of the wrist and appropriate portal placement greatly influences the surgeon's view of internal anatomy.[4] We must emphasize that all external anatomical landmarks and all portals must be marked after traction is applied but before starting the arthroscopic procedure. Important points to remember when creating the portals include (1) proper portal placement by careful palpation of the surrounding tendinous and bony landmarks, (2) incision only through the skin, and (3) blunt dissection to the capsule. To avoid iatrogenic cartilage injuries when entering the joint, the capsule should be distended by insufflating the joint with saline, and only blunt instruments should be used to pierce the capsule.[4] This technique can also provide some information on intercarpal ligamentous integrity if the fluid does not leak out of its respective compartment.

A systematic approach must be used when performing wrist arthroscopy to avoid missing any pathology and to properly view normal anatomy.[1] Certainly the order of visualizing structures is not critical, but one should develop a consistent pattern to avoid overlooking subtle abnormalities. Another important practice in wrist arthroscopy is switching viewing portals to visualize all structures from various angles. More than one viewing portal is always necessary during wrist arthroscopy. In contrast to knee and shoulder arthroscopy, there is an almost complete absence of in-and-out movement of the arthroscope when performing wrist arthroscopy. The inexperienced surgeon often makes the mistake of inserting the arthroscope too far so that the tip is against the volar capsule or of pulling the arthroscope back too much so that it is no longer in the joint. Because the anterior-posterior depth of the wrist joint is small, the arthroscope can only be moved in or out by approximately 1.5 cm. Pressurized saline irrigation maintains excellent viewing, especially through the small inflow available with wrist arthroscopes.

RADIOCARPAL ARTHROSCOPIC ANATOMY

In general, make the first portal away from the site of major symptoms to ensure that any pathology encountered will be untainted by portal entry injury. All portals are first checked with an 18-gauge needle to correctly determine angle of insertion and adequacy of traction. The 3-4 portal is created first and is usually the main viewing portal. The 4-5 portal is created next for instrumentation. The inflow tubing is attached to the arthroscope sheath to keep soft tissue away from the viewing field. Outflow is then created through the 6-U portal. This is done after the 6-U region is palpated from outside while viewing the prestyloid recess arthroscopically to confirm proper location.

The articular surfaces of the scaphoid and lunate, as well as the intervening scapholunate interosseous ligament are first visualized by rotating the field of view of the arthroscope to look distally (Figure 2.1). Be careful to maintain perspective with a visible horizon such as the distal radius and proximal carpal row. The volar and dorsal margins of the articular surfaces of the two bones can be inspected by flexing and extending the wrist slightly. The proximal articular surface of the lunate has two distinct segments. The lateral portion articulates with the lunate fossa of the

TABLE 2.1. Arthroscopic Portals for Various Diagnoses.

Diagnosis	Primary portals		Secondary portals		Treatment
	Viewing	Instrumenting	Viewing	Instrumenting	
Dorsal ligament injury/ganglion	1-2	3-4	6-R		Debride, excise
Radial styloiditis	3-4	1-2	1-2	3-4	Debride
Intra-articular distal radius fracture	3-4	4-5	4-5	3-4	Arthoscopically assisted reduction/pinning
Scaphoid fracture	3-4	1-2	1-2 RMC	3-4	Arthroscopically assisted reduction/fixation
Acute scapholunate ligament injury	3-4	4-5	4-5 RMC	3-4	Inspect/probe, debride, internal fixation
Volar radiocarpal ligament injury	3-4	4-5	—	—	Inspect/probe
Lunotriquetral ligament injury	4-5	6-U	6-U UMC	4-5	Inspect/probe, debride, internal fixation, ulnar shortening
TFCC tear					
Class IA	4-5	6-U	6-U	4-5	Debride
Class IB	6-U	4-5	—	—	Repair
Class IC	4-5	6-U	6-U	4-5	Debride
Class ID	6-U	3-4	6-U	3-4	Debride, repair
STT joint pain	RMC	STT	—	—	Inspect for staging, debride, fixation
Midcarpal pain	RMC	UMC	—	—	Inspect/probe, debride
DRUJ pain	DRUJ	DRUJ	—	—	Inspect, debride
Ulnar impaction syndrome	DRUJ	DRUJ	—	—	1. TFCC injury: Ulnar shortening 2. No TFCC injury: DRUJ arthroscopy
CMC arthritis/ fracture	TM (CMC) volar	TM (CMC) dorsal	TM (CMC) dorsal	TM (CMC) volar	Synovectomy, debridement, removal of loose bodies
Dorsal capsule contracture	Volar radial	Any dorsal port	—	—	Dorsal capsulotomy, inspect S-L volar ligament

distal radius, and the medial portion articulates with the triangular fibrocartilage complex (TFCC). The surface of the scaphoid can be followed radially up the wrist, at which point capsular attachments prevent further visualization. The articular cartilage should be off-white and smooth and should feel firm on palpation with a probe. Cartilage softening, fragmentation, or fissuring indicate chondromalacia and should be graded and recorded. The scapholunate interosseous ligament may not be immediately obvious in some cases because it has the appearance of cartilage. It can appear as a localized valley in an otherwise smooth cartilaginous surface. The location of the ligament is confirmed by palpating it with the probe, because the ligament is softer than the surrounding cartilage. The ligament has three distinct segments: (1) dorsal, (2) proximal or membranous, and (3) volar. Probing may also show tears that were not noticed initially (Figure 2.2). Partial tears often involve the proximal aspect of the ligament because it is fibrocartilaginous,

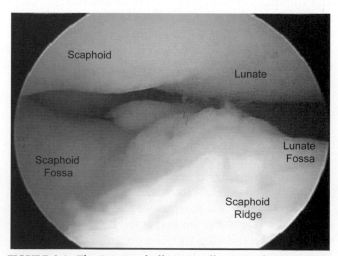

FIGURE 2.1. The 3-4 portal allows excellent visualization of the scapholunate ligament as well as the scaphoid and lunate fossae seen here.

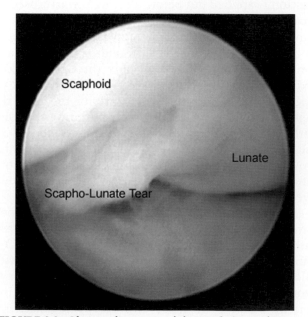

FIGURE 2.2. Obvious disruption of the scapholunate ligament.

unlike the dorsal and palmar aspects of the ligament.[5] It is impossible to fully visualize the volar aspect of the scapholunate ligament arthroscopically, but the membranous (proximal) and dorsal portions can be seen in their entirety.

The arthroscope is then rotated proximally, showing the lunate and scaphoid fossae of the distal radius (Figure 2.1). The two fossae are separated by a sagittal ridge. The scaphoid fossa can be followed radially up to the radial styloid (Figure 2.3). Air bubbles that obscure the view are frequently found in this region, because it is the highest portion of the radiocarpal joint with the forearm in the vertical position. Placing an egress needle here facilitates egress of bubbles.

The volar carpal ligaments are evaluated next and consist of the radioscaphocapitate (RSC), radiolunotriquetral (RLT), and radioscapholunate (RSL) ligaments. The latter two are also known as the long radiolunate (LRL) and short radiolunate (SRL) (Figure 2.3).[6] The RSC ligament is the most radial, arising from the radial styloid process and inserting onto the waist of the scaphoid as well as progressing distally to the capitate.[7] The orientation of the fibers is not longitudinal but oblique in the ulnar direction.[8,9] The ligament should feel taut on palpation with a probe because traction is being applied to the wrist.

The RLT ligament is just ulnar to the RSC ligament and is slightly broader and more obliquely oriented.[8] The ligament is also referred to as the radiolunate ligament because many question the importance of the lunotriquetral portion.[10,11] The RLT and RSC ligaments are separated by an interligamentous sulcus, which provides a useful arthroscopic landmark. The ulnar portion of the ligament may be covered with a synovial tuft, which originates from the radioscapholunate ligament.

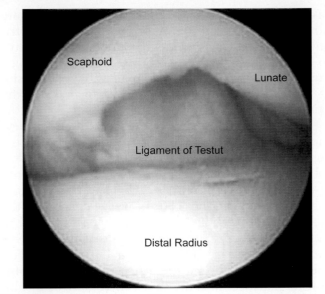

FIGURE 2.4. The ligament of Testut (radioscapholunate ligament) is a vestigial neurovascular structure just radial to the scapholunate ligament.

The radioscapholunate ligament (ligament of Testut) is visualized with the arthroscope pointed directly volar (Figure 2.4). The ligament can be identified by a synovial tuft covering a portion of it. There is a natural redundancy to the ligament that should not be mistaken for a tear. The fibers of the ligament course slightly in a radial direction and form a 60- to 80-degree angle to that of the RL ligament. The structure is weak and considered to be more of a neurovascular connection to the scaphoid and lunate rather than a ligament.[12]

The arthroscope is again directed at the articular surface of the lunate, which is then followed ulnarly to the triquetrum to view the lunotriquetral (LT) interosseous ligament (Figure 2.5). Deviating the wrist ulnarly can help in visualizing the triquetrum, but oc-

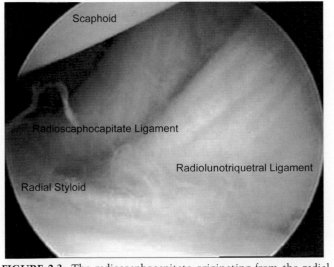

FIGURE 2.3. The radioscaphocapitate originating from the radial styloid lies just radial to the radiolunotriquetral ligament also known as the long radiolunate ligament.

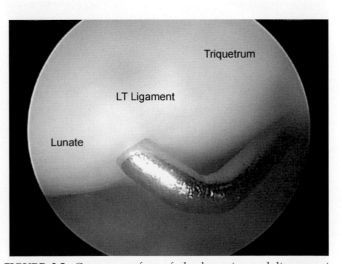

FIGURE 2.5. Concave surface of the lunotriquetral ligament is noted between the lunate and the triquetrum.

casionally the arthroscope must be moved to a more ulnar portal to see the triquetrum well. The lunotriquetral interosseous ligament is often more difficult to detect than the scapholunate interosseous ligament. There may again be a small valley at the site of the LT ligament, but probing the ligament is the best way to localize it.

The arthroscope is then rotated proximally to view the TFCC (Figure 2.6). The TFCC consists of the triangular fibrocartilage (TFC) or articular disk, the dorsal and palmar distal radioulnar ligaments, the floor of the extensor carpi ulnaris (ECU) sheath, and ulnocarpal ligaments. The TFC is wedge-shaped in the coronal plane with an ulnar base that is attached to the styloid process and a radial tip that merges with the articular surface of the distal radius. The junction between the TFCC and the distal radius can be difficult to visualize. In some cases, there may be a color change or crease at the junction. Palpation with a probe will show the junction with a change from the firm resistance of the lunate fossa to the softer resilience of the articular disk of the TFCC.[11] The resilient "trampolining" of the TFC on palpation (Figure 2.7) is an important finding because it indicates that the supporting structures are intact.[13] With a significant tear of the TFCC, this resilience is lost, and the TFC becomes soft and compliant with bulging in the middle.

Tears of the central avascular portion of the TFCC are common, particularly in older patients.[14] Ordinarily the ulnar head is not visible from the radiocarpal joint, but with a full-thickness tear of the TFCC, the ulnar head can be visualized through it (Figure 2.8). Congenital perforations of the central region are occasionally observed.[15] Also a ballooning buckethandle tear may obscure visibility here. Always use the probe to ascertain if a cleavage tear is present.

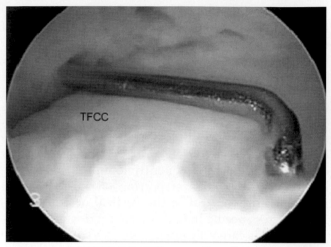

FIGURE 2.7. TFC trampoline effect.

The periphery of the TFCC should be examined and probed as well. The peripheral 15% to 20% of the TFCC is vascularized and therefore has healing potential if torn. The dorsal and palmar radioulnar ligaments are thickenings of the periphery of the TFCC and attach to the ulnar styloid and distal radius.[16] One has to differentiate deep radioulnar ligaments attaching to the fovea from superficial ones attaching to the styloid. Only foveal ligaments are seen. The palmar radioulnar ligament is taut in pronation, and the dorsal margin becomes taut in supination. The prestyloid recess (Figure 2.9) is located volar to the ulnar styloid and is a synovium-lined pocket that can be confused with a TFCC tear. It can also lead to confusion with imaging modalities because the recess fills with contrast in arthrography, and in wrists with effusions can appear as a bright signal on T2-weighted MRI. As noted earlier, the 6-U portal enters the joint above the

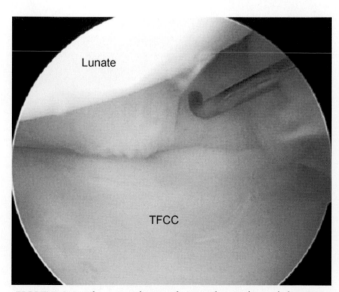

FIGURE 2.6. The normal smooth articular surface of the TFC.

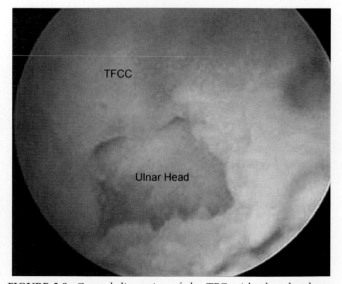

FIGURE 2.8. Central disruption of the TFC with ulnar head protrusion.

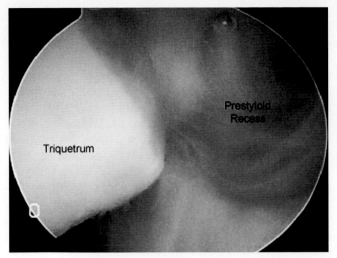

FIGURE 2.9. Prestyloid recess with adjoining articular surface of triquetrum and insertion of TFC.

prestyloid recess, and the surgeon must be certain that this is above the TFC articular disk.

The ulnocarpal ligaments (Figure 2.10) consist of the ulnolunate and ulnotriquetral ligaments. They both originate from the ulnar styloid, where they blend together with fibers of the TFCC.[15] They pass volar to the palmar distal radioulnar ligament and insert on the volar surfaces of the lunate and triquetrum, respectively. They limit wrist extension and radial deviation. These ligaments should be palpated with a probe to ensure their competence. It should be noted that the lunotriquetral interosseous ligament can be located by following distally the interval between the ulnolunate and ulnotriquetral ligaments.

The floor of the ECU sheath and the dorsal ulnotriquetral ligament are strong structures on the dorsal aspect of the TFCC. They are often covered with synovial tissue and therefore not immediately visualized arthroscopically. The synovial tissue should be removed and the structures inspected and followed along their course in patients with dorsoulnar wrist symptoms, because injuries are frequently seen, such as partial tears with surrounding synovitis.

When indicated, a new volar radial (V-R) portal can be used for specific indications such as viewing the dorsal capsule and palmar scapholunate (SL) ligament.[17] This may allow safer dorsal capsulotomies, assessment of scapholunate injuries, and perhaps volar carpal ganglionectomies. Slutsky recommends creating this portal from outside-in for any patient with radial-sided wrist pain.[18] The V-R portal can also be created from inside-out as described by Tham.[19] While viewing through the V-R portal and instrumenting the standard dorsal portals, a dorsal capsulotomy or bony debridement can be performed for dorsal capsule contracture or impingement.

MIDCARPAL ARTHROSCOPIC ANATOMY

The midcarpal joint is initially distended with 2 to 3 cc of saline injected through the radial midcarpal (RMC) portal to begin midcarpal arthroscopy. The depth of the midcarpal joint is less than half that of the radiocarpal joint, and great care must be taken when entering the joint. One must also be careful when creating this portal, because the space is tight and it is easy to create a furrow in the capitate.[20] Thus always triangulate this space with an 18-gauge needle prior to placing the blunt trocar. Sharp trocars should never be utilized in wrist arthroscopy. The ulnar midcarpal portal is created as well, for instrumentation and visualization of the ulnar portion of the midcarpal joint. The midcarpal joint space is smaller than that of the radiocarpal joint, and occasionally a smaller arthroscope is beneficial.[21]

The scaphocapitate joint is viewed through the radial midcarpal portal (Figure 2.11).[22] However, it is easiest to get one's orientation by visualizing the scapholunate joint ulnar to the insertion point of the arthroscope. One should first see the head of the capitate and the well-defined normal cleft between the scaphoid and lunate. This must always be probed through the companion ulnar midcarpal portal. The scapholunate interosseous ligament is present on the palmar, proximal, and dorsal edges but not the distal edge of the scapholunate joint; therefore, midcarpal arthroscopy usually gives the best view within the scapholunate joint. Marginal degenerative changes without an obvious static scapholunate dissociation may indicate a dynamic instability.[11] A fibrocartilaginous meniscus may extend into the joint from the membranous regions of the interosseous ligament. Intraoperatively, the stability of the joint can be assessed

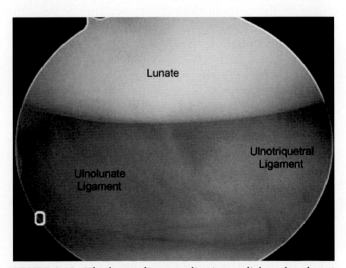

FIGURE 2.10. Ulnolunate ligament lies just radial to the ulnotriquetral ligament, both running in an ulnar to radial direction.

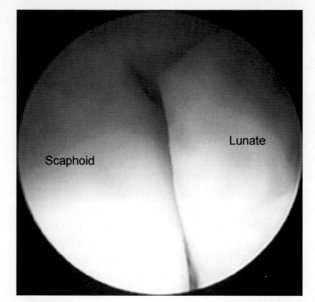

FIGURE 2.11. The radial midcarpal portal allows visualization of scaphoid and lunate pathology. The ulnar midcarpal portal (not shown) offers views of the lunate and triquetrum.

by performing the "scaphoid shift test."[23] While visualizing the joint arthroscopically, do not forget to move the wrist in the traction tower to provoke provocative stress when examining the scapholunate ligament.

The arthroscope is then brought back to the scaphocapitate joint. The articular surface of the capitate is convex, whereas that of the scaphoid is concave. If the arthroscope is advanced volarly, the scaphocapitate ligament can be seen. This ligament originates from the scaphoid tubercle and inserts onto the palmar aspect of the capitate.

The arthroscope is then brought distally along the scaphocapitate joint. The edge of the capitate-trapezoid joint can be seen. The arthroscope is further advanced over the scaphoid to enter the scapho-trapeziotrapezoidal (STT) joint. The trapezoid appears closer to the camera than the trapezium. Significant degenerative changes can be seen in the STT joint.[24] It is sometimes possible to see the palmar scapho-trapezial ligament on advancing the arthroscope volarly. This ligament is a strong structure reinforced by the flexor carpi radialis tendon sheath.[5,24] Bubbles tend to collect in this joint because it is higher than the RMC portal when the arm is held vertically in the traction device. If need be, the bubbles can be removed with a hypodermic needle placed through the STT portal.

The STT portal, located just ulnar to the extensor pollicis longus in line with the radial side of the second metacarpal, is utilized primarily for instrumentation of the STT joint. Located between the distal pole of the scaphoid, trapezium, and trapezoid, this portal can be created for better visualization or for instrumentation. When utilizing the radial midcarpal portal and visualizing the STT joint, evacuating bubbles with a needle inserted via the STT portal can be very beneficial.

The lunocapitate surface is then inspected and followed ulnarly. The distal ulnar aspect of the lunate should be evaluated for the presence of a medial facet. This facet, which articulates with the hamate, is present in approximately two-thirds of cases and is associated with degenerative changes of the hamate articular surface. In wrists with a medial facet of the lunate, the proximal articular surfaces of the capitate and hamate tends to form a biconvex curve, whereas in wrists with only a single facet on the lunate, the capitate and hamate generally form a single convex curve.[25] The arthroscope is then advanced further ulnarly and rotated proximally to view the lunotriquetral joint. It is possible to peer into this joint as with the scapholunate joint. A fibrocartilaginous meniscus may be present in this joint as well. A ballottement test can be performed while visualizing the joint to assess for instability.[11,26]

Rotating the arthroscope ulnarly shows the saddle-shaped triquetrohamate joint. Ordinarily the joint is held tightly by the volar triquetrohamate and triquetrocapitate ligaments.[24] Midcarpal laxity may be present if one can see across the joint to the volar capsule.

FIRST CARPOMETACARPAL JOINT ARTHROSCOPIC ANATOMY

Arthroscopic evaluation of the first carpometacarpal joint can be utilized in any instance where direct visualization of the first CMC intra-articular anatomy is desired and is a viable alternative to open arthrotomy. To date, the primary indication has been in osteoarthritis, but authors have advocated it both for the early treatment and partial resection of the trapezium, and for interpositional arthroplasty.[27,28]

After a 1.9-mm arthroscope has been inserted in either the 1-R (radial) or 1-U (ulnar) portal, most of the articular surface of the trapezium and the base of the first metacarpal articular surface can be visualized. With appropriate traction and anatomy, a 2.7-mm scope can be safely placed (Figure 2.12). The far lateral capsule and articular surfaces may be difficult to visualize from either portal. The 1-R (radial) portal allows visualization of the dorsoradial ligament (DRL), the posterior oblique ligament (POL), and the ulnar collateral ligament (UCL), while the 1-U (ulnar) portal provides for optimal viewing of the radial collateral ligament (RCL) and the anterior oblique ligament (AOL).[29]

DISTAL RADIOULNAR JOINT (DRUJ) ARTHROSCOPIC ANATOMY

Indications for diagnostic DRUJ arthroscopy include distal radius fracture involving the DRUJ; articular cartilage injury; partial-thickness, proximal-sided TFCC tear; and capsular contraction resulting in limitation

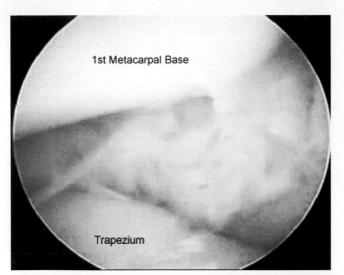

FIGURE 2.12. The 1-U (utilized here) or the 1-R portal allows visualization of most of the carpometacarpal articular surface and capsule.

of forearm rotation.[30] Therapeutic uses of DRUJ arthroscopy include arthroscopic distal ulnar resection for ulnocarpal abutment, removal of loose bodies, and synovectomy.[31] Arthroscopy of the DRUJ is more difficult than that of the radiocarpal or midcarpal joints because of the limited space. Occasionally, the 2.7-mm arthroscope cannot be inserted into the DRUJ, and a smaller arthroscope is required. In some wrists, however, it may be impossible to enter the joint even with a 1.9-mm arthroscope. Again, it is important to triangulate the entry portals with 18-gauge needles first. In these cases, one should abort the procedure or perform an arthrotomy instead rather than continue to struggle and risk iatrogenic injuries to the joint or surrounding soft tissue.

DRUJ arthroscopy is carried out with the forearm held vertically in the wrist traction device as in radiocarpal and midcarpal arthroscopy, but without any traction applied. After the joint is localized with the wrist in supination, 3 mL of saline are injected into it. A longitudinal incision is then made through the skin approximately 5 mm proximal to the proximal portion of the joint. After the soft tissue is spread down to the capsule with a hemostat, the arthroscopic sleeve with a blunt obturator is angled slightly distally and placed into the joint. If required, outflow can also be created by placing an 18-gauge needle into the distal portion of the joint. The sigmoid notch of the distal radius and the articular surface of the distal ulna are immediately seen through the arthroscope. Forearm rotation allows visualization of more of the distal ulna joint surface. Advancing the arthroscope distally allows inspection and brings the undersurface of the TFCC and dorsal and palmar radioulnar capsular ligaments into view. This is useful for lysis of adhesions, marginal debridement chondroplasty, exostectomy, or capsulotomy of the distal radioulnar joint.

CONCLUSION

Arthroscopic wrist anatomy is best learned from cadaveric bioskills first, and reinforced through experience. Correlating focal clinical findings with arthroscopic anatomy, both normal and pathologic, can expand the clinician's understanding and nuanced-interpretation of presenting complaints. Wrist arthroscopy has been shown to be more effective and predictable than all but the most sophisticated MRI and has an added benefit of real-time assessment of dynamic instability and partial cartilage lesions. Visualizing wrist pathology with the arthroscope is often more reliable than a physical examination or imaging studies such as MRI, arthrography, or plain radiographs. It is essential to alternate viewing and instrumentation portals to properly view normal and abnormal anatomy from various angles. Once arthroscopic wrist anatomy is understood and mastered, the surgeon can best plan and perform treatment based on the patient's internal wrist pathology.

References

1. Miyasaka KaR, MP. Diagnostic wrist arthroscopy. *Oper Tech Sports Med* 1998;6(1):42–51.
2. Geissler WB, Freeland AE, Weiss AP, et al. Techniques of wrist arthroscopy. *J Bone Joint Surg* 1999;81A:1184–1197.
3. Culp R. Wrist and hand arthroscopy. *Hand Clin* 1999;15:393–535.
4. Grechenig W, Peicha G, Fellinger M, et al. Anatomical and safety considerations in establishing portals used for wrist arthroscopy. *Clin Anat* 1999;12(3):179–185.
5. Bettinger PC, Cooney WP 3rd, Berger RA. Arthroscopic anatomy of the wrist. *Orthop Clin North Am* 1995;26(4):707–719.
6. North ER, Thomas S. An anatomic guide for arthroscopic visualization of the wrist capsular ligaments. *J Hand Surg Am* 1988;13(6):815–822.
7. Berger RA. Arthroscopic anatomy of the wrist and distal radioulnar joint. *Hand Clin* 1999;15(3):393–413, vii.
8. Stanley JSP. *Wrist Arthroscopy.* Philadelphia: Saunders, 1994.
9. Whipple TL, Cooney WP 3rd, Osterman AL, et al. Wrist arthroscopy. *Instr Course Lect* 1995;44:139–145.
10. Berger RA, Landsmeer JM. The palmar radiocarpal ligaments: a study of adult and fetal human wrist joints. *J Hand Surg Am* 1990;15(6):847–854.
11. Whipple TL. *Arthroscopic Surgery: The Wrist.* Philadelphia: Lippincott Williams & Wilkins, 1992:55–90.
12. Berger RA, Kauer JM, Landsmeer JM. The radioscapholunate ligament: a gross anatomic and histologic study of fetal and adult wrists. *J Bone Joint Surg* 1991;16:350–355.
13. Osterman AL, Terrill RG. Arthroscopic treatment of TFCC lesions. *Hand Clin* 1991;7:277–281.
14. Mikic Z. Age changes in the triangular fibrocartilage of the wrist. *J Anat* 1978;126:367–384.
15. Bowers W. The distal radioulnar joint. In: Green DP, (ed.) *Operative Hand Surgery*; 3rd ed. New York: Churchill Livingstone, 1993.
16. Kleinman WB, Graham TJ. The distal radioulnar joint capsule: clinical anatomy and role in posttraumatic limitation of forearm rotation. *J Hand Surg Am* 1998;23(4):588–599.
17. Abe Y, Doi K, Hattori Y, et al. A benefit of the volar approach for wrist arthroscopy. *Arthroscopy* 2003;19(4):440–445.
18. Slutsky DJ. Wrist arthroscopy through a volar radial portal. *Arthroscopy* 2002;18(6):624–630.

19. Tham S, Coleman S, Gilpin D. An anterior portal for wrist arthroscopy. Anatomical study and case reports. *J Hand Surg Br* 1999;24(4):445–447.

20. Hanker GJ. Diagnostic and operative arthroscopy of the wrist. *Clin Orthop* 1991;263:165–174.

21. Botte MJ, Cooney WP, Linscheid RL. Arthroscopy of the wrist: anatomy and technique. *J Hand Surg Am* 1989;14A:313–316.

22. Hofmeister EP, Dao KD, Glowacki KA. The role of midcarpal arthroscopy in the diagnosis of disorders of the wrist. *J Hand Surg Am* 2001;26(3):407–414.

23. Watson HK, Ashmead D IV, Makhlouf MV. Examination of the scaphoid. *J Hand Surg Am* 1988;13A:657–660.

24. Viegas SF. Midcarpal arthroscopy: anatomy and portals. *Hand Clin* 1994;10:577–587.

25. Viegas SF, Wagner K, Patterson R, et al. Medial (hamate) facet of the lunate. *J Hand Surg Am* 1990;15A:564–571.

26. Reagan DS, Linscheid RL, Dobyns JH. Lunotriquetral sprains. *J Hand Surg Am* 1984;9A:502–514.

27. Menon J. Arthroscopic management of trapeziometacarpal joint arthritis of the thumb. *Arthroscopy* 1996;12(5): 581–587.

28. Berger RA. A technique for arthroscopic evaluation of the first carpometacarpal joint. *J Hand Surg Am* 1997;22(6): 1077–1080.

29. Bettinger PC, Berger RA. Functional ligamentous anatomy of the trapezium and trapeziometacarpal joint (gross and arthroscopic). *Hand Clin* 2001;17(2):151–168, vii.

30. Zelouf DS, Bowers WH. Arthroscopy of the distal radioulnar joint. *Hand Clin* 1999;15(3):475–477, ix.

31. Whipple TL. Arthroscopy of the distal radioulnar joint. Indications, portals, and anatomy. *Hand Clin* 1994;10(4):589–592.

3

Evaluation of the Painful Wrist

Karl Michalko, Scott Allen, and Edward Akelman

Despite the increasing use and availability of newer imaging modalities, radiographs remain an important technique for evaluating the patient with wrist pathology. More advanced techniques and tests are available to further delineate abnormality, but are frequently unnecessary with properly executed plain films. The goal of this chapter is to present the various choices, including the advantages and disadvantages of each, that are available in the evaluation of the painful wrist.

ROUTINE RADIOGRAPHS

Following a thorough history and physical exam, radiographic evaluation of the wrist should be performed. The minimum studies that should be ordered include a posteroanterior (PA) and lateral view of the wrist. Additional studies that may be indicated, depending upon the clinical scenario, include the scaphoid view, or ulnar-deviated PA view, the PA 45-degree pronated oblique view, the carpal tunnel view, and the anteroposterior (AP) 30-degree supinated view. Adequate radiographic evaluation of the wrist is predicated upon standard positioning of the patient. The following explains the proper technique for obtaining the necessary views, as well as criteria for evaluating the adequacy of those views.

Posteroanterior View

TECHNIQUE

Consistency in how the PA radiograph is taken is important to assess the alignment of the carpal bones and to measure ulnar variance.[1] Ulnar variance has been shown to change with pronosupination. Supination will decrease the apparent length of the ulna, whereas pronation will increase the apparent length of the ulna as compared to the radius.[2] The convexity of the dorsal aspect of the hand makes AP positioning unreliable, but with the fingers in extension and the thumb in radial abduction, the PA position is stable and reproducible. The standard way to obtain a reproducible PA view is an X-ray with the shoulder abducted 90 degrees, the elbow flexed 90 degrees, and the hand flat on the plate with the fingers and thumb in the previously mentioned stable position. Changes in ulnar variance between exams and between patients may be assessed only when films are taken in this way.

ASSESSMENT

The ulnar styloid is at its most ulnar location when radiographed in this standard position. When it is located more radially, the wrist is likely pronated or supinated. At the distal radioulnar joint, there is no overlap of the articular surfaces, and the joint space is clearly outlined.[3] Distally, all the carpometacarpal joint spaces are well outlined, and all the intermetacarpal joint spaces are of equal width. The axis of the radius should be colinear with the long axis of the third metacarpal.

Clinical information available from a posteroanterior view of the wrist begins with evaluation of the joint surfaces. Parallelism is a normal condition of the joint surfaces of the wrist that is evident on a correctly performed study. Parallelism should be evident between the surfaces of the radius, scaphoid, and lunate; between the proximal and distal rows; and between the distal carpus and the metacarpals. Overlapping of these normally parallel surfaces should alert one to the possibility of subluxation or dislocation.[4] Gilula's arcs can be drawn on a normal PA view of the wrist. Arc I is formed by the proximal borders of the scaphoid, lunate, and triquetrum. Arc II corresponds to the distal borders of the same bones. Arc III is formed by the proximal borders of the capitate and hamate (Figure 3.1). These arcs should be smooth; if broken or not well delineated, this finding is suggestive of fracture, subluxation, or dislocation. The scaphoid fat pad is visible on a PA view, which parallels the radial surface of the scaphoid. This fat pad is located between the tendon sheaths of the extensor pollicis brevis, the abductor pollicis longus, and the radial collateral ligament. Obliteration, or bowing, of this line may be indicative of a subtle scaphoid fracture. The presence of a foreshortened scaphoid, or signet ring sign, on a PA view may signify a tear or attenuation of the scapholunate ligament. Abnormal widening of the scapholunate interval (>2 mm), known as the Terry Thomas sign, suggests this condition as well. In the wrist-neutral position, at least half of the lunate

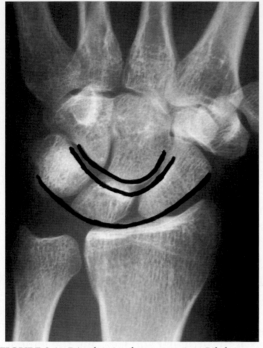

FIGURE 3.1. PA of wrist demonstrating Gilula's arcs.

should articulate with the distal radius. The relationship of the distal ulnar articular surface to the ulnar side of the distal radial articular surface is studied to measure ulnar variance.

Lateral View

TECHNIQUE

The lateral view is best taken with the arm adducted against the chest, the elbow flexed to 90 degrees, and the forearm and hand lying with their ulnar borders, especially the ulnar styloid and olecranon, against the radiographic plate.[3]

ASSESSMENT

To evaluate the adequacy of a lateral view, the ulnar head and distal radius should be superimposed, the ulnar styloid should be in the center of the ulnar head,[5] and the bases of the index, middle, and ring finger metacarpals should overlap.[3] Additionally, the pisiform should overlap the midportion of the scaphoid on a lateral view.

Special attention should be focused on soft-tissue shadows. The soft tissues of the distal wrist are normally concave, and therefore any convexity or straightening of the soft-tissue shadow is indicative of swelling. The pronator fat pad is visible as a straight line volar to the distal radius. Convexity of this line is associated with volar swelling and may be suggestive of a subtle fracture of the distal radius. The scapholunate and capitolunate angles may be calcu-

lated from the lateral view. For the scapholunate angle, a line is drawn that subtends the volarmost points on the proximal and distal poles of the scaphoid. A second line is drawn perpendicular to the line subtending the distalmost points of the dorsal and volar lip of the lunate. The scapholunate angle is the angle between these two lines and should be between 30 and 60 degrees. Any angle between 60 and 80 degrees is questionably abnormal, and greater than 80 degrees is abnormal. The capitolunate angle is calculated using the same line for the lunate and a second line drawn along the long axis of the capitate. This angle should be between 0 and 30 degrees. These two angles may be used to diagnose volar intercalated segment instability (VISI) or dorsal intercalated segment instability (DISI) types of instability patterns.

Other Views

SCAPHOID VIEW

The scaphoid view, which is also called the ulnar-deviated PA view, places the scaphoid in an extended position relative to the wrist. This aligns the long axis of this irregularly shaped bone perpendicular to the X-ray beam. The film is taken in the same manner as described for the PA view of the wrist, but with the hand in maximal ulnar deviation. This X-ray view's utility lies in its demonstration of the integrity of the scaphoid (Figure 3.2).

PA CLENCHED-FIST VIEW

This film is obtained by having the patient make a full fist with maximal force in the PA position. This X-ray effectively drives the capitate down into the acetabulum formed by the scaphoid and the lunate. If the scapholunate ligament is torn or attenuated, the scapholunate interval will widen when compared to a standard PA view.

CARPAL TUNNEL VIEW

This supplemental view of the wrist is obtained by placing the palmar surface of the wrist on the film cassette and maximally extending the wrist, using either the patient's opposite hand or a strap to hold the position. The beam is directed to the base of the hand angling approximately 15 degrees toward the carpus. This view affords an excellent projection of the hook of the hamate, the pisiform, and the volar aspect of the triquetrum.

AP 30-DEGREE SUPINATED OBLIQUE VIEW

The 30-degree supinated oblique view is the best way to assess the pisotriquetral joint for fracture or osteoarthritic changes. The ulnar side of the hand is

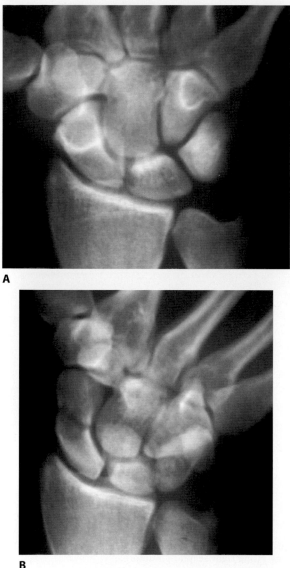

A

B

FIGURE 3.2. **A.** PA and **(B)** scaphoid view of wrist demonstrating scaphoid fracture.

placed against the film cassette at a 30-degree angle with the beam directed at the wrist. The pisotriquetral joint is seen in profile without bony overlap.

PA 45-DEGREE PRONATED OBLIQUE VIEW

This view is obtained by placing the ulnar border of the hand on the cassette and pronating the hand approximately 45 degrees. The beam is directed at the wrist. This view demonstrates the dorsal aspect of the triquetrum, the body of the hamate, the radiovolar border of the scaphoid, as well as the best view of the scaphotrapezial joint and the trapeziotrapezoid joint

CARPAL BOSS VIEW

This infrequently used view is obtained by taking a lateral view and slightly supinating the hand. This ef-

fectively places the boss directly in the path of the beam and allows for evaluation of the boss itself, as well as identification of secondary ossicles or fracture of the base of the second or third metacarpal.[4]

REVERSE OBLIQUE VIEW

Another infrequent view of the wrist is obtained by taking a PA view with the ulnar border of the hand elevated above the cassette. This can demonstrate avulsion fractures from the dorsoradial border of the scaphoid.[4]

Static Wrist Instability Series

If there is any suspicion from a patient's history, physical, or plain film evaluation, a wrist instability series may be indicated. This can be done with plain films or by fluoroscope, if available. The series consists of PA films taken of both wrists in neutral, radial, and ulnar deviation, as well as lateral views of the wrist in neutral, flexion, and extension.[6] These films allow scrutinization of all the carpal bones and assessment of their movement with different positions of the wrist. Comparison with the opposite side is important to differentiate pathologic motion from a patient's unique anatomy. The joint spaces should not change significantly with changes in wrist position. With the wrist in ulnar deviation, the scaphoid assumes an elongated posture, while in radial deviation the scaphoid flexes and appears rounded. The lunate should partially articulate with the distal radius in a neutral view whereas the surface contact increases more with ulnar deviation and less with medial deviation.

FLUOROSCOPY

As previously mentioned, the wrist instability series can be done fluoroscopically. This can be performed by the examining orthopaedist if in-office fluoroscopic equipment is available, or more commonly by the radiologist. Fluoroscopic evaluation is especially helpful in the patient with painful clicking or popping and for patients who have pain related to a specific motion. The wrist should be evaluated while watching the exact motion that causes pain. Motion between the carpal bones, especially between the scaphoid and lunate, lunate and triquetrum, and lunate and distal radius should be carefully evaluated. Midcarpal instability, in particular, can only be demonstrated reliably by using active motion studies.

CT SCANNING/TOMOGRAPHY

CT scanning has limited use in the routine evaluation of the painful wrist. Its role in evaluating healing scaphoid fractures has been demonstrated by numerous authors, and it is excellent for demonstrating occult fractures (Figure 3.3). It can be useful in evaluation of the distal radioulnar joint (DRUJ) with respect to subluxation. For this purpose, continuous 3 mm cuts are taken from Lister's tubercle to the distal carpal bones. The asymptomatic wrist can be scanned for comparison. Drawing arcs between the articular surface of the radius and the articular surface of the ulna assesses congruity of the DRUJ. These arcs should be congruent; loss of congruency is associated with subluxation or dislocation.[7]

BONE SCAN

A bone scan may be useful for evaluating the patient who has normal radiographs but unexplained pain. Its utility lies primarily in its specificity; however, a normal bone scan essentially rules out significant bone or joint pathology. A positive result is usually less diagnostic other than by confirming a pathological condition. Bone scans are generally performed by injecting an intravenous compound labeled with technetium 99m. Three-phase imaging is now standard. Phase 1, or the radionuclide angiogram, consists of multiple images taken in the first 1 to 2 minutes following injection while the isotope is still intravascular. Phase 2 is the soft-tissue pooling phase obtained 5 to 10 minutes after injection. This phase corresponds to the isotope diffusing into the extracellular fluid. Delayed bone images correspond to the third phase. These are taken 2 to 3 hours after injection when the

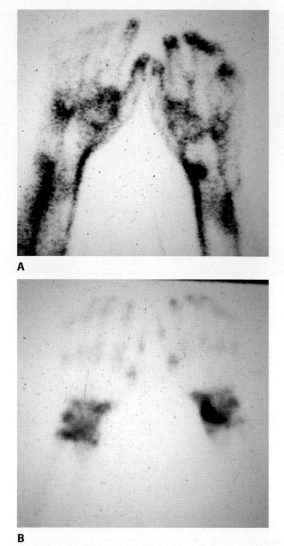

A

B

FIGURE 3.4. Bone scan soft tissue pool (**A**) and delayed (**B**) image demonstrating right scaphoid fracture.

isotope is bound to bone. Increased uptake or "hot spots" are displayed in areas of increased bony turnover (Figure 3.4).

MAGNETIC RESONANCE IMAGING

There is great interest in using magnetic resonance imaging (MRI) for the diagnosis of wrist pain, given its noninvasive nature and absence of ionizing radiation. Early enthusiasm for this diagnostic modality has been tempered by an understanding of its limitations. Standard MRI is unsurpassed in its ability to demonstrate osteonecrosis (ON), as early as 5 days following onset.[4] Imaging of the triangular fibrocartilage complex (TFCC) has generally been accepted as reliable using MRI, but concern has been raised regarding the sensitivity and specificity of MRI for the extrinsic and intrinsic ligaments. Ideally, MRI of the wrist should

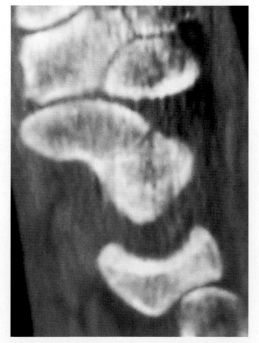

FIGURE 3.3. Sagittal CT scan demonstrating scaphoid fracture.

be performed using dedicated wrist surface coils and by a radiologist skilled in interpreting the images. Early studies showing the inferiority of MRI compared with other techniques were performed with coils not suited to wrist imaging. Current research is focused upon enhancing the ability to differentiate between symptomatic and asymptomatic lesions.

MRI is the gold standard for the diagnosis of ON, such as in Kienböck's disease. When evaluating cases for ON, it is important to look at both the T1-weighted and T2-weighted images, as osteonecrosis has an absent signal on both T1- and T2-weighted images. Other pathophysiologic processes, such as active bone healing, bone bruises, and marrow edema, have an absent or diminished signal on T1-weighted images but increased signal on T2-weighted images.[4]

MRI has been shown to be both sensitive and specific in identifying pathology in the TFCC.[8] The TFCC will appear as a band of low-signal intensity on both T1- and T2-weighted images. It arises from the ulnar aspect of the distal radius and inserts near the base of the ulnar styloid. The prestyloid recess is a constant perforation that is seen between the TFCC and the ulnocarpal meniscus.[9] On T1-weighted images, high signal intensity is normally seen here. Small fluid collections may be normal here as well, manifesting as high signal intensity on T2-weighted images. Tears of the TFCC will appear as discontinuities or fragmentation of the TFCC. Additionally, these discontinuities are highlighted by interposed high signal intensity. The vast majority of these tears will be found along the ulnar insertion. The major current limitation of identifying TFCC pathology with MRI is the inability to differentiate between lesions causing pain and those associated with the normal aging process. Up to 40% of patients over the age of 50 may have asymptomatic, degenerative tears of the TFCC, and this number increases to 50% for those over 60 years of age.[10] To aid in differentiating these lesions, most degenerative tears will be located centrally, where the substance of the complex is thinner.

The extrinsic ligaments can be seen on both sagittal and coronal sections as low-signal bands on both T1- and T2-weighted images. The radial and ulnar collateral ligaments are best seen on coronal images. Discontinuity of these ligaments, manifested as high signal intensity on T2-weighted images in the substance of the ligaments, is easily seen. Evaluation of the intrinsic ligaments of the wrist, specifically the scapholunate and lunotriquetral, is somewhat more difficult. This is due to their small size and curved shape. Normally, these ligaments should be seen as a continuous, low-signal band on at least two images when using 3 mm cuts.[9] Again, discontinuity, elongation, absence, or high signal intensity on T2-weighted images along or within the substance of the ligament is associated with a significant tear. The sensitivity and specificity for scapholunate tears has been reported as 86% and 100%, respectively. For lunotriquetral tears, it was reported as 50% and 100%, respectively. These numbers compare favorably with arthrography[9] (Figure 3.5).

WRIST ARTHROGRAPHY

Arthrography has been used most commonly to evaluate suspected lesions of the triangular fibrocartilage complex (TFCC) and the intercarpal ligaments—primarily the scapholunate (SL) and lunotriquetral (LT) ligaments. The technique involves injecting radiopaque contrast dye into the compartments of the wrist. Dye leakage between the compartments suggests the location of causative wrist pathology when correlated with a physical exam.

The three anatomically separate compartments of the wrist are the midcarpal, radiocarpal, and distal radioulnar joint (DRUJ) compartments. The midcarpal compartment lies between the carpal rows and is separated from the radiocarpal compartment by the intercarpal ligaments. The DRUJ compartment is separated from the radiocarpal compartment, which lies between it and the midcarpal compartment, by the TFCC. While the compartments are initially separate, it has been noted that communication between compartments due to attritional changes may be seen in asymptomatic wrists as early as the third decade of life, and that 50% of patients aged 50 years may have attritional tears.[10] In an evaluation of 30 patients with unilateral posttraumatic wrist pain, 30% had bilateral

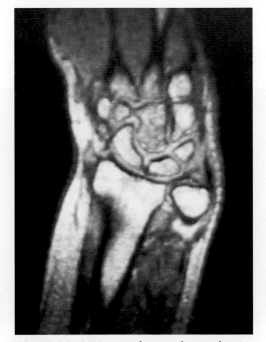

FIGURE 3.5. MRI coronal view of normal wrist.

compartment communication.[11] These findings emphasize the importance of the corresponding physical exam findings.

Single and triple compartment injection techniques have been advocated.[7,12–14] The passage of dye is monitored in both techniques by fluoroscopy during injection and subsequent range of motion, followed by a series of plain radiographs. In the single compartment technique, the dye is injected into the radiocarpal compartment and monitored. The triple compartment technique involves an initial injection with monitoring into the radiocarpal compartment (Figure 3.6) followed by injection into the midcarpal (Figure 3.7) and DRUJ (Figure 3.8) compartments. This technique requires approximately 3 hours between the radiocarpal and midcarpal/DRUJ injections to allow clearance of the contrast from the radiocarpal injection.[15] Digital image subtraction of the carpal bones may enhance interpretation and, when combined with subtraction of radiocarpal injection dye, may shorten waiting time in the triple technique.[12]

Some authors report increased lesion identification using the triple compartment injection technique. They suggest that a significant number of SL and LT tears are missed by the radiocarpal compartment injection alone, which may be blocked by flap tears of the ligaments.[13,14] In one large series of 300 consecutive wrist triple arthrograms, it was noted that of the total number of tears identified by the triple injection technique, 29% of LT, 43% of SL, and 14% of TFCC tears were missed by radiocarpal injection alone.[13] These authors also suggest that midcarpal injections better demonstrate SL and LT ligament tears, as 93% of LT and 87% of ST tears were seen after midcarpal injection alone, compared to 71% of LT and 57% of SL seen after radiocarpal injection alone. Of note, the 14% of TFCC tears picked up by the DRUJ injection were

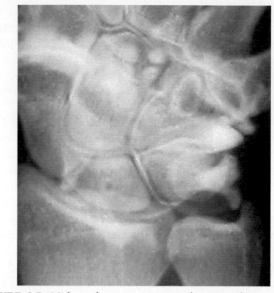

FIGURE 3.7. Midcarpal compartment arthrogram demonstrating lunotriquetral tear.

all at the ulnar attachment, none of which were seen on the radiocarpal injection alone.

Other authors advocate tailoring the arthrographic exam to the site of symptoms.[7,12] In a study of 50 wrist arthrograms, the author found that of the total lesions discovered by triple injection, 96% of midcarpal-radiocarpal communications and 83% of DRUJ-radiocarpal communications were demonstrated after radiocarpal injection alone.[12] One possible explanation for the difference between the aforementioned studies was a higher volume of contrast used to distend the radiocarpal joint. It was felt that in order to save time, money, and patient discomfort the exam should be stopped after radiocarpal injection if intercompartmental flow was noted at the site of pain on physical exam.

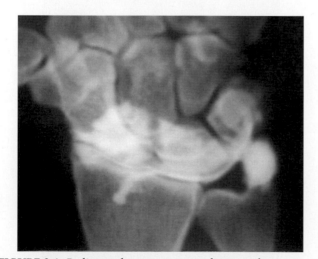

FIGURE 3.6. Radiocarpal compartment arthrogram demonstrating normal wrist.

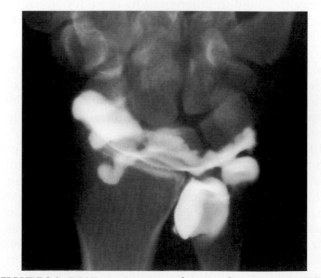

FIGURE 3.8. DRUJ compartment arthrogram demonstrating TFCC tear.

It is important to remember that results of an arthrogram may not correlate with traumatic injury to the intercarpal ligaments or the TFCC, due to the incidence of intercompartmental communication in asymptomatic wrists. It has also been shown that a negative arthrogram does not preclude a ligament tear. A subset of arthrogram study patients above had subsequent arthroscopy, and it was noted that only 69% of SL tears and 86% of LT tears were seen on arthrography.[13] In a study comparing arthrographic and arthroscopic findings, the sensitivity (56%), specificity (83%), and accuracy (60%) of the triple injection arthrograms were noted to be low when compared to arthroscopy.[16] Arthrography remains a useful technique, especially in the diagnosis of intercarpal ligament tears. It may ultimately be replaced by the MRI as a diagnostic intervention in evaluating the painful wrist as that imaging technique is refined and becomes more cost-effective.[15]

CONCLUSION

Numerous modalities are available for the evaluation of the painful wrist. Plain films will suffice in the vast majority of cases. Specialized views are ordered when the patient's history, physical exam, or plain film evaluation indicates the need. A static wrist instability series still has a place in diagnosis of the painful wrist. CT scanning is of limited utility for most wrist pathology except for DRUJ subluxation. Bone scans are less frequently indicated, given the increasing use of MRI, but are generally indicated when evaluating complex cases with minimal findings on other tests. MRI will become increasingly common in the place of arthrography, but currently is the gold standard for the diagnosis of carpal osteonecrosis. Its role in the diagnostic armamentarium is still being defined as technology improves.

References

1. Weiss AP, Akelman E. Diagnostic imaging and arthroscopy for chronic wrist pain. *Orthop Clin North Am* 1995;26(4):759–767.
2. Epner RA, Bowers WH, Guilford WB. Ulnar variance—the effect of wrist positioning and roentgen filming technique. *J Hand Surg Am* 1982;7(3):298–305.
3. Schernberg F. Roentgenographic examination of the wrist: a systematic study of the normal, lax and injured wrist. Part 2: stress views. *J Hand Surg Br* 1990;15(2):220–228.
4. Metz VM, Wunderbaldinger P, Gilula LA. Update on imaging techniques of the wrist and hand. *Clin Plast Surg* 1996;23(3): 369–384.
5. Bowers WH. The distal radial ulnar joint. In: Green DP, Hotchkiss RN, Pederson WC, (eds.) *Green's Operative Hand Surgery*. Philadelphia: Churchill Livingstone, 1999, pp. 986–1032.
6. Gilula LA, Destouet JM, Weeks PM, et al. Roentgenographic diagnosis of the painful wrist. *Clin Orthop* 1984;(187):52–64.
7. Bond JR, Cooney WP, Berger RA. Imaging of the wrist. In: Cooney WP, Linscheid RL, Dobyns JH, (eds). *The Wrist: Diagnosis and Operative Treatment*. New York: Mosby, 1998, pp. 262–283.
8. Golimbu CN, Firooznia H, Melone CP, Jr, et al. Tears of the triangular fibrocartilage of the wrist: MR imaging. *Radiology* 1989;173(3):731–733.
9. Zlatkin MB, Chao PC, Osterman AL, et al. Chronic wrist pain: evaluation with high-resolution MR imaging. *Radiology* 1989;173(3):723–729.
10. Mikic ZD. Age changes in the triangular fibrocartilage of the wrist joint. *J Anat* 1978;126:367–384.
11. Romaniuk CS, Butt WP, Coral A. Bilateral three-compartment wrist arthrography in patients with unilateral wrist pain: findings and implications for management. *Skeletal Radiol* 1995; 24(2):95–99.
12. Manaster BJ. The clinical efficacy of triple-injection wrist arthrography. *Radiology* 1991;178(1):267–270.
13. Levinsohn EM, Rosen ID, Palmer AK. Wrist arthrography: value of the three-compartment injection method. *Radiology* 1991;179(1):231–239.
14. Zinberg EM, Palmer AK, Coren AB, et al. The triple-injection wrist arthrogram. *J Hand Surg Am* 1988;13(6):803–809.
15. Linkous MD, Gilula LA. Wrist arthrography today. *Radiol Clin North Am* 1998;36(4):651–672.
16. Weiss AP, Akelman E, Lambiase R. Comparison of the findings of triple-injection cinearthrography of the wrist with those of arthroscopy. *J Bone Joint Surg* 1996;78(3):348–356.

4

Lasers and Electrothermal Devices

Daniel J. Nagle

A significant part of arthroscopic wrist surgery includes debridement of the triangular fibrocartilage (TFC), interosseous ligaments, synovium, cartilage, and even bone. Until the mid-1980s, these procedures were carried out using mechanical devices such as mini-banana blades, mini-suction punches, graspers, and motorized cutters and abraders. Good results were achieved with these instruments but with some difficulty because of the small size of the wrist joint. The small joint instruments were limited in variety and efficacy. This problem was first addressed by the holmium YAG (yttrium aluminum garnet) laser and later by radiofrequency (RF) devices, both of which are small, precise cutting and ablating tools.

LASERS

The bulk of the research on laser/RF assisted arthroscopy has been on the knee and shoulder. There has been some controversy on the use of lasers in the knee due to the report of four cases of femoral condyle avascular necrosis.[1] Whether the laser played a role in these cases remains to be seen. Avascular necrosis has also been reported after meniscectomy performed using mechanical devices.[2] Janecki et al. reviewed 504 laser-assisted knee arthroscopies and noted no new cases of avascular necrosis of the femur.[3]

There was also concern regarding the "sonic shock" produced by the vaporization of the water at the tip of the holmium YAG (Ho:YAG) laser. Gerber and his associates[4] have studied this issue and have concluded that there is no acoustic trauma associated with the use of the Ho:YAG laser.

The CO_2 laser was the first laser to be used in arthroscopy, but it proved difficult to use. The CO_2 laser energy cannot be transmitted through a fiberoptic cable and therefore requires a series of prisms in an articulated arm for delivery. Furthermore, the joint must be inflated with a gas (CO_2) because water strongly absorbs CO_2 laser light. This inflation often produces subcutaneous emphysema. Finally, the CO_2 laser produces a significant amount of char. The one advantage of the CO_2 laser is that its thermal effect remains very superficial (tissue

penetration of ± 50 microns) thus producing very little damage to adjacent tissue.

The shortcomings of the CO_2 laser contributed to the introduction of Ho:YAG laser-assisted arthroscopy. The holmium laser functions (as does the CO_2 laser) in the infrared region of the electromagnetic spectrum at 2.1 nm. In contrast to the CO_2 laser, the Ho:YAG energy can be transmitted through a quartz fiber and functions well underwater. Also, it is well absorbed by cartilage, fibrocartilage, synovial tissue, scar tissue, and hemoglobin. This last point explains the Ho:YAG's hemostatic capabilities.

Other types of lasers have been used in arthroscopy. The neodynium YAG laser has a wavelength of 1.064 nanometers, which, like the Ho:YAG and CO_2 lasers, is in the infrared region of the electromagnetic spectrum. Like the Ho:YAG laser, it can be used in a liquid medium. However, it has proved difficult to control the depth of penetration of the laser energy, and because of this the neodynium YAG laser is no longer used in arthroscopy.

Erbium lasers have also been used. Like the CO_2 and Ho:YAG lasers, the erbium is an infrared laser. The erbium laser combines the advantages of the Ho:YAG with the reduced collateral tissue injury seen with the CO_2 laser. Its use in the United Sates has been limited.

The excimer laser has also been used in arthroscopy. The wavelength of the excimer laser is in the ultraviolet region of the electromagnetic spectrum. This laser's ablative potential is based on its ability to resonate with and disrupt the covalent bonds of the tissues being ablated. This interaction produces no heat, and therefore thermal collateral injury is eliminated (hence the term *cold laser*). As mentioned, the excimer laser functions in the ultraviolet region of the electromagnetic spectrum; for this reason there is some concern it may be mutagenic. Hendrich et al. evaluated the mutagenic effect of ultraviolet light of the same wavelength (308 nm) as that used by the excimer laser and concluded that excimer laser energy is not mutagenic.[5] The excimer laser has not been used widely in arthroscopy, for two reasons. The first is that these lasers are extremely expensive. The second reason is that the fluence, or the amount of energy that can be transmitted through the quartz fiber carrying the laser energy, is barely sufficient to ablate fibrocartilage. Attempts to increase the fluence have resulted in destruction of the fiberoptic delivery system.

Let us return now for a closer look at the Ho:YAG laser. The Ho:YAG laser functions by superheating the tissues to be ablated. When the laser fires, it creates a small bubble of water vapor at its tip (the Moses effect). The tissue within this bubble absorbs the majority of the laser energy and is vaporized, leaving a layer of "caramelized" protein behind, but no char. Beyond the vapor bubble, the laser energy is quickly attenuated as it is absorbed by the water in the joint. This drop-off in energy allows the surgeon to titrate the amount of energy transmitted to the tissues in the joint. By "defocusing" the laser (pulling the tip away from the tissue), the tissue is taken out of the Moses bubble and less energy is imparted to the tissue. This allows the "melting" of chrondomalacic fronds and capsular shrinkage without injuring adjacent tissues. The water in the joint not only absorbs the laser energy but it also acts as a large, continually renewed heat sink. The problems of heat buildup and collateral tissue damage are also addressed by pulsing the laser light. The time between pulses allows the tissues outside the ablation zone to transmit the energy they absorb to the heat sink (water) and thus remain protected from thermal injury. Continuously applied laser energy does not permit the flow of heat energy away from the ablation site and results in significant collateral damage. Thus, with appropriate technique, one can modulate the energy imparted to the tissues by changing the laser pulse frequency, by changing the amount of energy per pulse, and finally, by focusing or defocusing the laser.

RADIOFREQUENCY DEVICES

Radiofrequency devices, like lasers, ablate/shrink tissue by heating the tissue. The RF devices transmit energy to the tissues via radiofrequency waves in the 100 to 450 kHz range. This electromagnetic energy causes the electrolytes within the tissue to oscillate very rapidly. This molecular oscillation creates friction within the tissue that, in turn, heats the tissue. The RF energy produces enough friction to either denature the collagen and cause shrinkage or vaporize the tissue. Monopolar and bipolar radiofrequency devices are available. Monopolar units require that a grounding pad be attached to the patient, while the bipolar devices do not. The RF devices oscillate the polarity of the active and passive electrodes to produce the RF energy. The energy of the monopolar devices flows from the active electrode *through* the tissue being treated to the passive, ground electrode. Bipolar devices have both the active and passive electrodes in the tip of the probe. The energy flows from the active

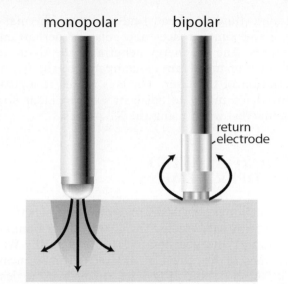

FIGURE 4.1. Monopolar: electrical current is conducted into the tissue to the grounding pad. Bipolar: current is conducted away from the tip to the return electrode on the probe shaft.

electrode back to the passive electrode, passing through the superficial layers of the tissue near the probe tip (Figure 4.1). The depth of penetration of the monopolar devices is greater than that noted with bipolar devices (4 mm vs 0.2 to 0.3 mm). With monopolar devices, the depth of tissue penetration also depends on the impedance of the tissue (see Table 4.1). It follows that the energy will penetrate deeper into a ligament than into cartilage. The RF current follows the path of least resistance.

Monopolar and bipolar devices both require a conductive milieu such as normal saline or lactated Ringer's. The tips of the RF probes are available in many shapes and sizes to accommodate the anatomy of the problem being treated.

While the following discussion focuses on the use of the Ho:YAG laser, radiofrequency (RF) devices can be used in place of the laser.[6] The only exception to this generalization is the ablation of bone, which is more readily accomplished with the laser. The RF probes can be used through the same portals described for the laser probes. Radiofrequency devices can ablate and shrink tissue. However, one must be careful while using RF wands to not overheat the joint or the structures adjacent to the joint. Adequate inflow/outflow is essential while using the RF devices. Prolonged use of the RF probes without an adequate

TABLE 4.1. Tissue Impedance.

Tissue/Substance	Impedance Ω
Saline	90–120
Ligaments	100–140
Cartilage	350–500
Bone	1100

heat sink (fluid flow) can lead to diffuse thermal injury of the joint surfaces and adjacent peri-articular structures. The RF energy penetrates the tissue to a depth of 4 or more mm as compared to the 0.5 mm penetration of the laser. There is therefore a greater potential for injury to adjacent extraarticular structures (nerves) when using the RF probes.

LASER/RF-ASSISTED TFCC DEBRIDEMENT

Andrew Palmer[7] devised a classification scheme for TFCC tears that divides TFCC tears into traumatic tears, type I and degenerative tears, type II.[7] While both types of tears can be treated arthroscopically, types I-A, II-C, and II-D lend themselves to laser-assisted debridement (Figure 4.2).

Before starting arthroscopic treatment of TFCC tears, the ulnar variance must be evaluated. This is done by taking an X-ray with the shoulder abducted to 90 degrees and the elbow flexed to 90 degrees with the hand flat on the X-ray cassette (the "90 × 90" view of Palmer).[8] Triangular fibrocartilage debridement in face of an ulnar-plus variance is doomed to fail, as the simple debridement of the TFCC is insufficient to decompress the ulnar side of the wrist. In such cases of ulnar abutment syndrome, an ulnar shortening is needed. The results of TFCC debridement in patients with an ulnar-zero variance can be good, but there lingers the possibility of having to perform an ulnar shortening later. It is recommended that this possibility be discussed with the patient preoperatively. In contrast to the patient with an ulnar plus variance, the patient who presents with an ulnar minus variance is very likely to respond to simple debridement of the central portion of the triangular fibrocartilage.[9,10]

The technique of laser-assisted triangular fibrocartilage debridement is similar to that of mechanical debridement of the triangular fibrocartilage with the exception that the arthroscope can be left in the 3-4 portal while the laser is kept in the 4-5 portal. The laser is set to 1.4 to 1.6 joules at a frequency of 15 pulses per second. With the help of a side-firing 70-degree laser tip, the triangular fibrocartilage can be

very rapidly and precisely debrided. The 70-degree laser tip permits ablation not only of the radial and palmar portions of the TFCC tear, but also the ulnar and dorsal components. There is no need to bring the laser probe in through the 3-4 portal. During the debridement, care must be taken not to injure the ulnar head. This is avoided by firing the laser tangentially to the head of the ulna or passing the probe beneath the triangular fibrocartilage and firing distally. This latter technique presents minimal danger to the lunate or triquetrum, in that the fluid used to expand the joint acts as a heat sink and absorbs the laser energy as it emerges from beneath the triangular fibrocartilage. The central portion of the TFCC is debrided back to stable edges, taking care not to injure the dorsal and palmar radioulnar ligaments.

The arthroscopic treatment of the ulnar abutment syndrome is facilitated by using the Ho:YAG laser.[11] Hyaline cartilage is very efficiently removed with the laser at higher energy settings (2.0 joules at 20 pulses per second). Not only are the ulnar head hyaline cartilage and subchondral bone rapidly removed, but, in contrast to burring, they are removed without producing much debris. Once the cancellous bone of the ulnar head is exposed, however, the bur becomes the most effective tool to complete the ulnar shortening. This is because it becomes very time consuming to focus the laser beam on each trabecula. During the ulnar head resection, care must be taken to not injure the sigmoid notch with either the laser or the bur. Also, care must be taken not to detach the insertion of the triangular fibrocartilage from the fovea at the base of the ulnar styloid. The successful arthroscopic ulnar shortening relies on teamwork. The assistant brings the surfaces of the ulnar head to be resected to the laser being held by the operating surgeon. By progressively supinating and pronating the forearm, an appropriate amount of ulnar head is excised. The goal is to resect sufficient ulna to produce a 2 mm negative ulnar variance. The amount of ulna resected must be verified with intraoperative fluoroscopy. Occasionally, complete visualization of the ulnar head requires that the scope be placed in the 4-5 portal with the laser entering the distal radioulnar joint through the distal radioulnar joint portal.

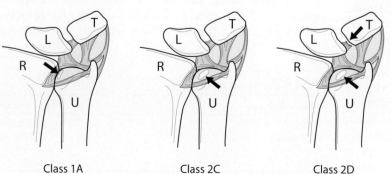

Class 1A   Class 2C   Class 2D

FIGURE 4.2. Palmer classification of TFCC tears. (Adapted with permission from Palmer AK. Triangular fibrocartilage complex lesions: a classification. *J Hand Surg Am* 1989;14:594–606.)

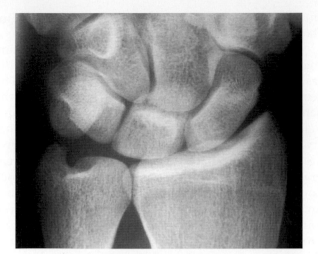

FIGURE 4.3. Ulnar abutment.

This portal is established just proximal to the 4-5 portal and TFCC.

An effort is made to leave a smooth surface on the remaining distal ulna. The trabeculae of the distal ulna always produce a somewhat rough distal ulna at the completion of the procedure. These irregularities, however, disappear during the months following the surgery (Figures 4.3 and 4.4). Large irregularities must be avoided, as they can catch on the proximal surface of the residual TFCC during supination and pronation.

The postoperative regimen after TFCC debridement, with or without ulnar shortening, includes providing the patient with a wrist splint to be worn as needed, as well as a home therapy program consisting of active and passive range of motion exercises. The sutures (wounds are closed using subcuticular sutures of 4-0 Prolene) are removed at 2 weeks. Strengthening exercises can be started at 6 weeks if needed. Premature resumption of heavy lifting or repetitive activi-

ties will lead to radiocarpal synovitis. Some patients feel so good after as little as 2 weeks that the surgeon must temper the patient's desire to return to full activity. In the case of an ulnar shortening, the recovery can be as long as 6 months, as suggested by Feldon.[12] However, the majority of patients will be improved long before 6 months.

OTHER INDICATIONS FOR LASER/RF-ASSISTED WRIST ARTHROSCOPY

Synovectomy

Synovectomy is probably the most frequently performed laser-assisted procedure. This procedure is often needed to permit complete joint visualization, particularly of the lunotriquetral and ulnocarpal joints. The laser, set at 1.2 to 1.5 joules and 15 pulses per second, vaporizes the inflamed synovium and scar tissue quickly and with minimal bleeding due to the hemostatic effect of the laser. The hemoglobin in the inflamed synovium absorbs the laser energy better than the adjacent capsule, thus providing an extra level of safety for the capsule. Scar tissue and synovitis in the radiocarpal, ulnocarpal, and midcarpal joints can be rapidly debrided. When performing a dorsal wrist synovectomy, or for that matter anytime the laser is being used, care should be taken to avoid aiming the laser at the arthroscope, as the laser energy will destroy the scope.

Partial Interosseous Ligament Tears

Partial tears of the scapholunate and lunotriquetral ligaments can be nicely treated with the laser set at 0.2

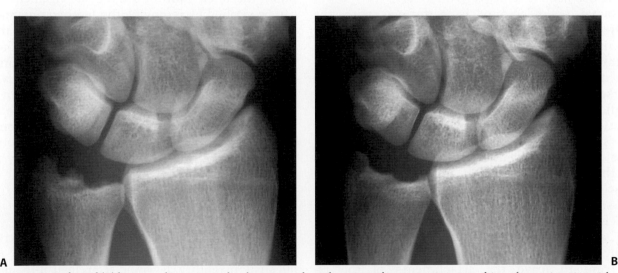

FIGURE 4.4. A. Early and **(B)** late post–laser-assisted arthroscopic ulnar shortening demonstrating smoothing of resection site with time. **A** is 6 weeks postoperative, and **B** is 6 months postoperative.

to 1.0 joule and 15 pulses per second. The ablation of these tears can be done very precisely without scuffing or injuring the adjacent intact articular cartilage.

Chondromalacia

Chondromalacia has been treated with the laser and RF devices. There is, however, evidence that at least in regard to the RF devices, significant injury to the underlying healthy cartilage can occur even when exercising caution and using low power settings.[13,14] Based on this information, it is difficult to recommend RF treatment of chondromalacia. Chondromalacic fronds can, however, be gingerly vaporized with the laser set at 0.2 to 0.8 joules and 15 pulses per second. The laser beam must be oriented tangentially to the joint surface so that only the fronds of frayed cartilage are treated. Great care must be taken to not injure the underlying healthy cartilage. Because the laser radiation can be directed selectively toward the chondromalacic fronds, sparing the underlying cartilage, it is safer in this situation than are RF devices. However, great care must be exercised. It should be kept in mind that the long-term effectiveness of debridement of chondromalacic fronds has not been established, and the potential for significant injury to healthy cartilage cannot be ignored even with the laser.

Bone Resection

We have seen that the Ho:YAG laser can be used to resect the distal ulna. Similarly, the laser can be used to perform radial styloidectomies, osteophytectomies, and complete resection of the ulnar head. The principles outlined in the section describing the laser-assisted arthroscopic Feldon procedure apply to these procedures as well. The articular cartilage and subchondral bone are vaporized with the laser, while the cancellous bone is removed with a bur.

Radial styloidectomy is performed with the arthroscope in the 4-5 portal and the laser and bur entering through the 1-2 and 3-4 portals. (The 1-2 portal is approached with caution, as the radial artery and branches of the superficial radial nerve course through this area. Only blunt dissection should be used in establishing the 1-2 portal.) A clear junction usually exists between the area of the radial styloid to be debrided (exposed subchondral bone) and the adjacent healthy cartilage. If this is not the case, a K-wire can be placed under both fluoroscopic and arthroscopic control through the radial styloid at the ulnar limit of the proposed bone resection. This provides an intra-articular landmark. The amount of styloid resected should be just enough to solve the problem being addressed, taking care to leave the attachments of the radioscaphocapitate and long radiolunate ligaments

intact. Postoperative care after this procedure is similar to that described for a TFCC debridement.

Laser-assisted arthroscopic Darrach procedures and matched ulnar resections are logical extensions of the laser-assisted arthroscopic Feldon procedure. The technique used for these procedures is essentially the same as that used for the laser-assisted arthroscopic Feldon procedure. One would anticipate less morbidity with this technique, though no published series are currently available. The use of the laser to treat grade IV chondromalacia has been successful in our hands in a limited number of cases. Two approaches are used, depending on the clinical presentation. If the joint surfaces involved cannot be unloaded (i.e., the proximal lunate), the laser is used to ablate the detached cartilage and subchondral plate. The laser debridement is extended to expose a healthy cartilage/bone interface. This "crater" margin is "freshened" with the bur. The subchondral bone is burred back to bleeding, cancellous bone. This last step is needed, as laser cauterization slows the fibrous tissue ingrowth necessary for the success of chondroplasty in this setting. Early range of motion is essential. The use of continuous passive motion has proven to be important.

The second approach is that applied to joint surfaces that can be unloaded through limited carpal shortening. A prime example of this is chondromalacia of the proximal pole of the hamate often seen in patients with a type II lunate.[15] In this situation the goal is not to promote soft tissue ingrowth but rather to unload the lunatohamate joint. This can be accomplished by establishing a viewing portal at the radial midcarpal port and an instrument portal at the ulnar midcarpal port. The proximal pole of the hamate is ablated using the laser. The resection is continued until the lunate no longer impinges on the hamate during ulnar deviation. (Care must be exercised not to injure the ulnar limb of the arcuate ligament.) This can be verified by removing the laser and manipulating the wrist while the arthroscope is still in the radial midcarpal joint. In this case the bur is not used to freshen the hamate defect, as cauterization produced by the laser seems to decrease postoperative discomfort. This effect is attributed to a decrease in postoperative bleeding and inflammation. Though early postoperative range of motion is promoted, continuous passive motion has not been needed. It should be noted that no clinical studies of chondroplasty using the Ho:YAG laser have been published.

Capsular Shrinkage

Wrist capsular shrinkage may offer an attractive alternative to more invasive treatments for subtle forms of carpal instability. It would seem logical to apply to the wrist what has been learned from shoulder capsular shrinkage. The basic science of capsular shrinkage should be the same for both joints. However, the wrist is not the shoulder, and extrapolation of shoulder data to the wrist may not be appropriate.

The biology of capsular shrinkage has been extensively studied in animal models. Capsular shrinkage is a refined "hot poker" technique. The triple helix of collagen unwinds when heated to 60 degrees C; maximum shrinkage is achieved between 65 and 75 degrees C (Figure 4.5). The hydrogen bonds holding the type I collagen triple helix together rupture as the collagen is heated beyond 60 degrees C. As the collagen triple helix unwinds, it shortens (Figure 4.6). This shortening can reach 50% of the resting length of the untreated collagen. The shortened, denatured collagen acts as scaffolding onto which new collagen is deposited.[16] The new collagen fibers maintain this shortened conformation, thus assuring the long-term maintenance of the shortening.

Biomechanical studies have demonstrated that the tensile strength of heated collagen decreases rapidly and does not return to normal values for 12 weeks.[17] The tensile strength returns to nearly 80% of normal by 6 weeks after heating (Figure 4.7). This transient loss of tensile strength would suggest that the application of stress to recently heated collagen is contraindicated. Premature loading of the shrunken collagen will lead to a lengthening of the collagen. This has been verified in an animal model.[18,19] Based on these data, it would seem reasonable to recommend at least 6 to 8 weeks of joint immobilization after capsular shrinkage. Clearly, heavy loading of the joint should be avoided for 12 weeks.

Shrinkage requires very low energy settings. The RF devices must be adjusted to heat the tissue to a temperature of between 65 and 75 degrees C. It is wise to start at low energy and slowly increase the energy output until the desired shrinkage is observed. The laser should be set to very low energy, i.e., 0.2 to 0.5 joules at 15 pulses per second (3 to 7.5 watts). The laser is held away from the target ligament and slowly advanced until the ligament is seen to shrink. Once

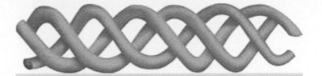

FIGURE 4.6. The normal collagen triple helix without shrinkage.

the shrinkage has stopped, continued laser exposure will only further weaken the ligament without increasing the shrinkage. The color of the ligament changes from white to light yellow during the shrinkage. Lu et al. have suggested that a cross-hatching shrinkage pattern optimizes the ingrowth of healthy tissue and hastens the recovery of the ligament.[20] During the shrinkage, traction on the wrist should be reduced as much as possible to permit optimal shrinkage.

Scapholunate Instability

Capsular shrinkage for mild scapholunate (SL) instability could be an attractive alternative to the currently available open procedures. The question is what can or should be shrunk to stabilize the SL axis. The SL interosseous ligament is a heterogeneous structure. Its central portion is composed of fibrocartilage, which is not shrinkable (Figure 4.8). The dorsal and palmar portions of the SL ligament are, however, composed of type I collagen and are shrinkable (Figure 4.9). Anecdotal reports would suggest that shrinkage of the dorsal and palmar aspects of the SL ligament can help patients with mild SL instability. No published studies are available, however, to substantiate these reports.

Capsular shrinkage of the dorsal intercarpal ligament (DIC) could potentially reinforce the stabilizing effect of SL ligament shrinkage. The DIC is attached to the distal dorsal aspect of the scaphoid and the dorsal triquetrum (Figure 4.10). Shrinkage of this

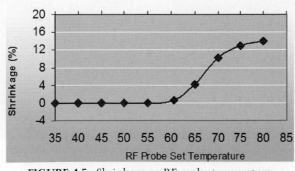

FIGURE 4.5. Shrinkage vs RF probe temperature.

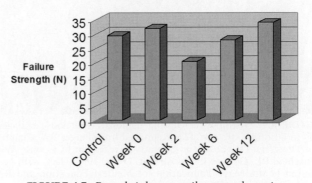
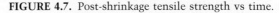

FIGURE 4.7. Post-shrinkage tensile strength vs time.

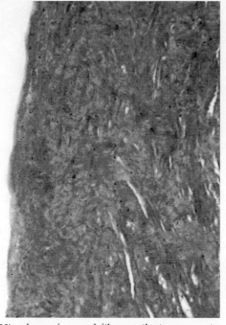

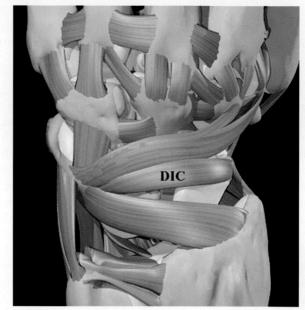

FIGURE 4.8. Histology of central fibrocartilaginous portion of the scapholunate ligament. (Reprinted from Berger RA, Chapter 5 of The Wrist Diagnosis and Operative Treatment by Cooney WP, Lilnscheid RL, Dobyns JH. Mosby: St. Louis, 1998. Used with permission of the Mayo Foundation for Medical Education and Research, Rochester, MN.)

FIGURE 4.10. Dorsal intercarpal ligament. Image from Primal Pictures, Ltd., www.primalpictures.com, with permission.

Lunotriquetral and Ulnocarpal Instability

ligament could simulate the tensioning of this ligament noted during open capsulodesis.[21] To accomplish this, the scope and laser would be placed alternately in the radial and ulnar midcarpal portals. Again, no published data are available that support this technique.

Mild forms of lunotriquetral instability can be treated with ulnocarpal ligament shrinkage. I have applied this technique in a limited number of cases with satisfying results. This procedure takes advantage of the anatomy of the ulnotriquetral and ulnolunate ligaments. These ligaments form a V as they diverge from their origin on the palmar distal radioulnar ligament and insert on the palmar aspect of the lunate or triquetrum (Figure 4.11). As the ligaments are

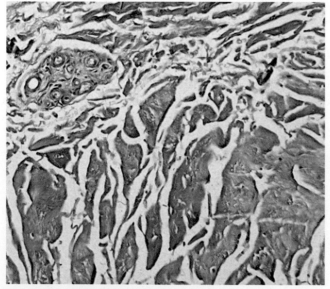

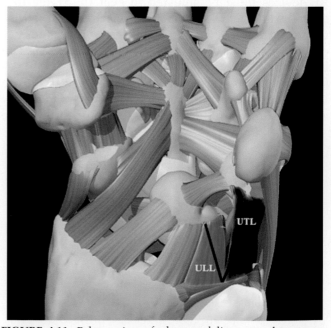

FIGURE 4.9. Histology of capsule demonstrating loose collagen (CF) in a fibrous stratum (FS). (Reprinted from Berger RA, Chapter 5 of The Wrist Diagnosis and Operative Treatment by Cooney WP, Lilnscheid RL, Dobyns JH. Mosby: St. Louis, 1998. Used with permission of the Mayo Foundation for Medical Education and Research, Rochester, MN.)

FIGURE 4.11. Palmar view of ulnocarpal ligaments demonstrating "V" configuration. Image from Primal Pictures, Ltd., www.primalpictures.com, with permission.

shrunk, the arms of the V shorten and approximate the lunate to the triquetrum thus stabilizing the LT joint. This stabilization can be further reinforced with the shrinkage of the LT interosseous ligament. The LT ligament histology is similar to that of the SL ligament and can therefore undergo dorsal and palmar but not central shrinkage. Isolated ulnocarpal ligament instability can also be treated with ulnocarpal ligament shrinkage. Ulnocarpal shrinkage is accomplished with the arthroscope in the 3-4 portal and the laser in the 4-5 or 6-U portal.

Midcarpal Instability

It is tempting to apply capsular shrinkage to the treatment of midcarpal instability. Midcarpal instability is associated with attenuation of the ulnar arcuate, triquetrohamate, dorsal intercarpal, and radiocarpal ligaments. All of these ligaments can be shrunk. The arthroscope would be placed in the radial midcarpal portal, while the laser probe would be placed in the ulnar midcarpal portal. Meaningful studies of the efficacy of this technique will be long in coming, in view of the rarity of this condition and the broad spectrum of pathology associated with midcarpal instability.

CONCLUSION

Our experience since 1990 with over 250 laser-assisted wrist arthroscopies using the Ho:YAG laser has been excellent. We have encountered no laser-related complications. We have noted no increase in postoperative wrist effusion or pain. These clinical findings echo those found in multiple articles reviewing the use of the Ho:YAG laser in the knee[22] and one article by Blackwell et al, which reviews the use of the Ho:YAG laser in the wrist.[23]

The Ho:YAG laser and RF devices should be viewed as additional tools in the wrist surgeon's armamentarium. The advantages of the laser/RF devices include their small size and the efficiency they bring to wrist arthroscopy, as well as their capability to cauterize and to precisely titrate the amount of power delivered to the operative site. The development of aggressive, 2.0 mm mechanical cutting devices has been slow and may be reaching its practical limits. This is not to say, however, that mechanical devices are obsolete. Certainly, the full-radius cutters and burs continue to be used routinely in wrist arthroscopy.

The future of lasers in wrist and joint surgery in general could be promising if the cost of the lasers decreases. Research is currently being done to evaluate the use of lasers to shrink the wrist capsule to correct subtle forms of carpal instability. Animal and tissue culture research has demonstrated that laser energy of the appropriate frequency can stimulate chonodroblast proliferation and cartilage production.[24,25] Perhaps one day the laser will help create tissue rather than ablate it.

References

1. Garino JP, Lotke PA, Sapega AA, et al. Osteonecrosis of the knee following laser-assisted arthroscopic surgery: a report of six cases. *Arthroscopy* 1995;11:467–774.
2. Johnson TC, Evans JA, Gilley JA, et al. Osteonecrosis of the knee after arthroscopic surgery for meniscal tears and chondral lesions. *Arthroscopy* 2000;16(3):254–261.
3. Janecki CJ, Perry MW, Bonati AO, et al. Safe parameters for laser chondroplasty of the knee. *Lasers Surg Med* 1998;23:141–150.
4. Gerber BE, Asshauer T, Delacretaz G, et al. Biophysical bases of the effects of holmium laser on articular cartilage and their impact on clinical application technics. *Orthopade* 1996;25:21–29.
5. Hendrich C, Werner SE. Mutagenic effects of the excimer laser using a fibroblast transformation assay. *Arthroscopy* 1997;13:151–155.
6. Osmond C, Hecht P, Hayashi K, et al. Comparative effects of laser and radiofrequency energy on joint capsule. *Clin Orthop* 2000;375:286–294.
7. Palmer AK. Triangular fibrocartilage complex lesions: a classification. *J Hand Surg Am* 1989;14:594–606.
8. Palmer AK, Glisson RR, Werner FW. Ulnar variance determination. *J Hand Surg Am* 1982;7:376–379.
9. Osterman AL. Arthroscopic debridement of triangular fibrocartilage complex tears. *Arthroscopy* 1990;6:120–124.
10. Minami A, Ishikawa J, Suenaga N, et al. Clinical results of treatment of triangular fibrocartilage complex tears by arthroscopic debridement. *J Hand Surg Am* 1966;21:406–411.
11. Nagle DJ, Bernstein MA. Laser-assisted arthroscopic ulnar shortening. *Arthroscopy* 2002;18(9):1046–1051.
12. Feldon P, Terrono AL, Belsky MR. The "wafer" procedure. Partial distal ulnar resection. *Clin Orthop* 1992;275:124–129.
13. Edwards RB 3rd, Lu Y, Nho S, et al. Thermal chondroplasty of chondromalacic human cartilage. An ex vivo comparison of bipolar and monopolar radiofrequency devices. *Am J Sports Med* 2002;30(1):90–97.
14. Lu Y, Edwards RB 3rd, Cole BJ, et al. Thermal chondroplasty with radiofrequency energy. An in vitro comparison of bipolar and monopolar radiofrequency devices. *Am J Sports Med* 2001;29(1):42–49.
15. Nakamura K, Patterson RM, Moritomo H, et al. Type I versus type II lunates: ligament anatomy and presence of arthrosis. *J Hand Surg Am* 2001;26(3):428–436.
16. Lopez MJ, Hayashi K, Vanderby R Jr, et al. Effects of monopolar radiofrequency energy on ovine joint capsular mechanical properties. *Clin Orthop* 2000;374:286–297.
17. Hecht P, Hayashi K, Lu Y, et al. Monopolar radiofrequency energy effects on joint capsular tissue: potential treatment for joint instability. An in vivo mechanical, morphological, and biochemical study using an ovine model. *Am J Sports Med* 1999;27(6):761–771.
18. Naseef GS 3rd, Foster TE, Trauner K, et al. The thermal properties of bovine joint capsule. The basic science of laser- and radiofrequency-induced capsular shrinkage *Am J Sports Med* 1997;25(5):670–674.
19. Hayashi K, Markel MD. Thermal capsulorrhaphy treatment of shoulder instability: basic science. *Clin Orthop* 2001;390:59–72.
20. Lu Y, Hayashi K, Edwards RB 3rd, et al. The effect of monopolar radiofrequency treatment pattern on joint capsular healing.

In vitro and in vivo studies using an ovine model. *Am J Sports Med* 2000;28(5):711–719.

21. Szabo RM, Slater RR Jr, Palumbo CF, et al. Dorsal intercarpal ligament capsulodesis for chronic, static scapholunate dissociation: clinical results. *J Hand Surg Am* 2002;27(6):978–984.

22. Lubbers C, Siebert WE. Holmium: YAG-laser-assisted arthroscopy versus conventional methods for treatment of the knee. Two-year results of a prospective study. *Knee Surg Sports Traumatol Arthrosc* 1997;5(3):168–175.

23. Blackwell RE, Jemison DM, Foy BD. The holmium:yttrium-aluminum-garnet laser in wrist arthroscopy: a five-year experience in the treatment of central triangular fibrocartilage complex tears by partial excision. *J Hand Surg Am* 2001;26(1):77–84.

24. Torricelli P, Giavaresi G, Fini M, et al. Laser biostimulation of cartilage: in vitro evaluation. *Biomed Pharmacother* 2001;55(2):117–120.

25. Morrone G, Guzzardella GA, Tigani D, et al. Biostimulation of human chondrocytes with Ga-Al-As diode laser: 'in vitro' research. *Artif Cells Blood Substit Immobil Biotechnol* 2000;28(2):193–201.

5

Repair and Treatment of TFCC Injury

James Chow

ANATOMY AND FUNCTION OF TFCC

The triangular fibrocartilage complex is a homogeneous structure composed of the articular disk, the volar and dorsal radioulnar ligament, the meniscal homolog, the ulnar collateral ligament, and the sheath of the extensor carpi ulnaris. The triangular fibrocartilage complex acts as an extension of the articular surface of the radius to support the proximal row and stabilize the distal radioulnar joint. The volar carpal ligaments assist in limiting wrist extension and radial deviation, as well as in stabilizing the volar-ulnar aspect of the carpus.

BIOMECHANICS

Approximately 20% of the actual load of the forearm is transferred through the ulnar side of the wrist and through the triangular fibrocartilage complex. The disk portion of the triangular fibrocartilage complex has thickening of the volar and dorsal margin, which are known as the volar and dorsal radioulnar ligaments. These ligaments help to stabilize the distal radioulnar joint. In 1989, Andrew Palmer of Syracuse, NY proposed a classification system for triangular fibrocartilage complex tear[1] that divides these injuries in two categories: traumatic (Class I) and degenerative (Class II) (Table 5.1). The four Class I subclassifications, which describe the location of injuries, clinical presentations, and suggested treatments, are outlined in Table 5.1. The five Class II subclassifications, which describe the severity of the wear to the triangular fibrocartilage complex, arthritic changes of the ulnar side of the wrist, and suggested treatments, are outlined in Table 5.2.

Class IA, IB, and IC

Class IA tears or perforations are horizontal tears of the triangular fibrocartilage complex that are usually 1 to 2 mm wide and are located 2 to 3 mm ulnar to the radial attachment on the sigmoid notch, where the articular disk is thinnest. The presenting symptoms usually are dorsal tenderness at the distal aspect of the ulna and pain with rotation of the forearm. A tri-compartmental arthrogram may demonstrate contrast medium leaking into the distal radioulnar joint. Arthroscopic debridement to remove the unstable flap of the tear is the preferred treatment for such an injury if the symptoms do not resolve after temporary splinting. The arthroscope is placed in the 3-4 portal. A small-joint banana blade is inserted through the 6-R portal, and the unstable flap is excised. The arthroscope is transferred to the 6-I portal, and a small-joint punch is inserted through the 3-4 portal to debride the most ulnar aspect of the tear, which is hard to reach from the 6-R portal. A small-joint shaver is used to smooth the remaining portion of the articular disk. Caution should be taken to avoid involving the volar and dorsal radioulnar ligaments, which serve to stabilize the distal radioulnar joint.

Class IB injuries are traumatic avulsions of the triangular fibrocartilage complex from its insertion into the distal aspect of the ulna; these avulsions may be accompanied by a fracture of the ulnar styloid process at its base.[1-3] These injuries are usually associated with distal radioulnar instability. The patient usually has tenderness around the 6-U portal, and the pain may be reproduced with ulnar deviation of the wrist. A triple arthrogram may demonstrate normal findings, and arthroscopic examination usually shows loss of tension of the articular disk of the triangular fibrocartilage complex.[4] There may be hypertrophic synovitis covering the torn part of the ulnar-dorsal portion of the articular disk, and debridement will help in locating the tear.[5,6] Various arthroscopic suturing techniques have been described for repair of ulnar peripheral tears.

For tears that extend dorsally, Whipple and associates[1-3] describe an outside-in technique that involves placing sutures longitudinally to reattach the central cartilage disk to the floor of the fifth and sixth extensor compartment. The arthroscope is normally inserted in the 3-4 portal. After establishment of a 6-R portal, fibrovascular tissue is debrided, and the dorsal margin of the central disk is freshened with a small motorized shaver. A longitudinal incision, approxi-

TABLE 5.1. Classification of Traumatic Injuries and Degenerative Lesions.

Type	Description	Clinical presentation	Suggested treatment
Class IA	Tears or perforations of the horizontal portion of the triangular fibrocartilage complex Usually 1–2mm wide Dorsal palmar slit located 2–3 mm medial to the radial attachment of the sigmoid notch	Dorsal tenderness of the distal ulna Pain with pronation/supination	Debridement to remove the unstable flap, taking care to avoid involving the volar and dorsal radioulnar ligament
Class IB	Traumatic avulsion of triangular fibrocartilage complex from insertion into the distal ulna May be accompanied by a fracture of the ulnar styloid at its base Usually associated with distal radiocarpal joint instability	Tenderness around the 6-U portal of the wrist Pain may be reproduced with ulnar deviation of the wrist Triple arthrogram may be negative	Arthroscopic examination may show loss of "trampoline sign" Debridement of hypertrophic synovitis will help locate tear Arthroscopic suturing of triangular fibrocartilage complex
Class IC	Tears of the triangular fibrocartilage complex that result in ulnocarpal instability, such as avulsion of the triangular fibrocartilage complex from the distal attachment of the lunate or triquetrum	Tenderness of palm over the pisiform Locking on ulnar side with firm grip	If no wrist instability, treat conservatively. Patients with ulnar carpal instability may need exploration and repair
Class ID	Traumatic avulsions of the triangular fibrocartilage complex from the attachment at the distal sigmoid notch	Diffuse tenderness along entire ulnar aspect of wrist Possible hemarthrosis of wrist	Past treatment: Immobilization for ~6 weeks Arthroscopic reattachment

mately 12 to 15 mm long, is then made incorporating the 6-R portal. The extensor carpi ulnaris tendon retinaculum is opened, and the tendon is retracted either ulnarly or radially. A curved cannulated needle and suture retriever are introduced through the extensor compartment floor, the needle at the distal radioulnar joint level, and the suture retriever at the radiocarpal level. The suture is advanced through the needle, brought through the dorsal capsule with the use of the suture retriever's wire loop, and tied over the dorsal capsule. Normally, two to three sutures are all that is needed to close the tear. The retinaculum can then be closed with a single suture and the skin edges closed. It is not necessary to disturb the extensor carpi ulnaris tendon for tears that lie over the ulnar styloid. For these, a 1.5 mm drill hole is made obliquely, under fluoroscopic control, through the base of the ulnar styloid. A straight needle is then used to pass a suture through the drill hole and then distally through the triangular fibrocartilage complex's ulnar edge. The suture is retrieved through a 6-U portal that has been made inside the surgical incision and tied around the volar edge of the styloid process. The patient is then placed in a long arm cast or sugar-tongs splint, in slight supination for 3 weeks; followed by a short arm cast or rigid splint for 3 weeks. The patient should avoid pronation and supination initially.

In Dr. Poehling's technique, the camera is placed

TABLE 5.2. Degenerative Lesions—Class II.

Subclassification	Description	Suggested treatment
Class IIA	Wear of the horizontal portion of the triangular fibrocartilage complex distally, proximally, or both; with no perforation Possible ulnar plus syndrome	Ulnar shortening if ulnar plus syndrome is present
Class IIB	Wear of the horizontal portion of the triangular fibrocartilage complex and chondromalacia of lunate and/or ulna	Ulnar shortening if ulnar plus syndrome is present
Class IIC	Triangular fibrocartilage complex perforation and chondromalacia of the lunate and/or ulna	Arthroscopic debridement Wafer procedure if ulnar plus syndrome is present
Class IID	Triangular fibrocartilage complex perforation and chondromalacia of the lunate and/or ulna Perforation of the lunotriquetrum ligament	Arthroscopic debridement Wafer procedure if ulnar plus syndrome is present
Class IIE	Triangular fibrocartilage complex perforation and chondromalacia of the lunate and/or ulna Perforation of the lunotriquetrum ligament Ulnocarpal arthritis	Arthroscopic debridement Wafer procedure if ulnar plus syndrome is present

in the 4-5 portal and a 20-gauge Tuohy needle is placed in the radiocarpal joint through either the 1-2 or 3-4 portal. Under direct visualization, the needle is passed through the torn edge of the triangular fibrocartilage complex, then through the ligamentous tissue above the ulnar styloid, and out through the soft tissue and skin. A 2-0 absorbable suture is threaded through the entire needle and anchored at each end with hemostats. The needle is then brought back into the joint space and passed through the edge of the tear again, advanced through the ligamentous tissue on the ulnar side of the joint, and out through the soft tissue and skin, with the suture traveling through the soft tissue both inside and outside the needle. The suture is pulled out of the needle on the ulnar side of the wrist. The needle is then withdrawn back into the joint space. Both ends of the suture are anchored in the same manner as before. This is repeated until three sutures are in place; then the needle can be removed from the wrist. Blunt subcutaneous dissection is then carried out, and, under direct visualization from the 4-5 portal, all sutures are pulled back through the skin and out the single incision. They are tied firmly so that the triangular fibrocartilage complex is pulled against the ulnar side of the wrist. The skin can then be closed over the knots so that they stay subcutaneous. The patient is then placed in a splint for 1 month and allowed to move the fingers and pronate/supinate the forearm.

The Chow technique uses a meniscus mender instrument set, along with a 25-gauge needle as a guide for insertion of the sutures to reattach the triangular fibrocartilage complex to the joint capsule. The arthroscope is engaged in the 3-4 portal, using the 6-U portal for assistance. A shaver is introduced to remove the synovium and allow better visualization of the dorsal aspect between the 3-4 and 4-5 portals. The peripheral tear is identified, and the shaver used to refresh the edges of the torn tissue, preferably to bleeding tissue but taking care to avoid debriding too much of the joint capsule. Following this, a 25-gauge needle,

with the head removed to gain access from the outside, is used as a guide for the insertion of the repair sutures. The straight needle is then checked to be sure that the wire loop is easy to open and that the sharp-tipped side is pointing down.

The 4-5 and 6-R arthroscopy portals are the most common suturing sites and, if the patient has a large hand, it is recommended that the portals be made at this time to allow easier movement of the needle inside the joint (Figure 5.1). The wire loop is brought back inside the straight needle, and the needle is inserted on the distal side of the triangular fibrocartilage complex, following the guide of the 25-gauge needle and being careful that the bevel of the needle is facing up to avoid damage to the articular surface. The second straight needle, containing the suture, is inserted 4 to 5 mm inferior to the first needle, with the bevel face inserted face down and with the sharp-tipped edge pointing upwards, for ease in puncturing the torn triangular fibrocartilage complex.

Once the needle has passed through the triangular fibrocartilage complex, the wire loop is advanced from the first needle to loop around the second needle. Turning the second needle gently so that the bevel face is face up will engage the wire loop further while the wire loop is gently pulled to further engage the triangular fibrocartilage complex with the second needle. The suture is then passed through the second needle. Following this, the second needle is retreated gently through the triangular fibrocartilage complex to avoid cutting the suture (Figure 5.2). If there is difficulty in

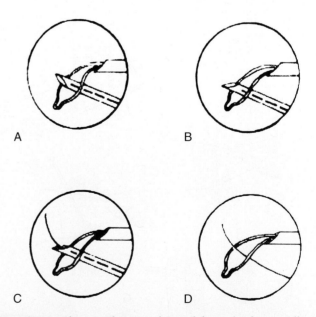

FIGURE 5.2. The wire loop is advanced from the first needle to loop around the second needle **A**. Turning the second needle gently so that the bevel face is up will engage the wire loop further **B**. The suture is passed through the second needle (**C**), and the second needle is retreated gently through the triangular fibrocartilage complex to avoid cutting the suture **D**.

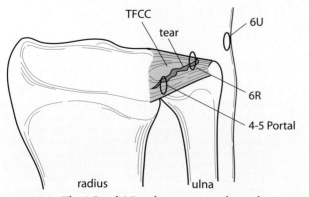

FIGURE 5.1. The 4-5 and 6-R arthroscopy portals are the most common for suturing.

placing the wire loop over the second needle, the grasper can be advanced to grasp the suture and pull it through the 6-U portal.

The end of the suture is secured to the second needle with a hemostat, and the wire loop is retracted, pulling the suture back through the 6-U portal and out the dorsal aspect of the wrist, where it is secured. A small incision is made between the sutures and blunt dissection to the joint capsule is performed with a hemostat, under direct visualization of the scope, taking care not to trap any tendons or puncture the joint capsule.

A probe is inserted into the incision and looped around the suture, above and below, to bring it out of the center incision. The probe is then used to ensure that no tendons or tissue are caught, and hemostats are used to tack down the suture for future tying. A second suture can be placed in the same fashion. When all of the sutures are in place, the tying process begins. The surgeon's knot is preferred for the first knot, followed by insertion of the probe under arthroscopic visualization to ensure that the suture is tight before tying the second knot.

If the tear involves the 6-R or 6-U portal, an alternative method of the Chow technique can be used. As the flat edge of the triangular fibrocartilage complex tear should be easily identified, a grasper is brought in through the portal to hold the triangular fibrocartilage complex. A simple straight needle is passed through the triangular fibrocartilage complex without difficulty with the bevel face down. Once through, the needle is turned bevel face up, and the suture is passed through to be retrieved by the grasper. The needle is backed out to avoid severing the suture, while the grasper gently pulls the arm of the suture through the portal. A nerve probe is then used to loop the other suture arm and bring it through the portal (Figure 5.3). Now the suture is freely tacked onto the triangular fibrocartilage complex, and the ends of the sutures are free to tack to the joint capsule. The rest of the suturing procedure is as described above.

Class ID

Recently, Scott Sagerman and Walter Short have suggested arthroscopic reattachment. Following debridement of the bony rim of the sigmoid notch, the radial edge of the horizontal disk is reattached to the bone by means of drilling two holes with small K-wires percutaneously into the joint from the sigmoid notch across the distal radius.[7] Long meniscal repair needles are inserted through the drill holes to place two nonabsorbable sutures into the horizontal disk and out the radial aspect of the wrist. These sutures are tied directly over the radius by means of a small incision. The distal radioulnar joint is then pinned in neutral position using one 0.062″ K-wire percutaneously.

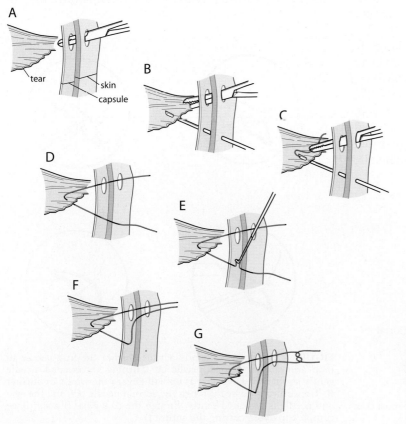

FIGURE 5.3. A grasper is brought in through the portal to hold the triangular fibrocartilage complex **A**. A straight needle is passed through the triangular fibrocartilage complex with the bevel face down **B**. Once through, the needle is turned bevel face up and the suture is passed through and retrieved by the grasper **C**. The needle is backed out gently while the grasper gently pulls the arm of the suture through the portal **D**. A nerve probe is then used to loop the other suture arm and bring it through the portal **E–G**.

Class IIC, IID, and IIE

Arthroscopic debridement is the recommended treatment of these lesions; however, if ulnar pulse is present, the wafer procedure can be performed through the arthroscope.[8] This involves using a bur to resect 2 to 3 mm of the ulnar head; visualization is gained through the triangular fibrocartilage complex tear by supinating or pronating the wrist. The most common question regarding the wafer procedure is how much bone needs to be resected. Under normal conditions less than 4 mm of resection should be undertaken. Precautions should be taken to preserve the stability of the distal radioulnar joint and the origins of the ulnar carpal ligament. Some surgeons recommend the use of the laser to resect the ulnar head to the bony section before using the bur.[9,10] However, I do not have enough experience with this technique to comment on its success.

In patients with Class IIA or B type pathology, where the articular disk is eroded but not perforated, open ulnar shortening may be considered. This is indicated in patients with chronic ulnar-sided wrist pain who are ulnar positive. It is important not to perforate the articular disk to perform an arthroscopic ulnar shortening. An oblique ostectomy is made in the ulna, and a 7-hole, 35 mm plate is placed on the volar surface of the ulna. The patient is less likely to feel the plate on the volar surface of the ulna or to require eventual metal removal. It is important not to make the screws too long, or the patient may feel them dorsally.

It is helpful to place three saw blades together in the saw when making the cut to ensure a perfect parallel ostectomy. Also, one screw placed on the distal portion of the plate prior to cutting the bone helps to control the ostectomy. A lag screw is placed through the fourth screw hole across the oblique ostectomy.

References

1. Whipple, TL. TFCC Injury-Biomechanics, classification and treatment with Whipple technique. In: James Chow, (ed.) *Advanced Arthroscopy*, New York: Springer-Verlag, *to be published*.

2. Whipple, TL (ed). *Arthroscopic Surgery: The Wrist*. Philadelphia: Lippincott, 1992, pp. 103–105.

3. Corso SJ, Savoie FH, Geissler WB, et al. Arthroscopic repair of peripheral avulsions of the triangular fibrocartilage complex of the wrist: a multicenter study. *Arthroscopy* 1997;13:78–84.

4. Roth JH, Haddad RG. Radiocarpal arthroscopy and arthrography in the diagnosis of ulnar wrist pain. *Arthroscopy* 1986;2(4):234–243.

5. Richards RS, Bennet JD, Roth JH, et al. Arthroscopic diagnosis of intra-articular soft tissue injuries associated with distal radius fractures. *J Hand Surg Am* 1997;22A:772–776.

6. Palmer AK. Triangular fibrocartilage complex lesion: a classification. *J Hand Surg Am* 1989;14A:494–606.

7. Hermansdorfer JD, Kleinman WB. Management of chronic peripheral tears of the triangular fibrocartilage complex. *J Hand Surg Am* 1991;16A:340–346.

8. Sagerman SD, Short W. Arthroscopic repair of radial-sided triangular fibrocartilage complex tears. *Arthroscopy* 1996;12:339–342.

9. Wnorowski DC, Palmer AK, Werner FW, et al. Anatomic and biomechanical analysis of the arthroscopic wafer procedure. *Arthroscopy* 1992;8(2):204–212.

10. Nagle DJ. *The Use of Lasers in Wrist Arthroscopy*. Presented at the AANA Fall Meeting, Orthopaedic Learning Center, Rosemont, IL, November 7, 1997.

6

Repair of Peripheral Ulnar TFCC Tears

Sanjay K. Sharma and Thomas E. Trumble

The use of the arthroscope in hand surgery has greatly advanced the diagnosis, evaluation, and management of ulnar-sided wrist pain. One cause of ulnar-sided wrist pain stems from an injury to the triangular fibrocartilage complex (TFCC), an integral component to rotation of the carpus about the ulna. This motion is quite complex, as it involves combinations of rotation, translation, and load transmission. Hence, injury to this region can cause persistent pain, limited hand function, and patient unhappiness. An understanding of the complex anatomy of the TFCC has allowed practitioners to use the arthroscope effectively in treating TFCC injuries. In the last 10 years, studies have shown arthroscopic repair of TFCC injuries to be safe, effective, and long-lasting. Though much has been written about treatment of TFCC injuries, the focus of this chapter will be arthroscopic repair of peripheral ulnar-sided TFCC tears.

CLASSIFICATION

The most commonly used classification system used to describe TFCC injuries was developed by Palmer.[1] This classification helps differentiate between traumatic lesions and degenerative lesions. Understanding the Palmer classification determines the course of treatment, so it is essential to understand it.

Class 1

These acute, traumatic injuries are subdivided into 4 types based on the site of injury (Figure 6.1). Type 1A lesions involve the central avascular portion and are generally not suitable for direct repair. Arthroscopic treatment is limited to debridement of the central tear to remove any flaps that may impede movement. Type 1B (ulnar avulsion) injuries occur when the ulnar side of the TFCC complex is avulsed from its insertion. These injuries can be associated with ulnar styloid fractures. The type 1C (ulnar distal) injury involves rupture of the volar attachment of the TFCC or distal ulnocarpal ligaments; this is variably amenable to repair. Finally, type 1D (radial avulsion) injuries occur

when the radial attachment of the TFCC ruptures; this can happen with or without a fracture of the radial sigmoid notch.

Class 2

Degenerative TFCC lesions all involve the central portion and are staged from A to E depending on the presence or absence of TFCC perforation, lunate and ulnar chondromalacia, lunotriquetral ligament perforation, and degenerative radiocarpal arthritis. These degenerative lesions usually arise from ulnar abutment. Generally, class 2 lesions are not amenable to surgical repair.

We have subdivided TFCC tears further by their time course.[2] Acute tears have occurred less than 3 months from the time of injury to repair and result in the recovery of 80% of the grip strength and range of motion of the contralateral side. Acute injuries have a better prognosis than subacute injuries (3 months to 1 year) and chronic injuries (greater than 1 year).[3,4] Subacute injuries are still amenable to direct repairs of the TFCC, but in general regain less strength. Occasionally, the TFCC tear in a chronic injury is repairable, but the result is not as good as in acute repairs, presumably due to contraction of the ligaments and degeneration of the torn fibrocartilage margins.[4] Chronic injuries frequently require ulnar shortening with or without TFCC debridement.

DIAGNOSIS

History

Injuries to the TFCC commonly occur with extension and pronation of the axially loaded carpus, as commonly occurs with a fall on the outstretched hand. Another common mechanism involves traction forces to the ulnar side of the wrist or forearm. Athletic activities involving rapid twisting of the wrist with ulnar-sided loading, such as in racquet sports or golf are common injury mechanisms. Patients often delay treatment or are misdiagnosed as having a wrist sprain that fails to get better.

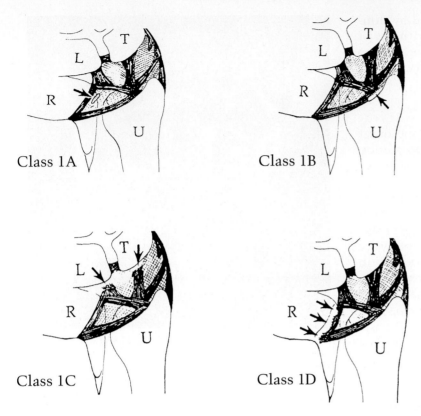

Class 1A   Class 1B

Class 1C   Class 1D

FIGURE 6.1. Palmer classification for class 1 triangular fibrocartilage complex lesions. Class 1B and 1C represent ulnar and distal injuries, respectively. (Modified and reprinted from J. Hand Surg. (WB Saunders Co.) Triangular Fibrocartilage Complex Lesions: A Classification,' Palmer, AK, 1988, Vol. 14A, No. 4, Figures 5, 7, 9, and 11 from p. 598–601 with permission from Elsevier Science.)

Symptoms of a TFCC injury include ulnar-sided wrist pain characterized by diffuse, deep aching, sometimes burning in nature, that can radiate dorsally but rarely volarly. Pain is also elicited with firm grasp. A clicking sensation may be present with wrist pronation and supination. Patients may also complain of generalized weakness both with and without wrist loading.

Physical Examination

Acute TFCC injuries are accompanied by ulnar-sided wrist swelling. A reversal of the normal convex shape of the ulnar border of the wrist is noted in many cases. Point tenderness is present when palpating the ulnar side of the wrist in the ballotable region between the ulnar styloid and the triquetrum (Figure 6.2). Passive motion of the wrist through its range can reveal a clicking sensation resulting from a fibrocartilage flap trapped in the radiocarpal joint or lunotriquetral ligament.

Several tests have been described that are helpful in the diagnosis of ulnar-sided wrist pain. The TFCC compression test is positive if axial loading of the TFCC with ulnar deviation results in significant pain. Similarly, de Araujo et al. described the ulnar impaction test that elicits pain by wrist hyperextension and ulnar deviation with axial compression.[5] The piano key test reveals distal radioulnar joint instability if the distal ulna is found to freely move in the dorsal-volar plane. Volar sublux-

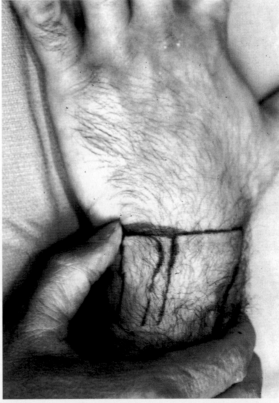

FIGURE 6.2. Pain elicited with pressure applied between the ulnar styloid and triquetrum correlates with TFCC injury. (Reproduced from Trumble TE: 'Principles of Hand Surgery and Therapy,' (W.B. Saunders Co,) (© July 2000), Chapter 6, 'Distal Radioulnar Joint and Triangular Fibrocartilage Complex,' Fig. 6–7 with permission from Elsevier Science.)

ation of the distal ulna can be represented by dimpling along the dorsal wrist surface with wrist supination. Finally, the shuck test[6] can be used to diagnose lunotriquetral ligament instability.

Diagnostic Modalities

All patients presenting with acute or chronic onset ulnar-sided wrist pain should have anteroposterior, lateral, and oblique radiographs taken of the wrist. While this does not directly diagnose soft tissue pathology, indirect information can be obtained from the relationships of ulnar variance, the distal radioulnar joint, and the presence or absence of an ulnar styloid or distal radius fracture. The presence of cystic changes in the lunate and distal ulna, especially in conjunction with ulnar neutral or positive variance, implies excessive loading through the ulnar carpus and suggests additional offloading treatments be considered for this region.

Triple-injection wrist arthrography as described by Zinberg et al has been useful in diagnosing certain aspects of TFCC tears.[7] Arthrography reliably diagnoses TFCC radial detachment and lunotriquetral ligament tears; however, other ulnocarpal ligament injuries and ulnar TFCC detachments are often missed.[2,3] Peripheral TFCC tears are not well differentiated from central tears.[8] Several reports of positive arthrograms in asymptomatic patients raise the question of false positive results.[9–15]

The usefulness of magnetic resonance imaging (MRI) for the diagnosis of TFCC injuries is a contentious issue. Golimbu et al[16] and Skahen et al[17] stated that MRI detects central and radial detachment lesions well. T2-weighted images enhance synovial fluid, thus detecting TFCC injuries with an accuracy of 95% (Figure 6.3). Bednar was less enthusiastic, stating that MRI is 44% sensitive and 75% specific for TFCC injuries.[18] Corso et al found a sensitivity of 76% in a study of ulnar TFCC lesions.[8] Fulcher and Poehling felt that MRI understaged some TFCC pathology while overstaging others, and recommend the use of arthroscopy for definitive diagnosis.[19] Pederzini et al performed arthrography, MRI, and arthroscopy on 11 patients with TFCC injuries.[20] Using arthroscopic findings as the gold standard, they found 100% specificity of both techniques and 80% and 82% sensitivity, respectively, of arthrography and MRI. It is important to note that these were chronic injuries (average 18 months old), and 9 of 11 demonstrated chondromalacia.

Studies comparing arthroscopy with arthrography confirm arthroscopy to be the gold standard in detecting and characterizing TFCC injuries.[11,21,22] The principal advantage in proceeding with arthroscopy is that one procedure has both diagnostic and therapeutic capabilities. Irreparable or degenerative TFCC tears can be debrided, while repairable tears can be ad-

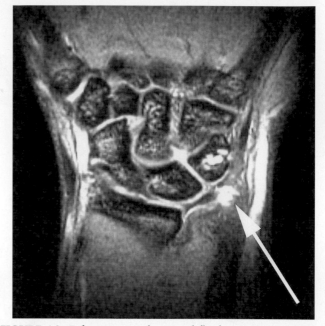

FIGURE 6.3. Enhancement of synovial fluid seen on T2-weighted image MRI can delineate ulnar-sided tears of the TFCC. (Reproduced from Orthopedic Clinics of North America, (WB Saunders Co.) Arthroscopic Repair of Triangular Fibrocartilage Complex Injuries. Cober, SE and Trumble, TE. © 2001, Vol 30, No. 2, figure 8, p. 284 with permission from Elsevier Science.)

dressed immediately. The prudent surgeon is advised to consider the patient's history, mechanism of injury, and findings on physical examination to help guide the choice of immediate arthroscopy versus advanced imaging studies.

TREATMENT

Nonoperative Intervention

The appropriate treatment for TFCC injuries is variable and dependent on the type of injury. The initial decision for operative vs. nonoperative intervention is based on ulnar-sided carpal and distal radioulnar joint stability. If a patient presents with a history and exam consistent with a TFCC injury, has normal radiographs, and is clinically stable, 4 weeks of long arm cast immobilization is usually successful. If no improvement is noted after 1 month, further diagnostic studies such as arthrograms, MRI, or arthroscopy are warranted. If a patient presents with radiographic or clinical instability, primarily arthroscopic evaluation and repair should be considered.

Ulnar Recession

Another confounding variable facing the surgeon repairing the TFCC, especially in the chronic setting, is whether to shorten the ulna. Numerous articles elucidate the importance of ulnar variance in the outcomes of TFCC repair.[23–25] The senior author believes it is appropriate to perform ulnar recession when symptoms have been present for more than one year and an ulnar neutral or positive variance is present.[4]

Class 1B

These lesions will likely heal with suture repair since they occur in the peripheral, well-vascularized portion of the TFCC. Repairs of this class of ulnar-sided avulsion injuries can be divided into inside-out or outside-in types. The inside-out repair enjoyed early recognition. Several authors describe using a 6-inch, 20-gauge Tuohy (Becton Dickinson, Franklin Lakes, New Jersey) needle with a blunt tip originally designed for epidural placement.[19,26] The technique described by de Araujo et al introduces the needle into the radiocarpal joint from the 1-2 portal, passing it through the free edge of the TFC tear, and out the volar skin of the ulnar carpus.[5] Once a 2-0 PDS is completely through the needle, the Tuohy is withdrawn into the radiocarpal joint, and the TFC is repunctured 3 to 5 mm from the first site and back out the skin. Next, a horizontal mattress suture is placed in the TFC and tied on the ulnar wrist capsule through a small skin incision. Patients are immobilized in supination for 3 to 4 weeks and progress gently to activity as tolerated at 6 weeks.[19] These authors reported a 70% satisfaction rate at 16 to 24 months in 17 patients. Skie et al. describe a variation on this technique using "zone-specific" cannulas from knee arthroscopic kits which enabled long, flexible meniscal needles to be introduced from the 4-5 portal and directed through the torn region in a horizontal mattress manner.[27]

The outside-in repair techniques all involve puncturing the ulnar wrist capsule through the torn edge of the TFCC. The suture is then retrieved and brought out the ulnar side of the wrist. Several authors describe using a TFCC repair kit (Linvatec, Largo, Florida).[8,26] A curved, cannulated suture passer is inserted through the extensor carpi ulnaris (ECU) sheath and the edge of the TFCC tear. A loop suture retriever is then inserted with the loop end over the tip of the suture passer. Using a 2-0 PDS suture, a simple tie secures the TFCC across the tear. Several sutures are passed as needed. Taking the wrist through its range of pronation and supination with the sutures pulled tight will help find the best position for coaptation of TFCC edges. The sutures are then tied in this position either over a bolster or on the wrist capsule through a small skin incision. The postoperative regimen includes immobilizing patients for 4 weeks in a long arm cast, then advancing to a short arm splint with progressive range of motion.[8] In a multicenter study, Corso et al. reported 41 of 45 patients with good or excellent results using the Mayo modified wrist score and return to normal activity by 3 months.

Other methods of TFCC repair are modifications of a meniscal repair described by Clancy, Graf, and Warren.[28,29] Zachee repairs ulnar-sided TFCC avulsions by extending an 18-gauge needle across the tear from the ulnar side of the wrist.[30] A suture is then passed through the needle and retrieved through a radial port. After an external knot is tied, the suture is pulled back into the joint, leaving the internal knot as an anchor to coapt the edges of the tear. A number of sutures are passed in this manner so as to complete the repair.

Our preferred repair method of ulnar-sided TFCC injuries is an outside-in technique. The arthroscopy is performed using distraction with a wrist traction tower. Ten to 15 pounds of traction are applied depending on the size of the extremity. After initial debridement is completed, a small probe is inserted to diagnose peripheral detachment of the TFCC, using the trampoline test as described by Hermansdorfer and Kleinman (Figure 6.4).[31] The repair suture is threaded into an 18-gauge needle and inserted into the wrist joint just inferior to the 6-U portal under arthroscopic guidance (Figure 6.5). The needle passes just radial through the torn edge of the TFCC. The suture is

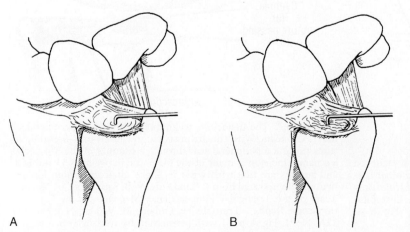

A   B

FIGURE 6.4. Trampoline test to detect lax peripheral detachment of the TFCC. An intact TFCC is firm and tense (**A**) whereas the torn TFC is loose and slack (**B**). (Reproduced from Trumble TE: Principles of Hand Surgery and Therapy, (W.B. Saunders Co.) (© July 2000) Chapter 6, 'Distal Radioulnar Joint and Triangular Fibrocartilage Complex,' Fig. 6–18 with permission from Elsevier Science.)

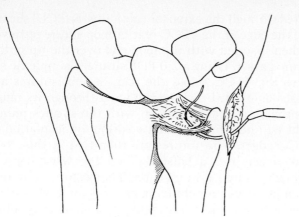

FIGURE 6.5. The outside-in technique of repairing ulnar-sided TFCC injuries. Using a passing needle, such as an 18-G needle, a suture is introduced through the ulnar wrist capsule, which has been guided through the detached edge and out the other side of the TFCC. (Reproduced from Trumble TE: *Principles of Hand Surgery and Therapy*, W.B. Saunders Co., © 2000 Chapter 6, 'Distal Radioulnar Joint and Triangular Fibrocartilage Complex,' Fig. 6–19 with permission from Elsevier Science.)

threaded out through the needle and grasped using a small arthroscopic grasping forceps or wire suture grasper placed through the 6-U portal (Figure 6.6). Two or three sutures are passed using this technique. To help identify the dorsal sensory branch of the ulnar nerve, the 6-U portal is made larger. This portal is bounded radially by the ECU tendon and ulnarly by the ulnar sensory branch. Thus, care must be taken to identify the branches of the dorsal ulnar sensory nerve while placing and tying the repair sutures. Tension is then placed on the sutures to ensure that there is reestablishment of TFCC tension and obliteration of any gapping between the articular disk and the peripheral capsular tissue. The hand is then taken out of the traction device, and the sutures are tied with the wrist in slight ulnar deviation and the forearm in neutral rotation.

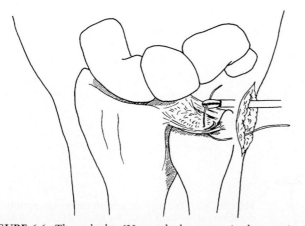

FIGURE 6.6. Through the 6U portal, the suture is then retrieved using a grasping forceps and tied taking care to avoid the ulnar sensory nerve. (Reproduced from Trumble TE: *Principles of Hand Surgery and Therapy*, W.B. Saunders Co., © 2000 Chapter 6, 'Distal Radioulnar Joint and Triangular Fibrocartilage Complex,' Fig. 6–20 with permission from Elsevier Science.)

Class 1C

Injuries that are directly along the volar side of the wrist are often not amenable to arthroscopic repair, but can be improved by debridement. When a repair can be accomplished, we prefer an inside-out technique (Figure 6.7). A straight #12 French suction tip is placed into the 3-4 portal as a cannula for 2-0 Maxon meniscal repair sutures (Davis & Geck, Wayne, NJ). The ulnar nerve is identified and protected using a retractor. The sutures are then placed through the cannula and brought out through the ulnar incision. Two or three sets of sutures are normally required.

CONCLUSION

The use of arthroscopy in the management of TFCC lesions has changed and improved the outcomes of pa-

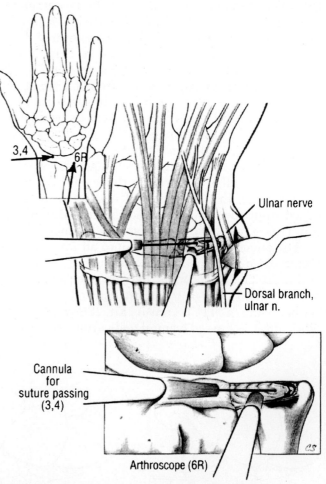

FIGURE 6.7. The inside-out technique for repairing peripheral ulnar TFCC tears. With the arthroscopic in the 6R or 4–5 portal, sutures transfix a peripheral tear through a cannula in the 3–4 portal; a separate incision is made at the 6U portal between FCU and ECU and sutures are tied with wrist in slight ulnar deviation, forearm neutral. (Reproduced from J. Hand Surg. W.B. Saunders Co. "Isolated Tears of the Triangular Fibrocartilage: Management by Early Arthroscopic Repair," Trumble TE, Gilbert, M, Vedder, N. 1997, Vol. 22A, No. 1, Fig. 4, p. 61 with permission from Elsevier Science.)

tients with this spectrum of wrist injuries. Ulnar-sided TFCC lesions, even the rare type IC tears, can be effectively treated with arthroscopic assistance. Less scarring and less need for postoperative immobilization help patients return to work with greater functional capacity. Further refinements in repair of the distal ulnar TFCC lesions will enhance the treatment of these injuries and improve patient satisfaction and outcomes.

References

1. Palmer A. Triangular fibrocartilage complex lesions: a classification. *J Hand Surg* 1989;14A:594–606.
2. Trumble T, Gilbert M, Vedder N. Isolated tears of the triangular fibrocartilage: management by early arthroscopic repair. *J Hand Surg* 1997;22A:57–65.
3. Trumble T, Gilbert M, Vedder N. Arthroscopic repair of the triangular fibrocartilage complex. *Arthroscopy* 1996;12:588–597.
4. Trumble T, Gilbert M, Vedder N. Ulnar shortening combined with arthroscopic repairs in the delayed management of triangular fibrocartilage complex tears. *J Hand Surg* 1997;22A:807–813.
5. de Araujo W, Poehling G, Kuzma G. New Tuohy needle technique for triangular fibrocartilage complex repair: preliminary studies. *Arthroscopy* 1996;12:699–703.
6. Nagle D. Arthroscopic treatment of degenerative tears of the triangular fibrocartilage. *Hand Clin* 1994;10:615–624.
7. Zinberg E, Palmer A, Coren A, et al. The triple-injection wrist arthrogram. *J Hand Surg* 1988;13A:803–809.
8. Corso S, Savoie F, Geissler W, et al. Arthroscopic repair of peripheral avulsions of the triangular fibrocartilage complex of the wrist: a multicenter study. *Arthroscopy* 1997;13:78–84.
9. Brown J, Janzen D, Adler B, et al. Arthrography of the contralateral, asymptomatic wrist in patients with unilateral wrist pain. *Can Assoc Radiol J* 1994;45:292–296.
10. Cantor R, Stern P, Wyrick J, et al. The relevance of ligament tears or perforations in the diagnosis of wrist pain: an arthrographic study. *J Hand Surg* 1994;19A:945–953.
11. Cooney W. Evaluation of chronic wrist pain by arthrography, arthroscopy, and arthrotomy. *J Hand Surg* 1993;18A:815–822.
12. Kirschenbaum D, Sieler S, Solonick D, et al. Arthrography of the wrist: assessment of the integrity of the ligaments in young asymptomatic adults. *J Bone Joint Surg Am* 1995;77A:1207–1209.
13. Koman L, Poehling G, Toby E, et al. Chronic wrist pain: indications for wrist arthroscopy. *Arthroscopy* 1990;6:116–119.
14. Levinsohn E, Rosen I, Palmer A. Wrist arthrography: value of the three-compartment injection method. *Radiology* 1991;179:231–239.
15. Osterman A. Arthroscopic debridement of triangular fibrocartilage complex tears. *Arthroscopy* 1990;6:120–124.
16. Golimbu C, Firooznia H, Melone CJ, et al. Tears of the triangular fibrocartilage of the wrist: MR imaging. *Radiology* 1989;173:731–733.
17. Skahen JI, Palmer A, Levinsohn E, et al. Magnetic resonance imaging of the triangular fibrocartilage complex. *J Hand Surg* 1990;15A:552–557.
18. Bednar M, Arnoczky S, Weiland A. The microvasculature of the triangular fibrocartilage complex: its clinical significance. *J Hand Surg* 1991;16A:1101–1105.
19. Fulcher S, Poehling G. The role of operative arthroscopy for the diagnosis and treatment of lesions about the distal ulna. *Hand Clin* 1998;14:285–296.
20. Pederzini L, Luchetti R, Soragni O, et al. Evaluation of the triangular fibrocartilage complex by arthroscopy, arthrography, and magnetic resonance imaging. *Arthroscopy* 1992;8:191–197.
21. Chung K, Zimmerman N, Travis M. Wrist arthrography versus arthroscopy: a comparative study of 150 cases. *J Hand Surg* 1996;21A:591–594.
22. Weiss A, Akelman E, Lambiase R. Comparison of the findings of triple-injection cinearthrography of the wrist with those of arthroscopy. *J Bone Joint Surg Am* 1996;78A:348–356.
23. Hulsizer D, Weiss AP, Akelman E. Ulna-shortening osteotomy after failed arthroscopic debridement of the triangular fibrocartilage complex. *J Hand Surg Am* 1997;22:694–698.
24. Minami A, Ishikawa J, Suenaga N, et al. Clinical results of treatment of triangular fibrocartilage complex tears by arthroscopic debridement. *J Hand Surg Am* 1996;21:406–411.
25. Minami A, Kato H. Ulnar shortening for triangular fibrocartilage complex tears associated with ulnar positive variance. *J Hand Surg Am* 1998;23:904–908.
26. Gan B, Richards R, Roth J. Arthroscopic treatment of triangular fibrocartilage tears. *Orthop Clin North Am* 1995;26:721–729.
27. Skie M, Mekhail A, Deitrich D, et al. Operative technique for inside-out repair of the triangular fibrocartilage complex. *J Hand Surg* 1997;22A:814–817.
28. Clancy WJ, Graf B. Arthroscopic meniscal repair. *Orthopedics* 1983;6:1125.
29. Warren R. Arthroscopic meniscus repair. *Arthroscopy* 1985;1:170–172.
30. Zachee B, DeSmet L, Fabry G. Arthroscopic suturing of TFCC lesions. *Arthroscopy* 1993;9:242–243.
31. Hermansdorfer J, Kleinman W. Management of chronic peripheral tears of the triangular fibrocartilage complex. *J Hand Surg* 1991;16A:340–346.

7

Repair of Peripheral Radial TFCC Tears

William B. Geissler and Walter H. Short

Arthroscopy has revolutionized the practice of orthopaedics by providing the technical capability to examine and treat intra-articular abnormalities. The development of wrist arthroscopy was a natural progression from the successful application of arthroscopy to other, larger joints. The wrist is a labyrinth composed of 8 carpal bones, multiple articular surfaces with 28 intrinsic and extrinsic ligaments, and the triangular fibrocartilage complex (TFCC), all within a 5-cm interval. This perplexing joint continues to challenge clinicians with an array of potential diagnoses and treatments. Wrist arthroscopy allows direct visualization of the cartilage surfaces, synovial tissue, and the triangular fibrocartilage complex under bright light and magnification.

Ulnar-sided wrist pain is a common complaint that encompasses a broad range of potential differential diagnoses. One potential cause of ulnar-sided wrist pain is a tear or degeneration of the TFCC. Tears of the TFCC can occur centrally or at the radial or ulnar attachment. This chapter addresses the arthroscopic management of radial-sided tears of the triangular fibrocartilage complex.

ANATOMY OF THE TFCC

The anatomy of the TFCC is quite complicated. It includes the articular disk, meniscus homologue, both the volar and dorsal radioulnar ligaments, and the tendon sheath of the extensor carpi ulnaris tendon. The disk portion of the triangular fibrocartilage complex is thicker at its volar and dorsal margins, which are known as the volar and dorsal radioulnar ligaments. These ligaments function as important stabilizers to the distal radioulnar joint. Approximately 20% of the load of the forearm is transferred through the ulnar side of the wrist and the TFCC. The TFCC acts as an extension of the articular surface of the radius to support the proximal carpal row.

Chidgey et al evaluated the collagen structure of the triangular fibrocartilage complex, attempting to correlate its biomechanic function.[1] He found that short, thick collagen fibers extended from the radius

1 to 2 mm into the articular disk. It is this area where there is a change in collagen arrangement and where many traumatic tears are found (Palmer Class 1A).

The arterial anatomy of the TFCC has also been well studied. Thiru et al. evaluated 12 cadaveric specimens with latex injection and determined three main blood supplies to the triangular fibrocartilage complex.[2] The ulnar artery supplies most of the blood to the TFCC, supporting the ulnar portion through both dorsal and palmar radiocarpal branches. Dorsal and palmar branches of the anterior interosseous artery supply the more radial part of the TFCC. Histological examination of the triangular fibrocartilage complex found vessels filled with latex dye in the outer 15 to 20% of the articular disk. Similarly, Bednar et al. examined 10 cadavers with an ink injection technique and found penetration of the vessels from the peripheral 10 to 40% of the disk.[3] In both studies, there was a relative paucity of vessels found supplying the radial attachment of the triangular fibrocartilage complex. This has significant clinical applications, in that a sufficient blood supply is necessary for successful healing of a repaired peripheral tear. This would be similar to arthroscopic repair of the knee meniscus in its vascular zone. However, several studies have shown clinical improvement and healing following repair of radial-sided TFCC tears, perhaps secondary to stimulating a vascular response from the radius by abrading the bony surface of the sigmoid notch.[4–12] Cooney et al. evaluated 5 patients by MRI evaluation 2 years or more after open repair of a radial-sided tear of the triangular fibrocartilage complex.[5] He documented a solidly healed edge by MRI evaluation.

CLASSIFICATION OF TFCC TEARS

In 1989, Palmer proposed a classification system for tears of the triangular fibrocartilage complex that divides these injuries into two basic categories: traumatic (Class 1) and degenerative (Class 2) (Table 7.1).[13] Traumatic tears of the triangular fibrocartilage complex from its radial attachment are classified as Type

TABLE 7.1. Classification of TFCC Tears.

Class 1: Traumatic

A	B	C	D
Central Perforation	Ulnar Avulsion with distal ulnar fx without distal ulnar fx	Distal Avulsion	Radial Avulsion with sigmoid notch fx without sigmoid notch fx

Class 2: Degenerative (Ulnocarpal Abutment Syndrome)

A	B	C	D	E
TFCC Wear	TFCC Wear lunate/ulnar chondromalacia	TFCC Perforation lunate/ulnar chondromalacia	TFCC Perforation lunate/ulnar chondromalacia lunotriquetral ligament perforation	TFCC Perforation lunate/ulnar chondromalacia lunotriquetral ligament perforation ulnocarpal arthritis

ID lesions (Figure 7.1). These tears are traumatic avulsions of the triangular fibrocartilage complex from its attachment on the sigmoid notch, which may or may not include a fracture. It is vital to understand the difference between a Class 1A central perforation and a Class 1D radial avulsion without a bony fragment. A Class 1A central perforation usually runs in a longitudinal volar to dorsal direction and occurs just ulnar to the attachment of the articular disk to the sigmoid notch of the radius. The important distinction between a Class 1A central perforation and Class 1D radial avulsion is involvement of the volar and/or dorsal radioulnar ligaments. When the volar and dorsal radioulnar ligaments are involved in the tear, it affects the stability to the distal radioulnar joint (Figure 7.2) and would be classified as a Class 1D tear.

The articular disk has variable thickness throughout its dimension from radial to ulnar. Near its radial attachment, the articular disk is approximately 2 mm thick as compared to its peripheral ulnar attachment, which is up to 5 mm in thickness. Adams has shown

that the peak load occurs along the radial aspect to the articular disk, which is maximized with pronation.[14] The peak strain runs from volar to dorsal in this same area. This is in the area where Chidgey found a change in the collagen arrangement to the articular disk. This is a potential explanation why the prevalence of TFC articular disk injuries occurs along the radial aspect.

DIAGNOSIS

History

Patients with radial sided tears of the triangular fibrocartilage complex commonly report ulnar-sided wrist pain. This may limit work or sports activities. Patients frequently report a single traumatic event, usually a hyperextension injury with the wrist in ulnar deviation, with an acute onset of pain. A common

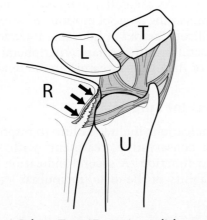

FIGURE 7.1. A Palmer Type 1D tear is a radial tear of the articular disk from the sigmoid notch of the radius with or without a bony avulsion and involvement of the radioulnar ligaments. R = radius, T = triquetum, U = ulnar, L = lunate.

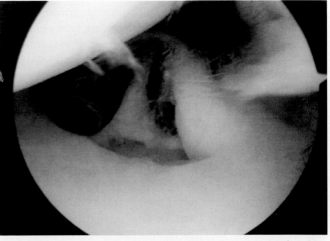

FIGURE 7.2. Arthroscopic view of a Palmer Type 1D peripheral radial tear of the TFCC. The articular disk is torn from its insertion onto the sigmoid notch of the radius, and the volar radioulnar ligament is involved as well.

history is the driver with hands on the steering wheel involved in a motor vehicle accident. Occasionally, patients report a history of a hypertwisting injury to the wrist as well.

Physical Examination

Physical examination of the wrist frequently reveals ulnar-sided wrist swelling. Patients are tender to palpation over the area of the triangular fibrocartilage complex between the triquetrum and the ulnar styloid. Patients complain of pain with radial and ulnar deviation, as ulnar deviation compresses the TFCC, and radial deviation applies tension to a peripheral tear. Patients may complain of a click when the wrist is pronated passively and supinated in maximum ulnar deviation. This click often represents a tear in the triangular fibrocartilage complex interposed between the head of the ulna and the proximal row of the carpus. Occasionally, when both wrists are flexed, there may be an increased dorsal prominence of the head of the ulna as compared to the unaffected side.

Diagnostic Modalities

Standard radiographic posterior, anterior, and lateral views may reveal a bony avulsion, and also evaluate ulnar variance. Oblique radiographs are helpful when a bony avulsion is seen. The position of the extremity with the wrist in neutral flexion/extension, the forearm in neutral pronation/supination with the elbow flexed 90 degrees, and the shoulder abducted 90 degrees is used as a standard to measure ulnar variance. Patients with positive ulnar variance may have ulnar impingement syndrome, which is more likely to be associated with a triangular fibrocartilage complex tear. It is important to shorten the ulna at the same sitting with a peripheral repair in a patient with an ulnar-positive wrist.

The use of MRI has become more common in diagnosing tears of the triangular fibrocartilage complex. T2-weighted images are best for evaluation of traumatic tears. The synovial fluid has a high signal intensity on T2-weighted images, allowing it to act as a contrast material. In T1-weighted images, traumatic tears and degenerative changes appear as an intermittent signal. The articular cartilage of the distal radius as it continues as the articular cartilage of the sigmoid notch may be misinterpreted as a radial-sided tear of the triangular fibrocartilage complex on T1-weighted images.

Triple-injection wrist arthrography is the most accurate technique for wrist arthrography if this is chosen to evaluate for tears of the triangular fibrocartilage complex.[15,16] This technique involves an initial injection of the radial carpal joint under fluoroscopic evaluation, followed by injection and evaluation of the midcarpal and distal radioulnar joints. Approximately 25% of triangular fibrocartilage complex abnormali-

ties may be missed by a single-injection wrist arthrography. The distal radioulnar joint injection is important for evaluation of ulnar-sided attachment and partial tears of the proximal surface of the TFCC. Patients with persistent symptoms and a negative arthrogram may still have a peripheral tear of the triangular fibrocartilage complex. This is due to synovitis that forms over the tear, blocking the flow of contrast material. Also, a positive arthrogram must have a strong clinical correlation, as there is a high rate of false positive arthrograms in asymptomatic patients.[17] The natural history of TFCC tears shows that asymptomatic, age-related attrition occurs in more than half of patients over the age of 50. Brown et al. found perforation of the TFCC in 59% of symptomatic patients and in 51% of asymptomatic patients undergoing arthrography for lateral wrist pain.[17]

Wrist arthroscopy continues to be the gold standard for the diagnosis of triangular fibrocartilage complex tears. This technique allows evaluation of the articular disk under bright light and magnified conditions. A probe may be used to palpate the tension to the articular disk using the trampoline test. The articular disk should have a normal taut appearance when palpated by the probe. In a patient with a peripheral tear of the articular disk, the disk is boggy and redundant. In particular, wrist arthroscopy is extremely useful to differentiate between a Palmer Class 1A tear and a radial sided Palmar 1D peripheral tear with involvement of the volar and/or dorsal radioulnar ligaments. The treatment for these two different types of traumatic tears varies significantly.

TREATMENT

Nonoperative Management

The nonoperative management for patients with traumatic tears of the articular disk includes a trial of immobilization. Occasionally, a physical therapy program encompassing range of motion and strengthening may be utilized. Steroid or lidocaine injections are extremely useful to differentiate a peripheral tear from tendinitis of the extensor carpi ulnaris tendon.

Indications for Surgery

Surgical indications include failure to improve after 3 months of conservative treatment, with symptoms that impair function. A second indication would include instability of the distal radioulnar joint.

SURGICAL TECHNIQUE

The patient is positioned supine on the operating room table with the affected arm on a hand table and a padded tourniquet proximal to the arm. A tourniquet is applied but rarely inflated during the procedure. After general endotrachial anesthesia has been obtained, the wrist is suspended in a traction tower with approximately 10 pounds of traction. The wrist is systematically evaluated, with the arthroscope initially placed in the 3-4 viewing portal. A probe is utilized in the 6-R portal to palpate the articular disk and to assess the tension to the articular disk. If the tear is ulnar to the attachment of the articular disk to the radius with no loss of tension and does not involve the volar or dorsal radioulnar ligaments, the tear is arthroscopically debrided as described in Chapter 9. When the tear involves the entire length of the sigmoid notch with involvement of the volar and/or dorsal radioulnar ligament and the disk is soft with loss of tension, this would be consistent with a Palmer Class 1D radial-sided tear of the triangular fibrocartilage complex. A number of arthroscopic repair techniques for radial-sided tears of the triangular fibrocartilage complex have been described in the literature.[4,6,7,9–12,18,19]

Patients who have a bony avulsion of the articular disk from the sigmoid notch to the radius are arthroscopically pinned. The wrist is removed from traction. Under fluoroscopic control, two 0.045 Kirschner wires are placed just proximal to the articular surface from the radial styloid across the radius into the avulsed fragment. The starting position for the Kirschner wire just beneath the articular surface of the radial styloid is visualized under fluoroscopy. It is important to make approximately a 1 cm skin incision and insert the Kirschner wires through a soft tissue protector to protect the soft tissues, particularly the dorsal sensory branch of the radial nerve. Under fluoroscopic control, the Kirschner wires are started into the radius and advanced ulnarly just short of crossing the avulsed fracture fragment. The wrist is then placed back in traction. The arthroscope is then placed in the 3-4 portal, and a probe is utilized in the 6-R portal. Under direct arthroscopic visualization, the fracture fragment is reduced and potentially stabilized with the probe in the 6-R portal. Once the fracture is anatomically reduced under direct observation with the arthroscope, the Kirschner wires are advanced across the fracture fragment. Following placement of the Kirschner wires, the wrist is removed from traction and viewed under fluoroscopy. Two Kirschner wires are usually inserted. It is important to view this under fluoroscopy to determine that the pins have not violated the distal radioulnar joint or the articular surface. Once this has been confirmed fluoroscopically, the wrist is pronated and supinated to note any crepitance. If crepitance is noted, the pins are backed up slightly, as they are impinging upon the distal radioulnar joint. Following successful pinning, the wrist is immobilized. The pins may then be removed in the office approximately 6 weeks later. If the fracture fragment is relatively large, consideration can be given to potentially using a head-

less cannulated screw. Generally, one screw would be used. The technique for using a headless cannulated screw is similar to using Kirschner wires. Two cannulated guidewires are placed, from radial to ulnar, similar to the Kirschner wire technique. One cannulated guidewire is for placement of the screw, and the second is to control rotation while the fracture fragment is drilled and the screw is inserted. Once the guidewires have been advanced into the fracture fragment as viewed arthroscopically, the wrist is taken out of traction. The radius and avulsion fragment are drilled with a cannulated reamer, and a headless cannulated screw is then placed under fluoroscopic control across the radius into the avulsion fragment. Following placement of the screw, the wrist is placed in pronation and supination to confirm that the distal radioulnar joint has not been violated and that there is no impingement of the screw against the articular surface of the ulna. Once this has been confirmed, the wrist is again suspended in traction, and the reduction is checked under arthroscopic control to make sure the fragment is not rotationally malpositioned. After anatomic reduction of the avulsion fragment is confirmed arthroscopically, the secondary guidewire used to protect against rotation is removed. The wrist is then immobilized.

Several arthroscopic techniques have been developed for repair of a Palmer Type 1D radial-sided tear of the triangular fibrocartilage complex that does not involve bone.[4,6,7,9–12] Sagerman and Short have described an arthroscopic technique for reattachment of radial-sided tears of the articular disk.[7] Utilizing their technique, the wrist is suspended in a traction tower with 10 pounds of traction. The arthroscope is introduced into the 3-4 portal, and working portals are made in the 6-R and 6-U portals. Particularly when making the 6-U portal, it is vital to excise only the skin, with just the tip of the knife blade. This is performed by pulling the tip of the knife blade against the skin with the thumb. Blunt dissection is then continued with a hemostat to level the capsule, and an arthroscopic wrist cannula is then introduced into the 6-U portal. It is important to protect the dorsal sensory branch of the ulnar nerve when utilizing these techniques. Prior to making the 6-U portal, a needle is inserted into the proposed location and viewed intraarticularly with the arthroscope in the 3-4 portal. It is important to determine the ideal location of the 6-U portal so that it is not too proximal or distal to violate the carpus of the wrist or too proximal to pass through the articular disk itself.

An arthroscopic bur is brought in through the 6-R portal. The sigmoid notch of the distal radius is then abraded with the bur (Figure 7.3). The purpose of this is to help stimulate a vascular response to facilitate healing of the radial triangular fibrocartilage complex. This is similar in principle to abrading the greater tuberosity of the humerus while repairing a tear of the

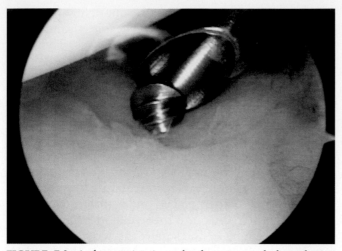

FIGURE 7.3. Arthroscopic view of a burr inserted through 6-R working portal being used to abrade lightly the sigmoid notch of the radius to facilitate revascularization of the radial TFCC tear that is to be repaired

rotator cuff. The key in this technique is not to overabrade the sigmoid notch of the radius. If the sigmoid notch is aggressively abraded and too much bone is taken, the articular disk may not reach the radius. It is best to slightly abrade the sigmoid notch until cancellous bone is visualized. Following abrasion of the sigmoid notch, a 0.062 Kirschner wire is brought in through the 6-U portal in the cannula (Figure 7.4). The cannula is important to protect the soft tissues, particularly the dorsal sensory branch of the ulnar nerve. The 0.062 Kirschner wire is used to make the drill hole, rather than a drill bit. There is less tendency for the Kirschner wire to travel when initially making the drill hole. Three drill holes are then made, starting at the sigmoid notch and exiting across the radius. The wires should exit on the distal third of the

radial side of the forearm. The three drill holes are spaced equally, volar to dorsal. Double-armed, long meniscus repair needles with nonabsorbable suture are then utilized. The first limb of the needle is placed through the cannula (Figure 7.5). The needle is placed through the articular disk and into the volarmost drill hole made by the Kirschner wire. A trick to help the needle penetrate the articular disk is to flip up the torn edge of the articular disk with a probe inserted through the 6-R portal. Another option is to take a grasper through the 6-R portal and grab the torn edge of the articular disk and invert this. This makes it easier for the needle to penetrate through the articular disk. There is always concern about finding the drill hole made in the sigmoid notch and across the radius with the Kirschner wire with the needle after it has penetrated through the articular disk. This is usually not a problem. The drill hole made by a 0.062 Kirschner wire is considerably larger than the meniscus repair needle. It is usually relatively easy and straightforward to find this hole with a needle. A grasper inserted through the 6-R portal can further help to direct the needle into the drill hole, as these needles are quite flexible and may be hard to control inserting through the 6-U portal and a cannula. The meniscus repair needle is then advanced through the drill hole in the radius and advanced out the skin. A second arm of the meniscus repair needle is then brought in through the 6-U portal and advanced through the articular disk in a horizontal mattress fashion (Figure 7.6). The wire is then passed through the middle drill hole of the sigmoid notch and out the radius. The sutures are tagged with a hemostat.

The procedure is repeated with a second set of meniscus repair needles. The first arm of the needle is passed through the articular disk and through the

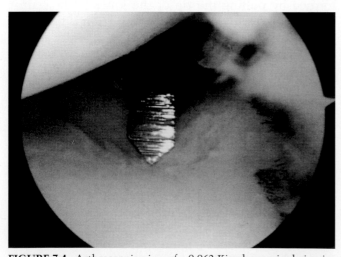

FIGURE 7.4. Arthroscopic view of a 0.062 Kirschner wire being inserted through a cannula in the 6-U portal to drill 3 holes volar to dorsal from the sigmoid notch across the radius and exiting at the distal radial portion of the radius.

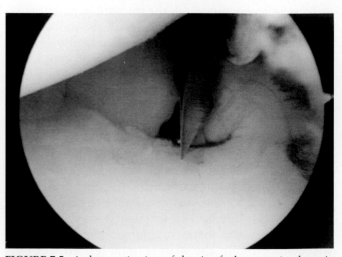

FIGURE 7.5. Arthroscopic view of the tip of a long meniscal repair needle inserted through a cannula in the 6-U portal as it is about to be inserted through the radial articulate disk.

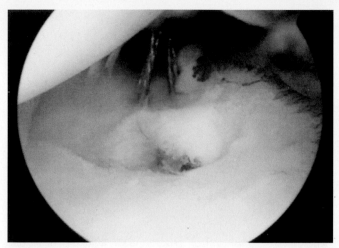

FIGURE 7.6. Arthroscopic view of the 2-0 braided suture being pulled through the articular disk to reattach it to the sigmoid notch.

central drill hole. The last arm of the meniscus repair needle is passed through the articular disk into the dorsalmost drill hole in the sigmoid notch (Figure 7.7). Following placement of the sutures, a small skin incision is made over the radius. Dissection is carried down to identify the suture. The suture is then tied down directly on bone. It is important to visualize that the knot is tied directly down to the bone so that no soft tissue is impaled in the repair, such as the tendons of the extensor carpi ulnaris longus or, particularly, the dorsal sensory branch of the radial nerve. Previous attempts have been made to tie the sutures over a 3.5 mm screw by the lead author. However, this screw frequently caused a painful bursa over the extensor carpi radialis brevis tendon, and this technique is no longer utilized. The distal radioulnar joint may then be pinned in neutral position with a 0.062 Kirschner wire, depending on the surgeon's preference.

Trumble et al described a similar technique.[4] In his technique, the arthroscope is again placed in the 3-4 portal and meniscus repair sutures (2-0 Maxon, Davis & Geck, Manati, PA) are placed into the 6-U cannula and into the radial edge of the TFCC tear under arthroscopic guidance. The needles are then driven across the radius using a power wire driver, aiming to exit between the first and second dorsal compartments of the radial aspect of the wrist. He notes that care must be taken to avoid coiling of the double-arm sutures, which is accomplished when drilling the first needle by loosely holding the suture, and allowing the second needle to rotate. The first suture is brought out through the skin, and a second suture is placed. To avoid coiling as the second needle is passed, Trumble advised placing the wire driver with the suture folded next to the needle and placing a curved retractor around the loop of the suture between the tip of the wire driver and the patient. As the wire advances, the suture coils around the needle until it reaches the

length of the needle, when the driver wire is reversed. The coiling and uncoiling of the sutures continue until the needle exits the skin along the radial side of the wrist. Trumble recommends two sets of repair sutures be placed to secure the triangular fibrocartilage complex to the radius. In a modification of Trumble's technique, long Keith needles may be placed through the 6-U portal into the articular disk and advanced with a power driver across the radius. Once the needle exits the skin on the radial side of the wrist, a nonabsorbable suture may be placed through the eye of the Keith needle and the needle then pulled through the articular disk and out the radius. In this technique, the coiling and uncoiling of the suture is minimized.

Plancher describes his surgical technique for arthroscopic repair of radial-sided tears of the triangular fibrocartilage complex.[12] In his technique, he utilizes a small-joint arthroscopic guide inserted with a point through the 4-5 portal. A guidewire is then brought in from radial to ulnar through the articular disk. This guidewire is then used to pass a 2-0 PDS suture through the radius. A Mulberry knot is then tied in the PDS suture to stabilize the articular disk.

Similarly, Jantea has developed a specialized jig for radial-sided TFC repair.[9,10] With this specialized jig, the meniscus repair needle is brought in through the 6-U portal and out the distal radius. This jig helps to identify the location of the needle as it exits the radial side of the wrist.

New arthroscopic techniques to simplify the repair of radial- and ulnar-sided tears of the triangular fibrocartilage complex are currently being developed. One such technique currently being developed by Geissler utilizes technology similar to the DePuy Mitek RAPIDLOC™ (Norwood, MA), a hybrid suture device for meniscus repair of the knee. In this technique, the arthroscope is placed in the 3-4 portal and two drill holes are made in the sigmoid notch with a Kirschner

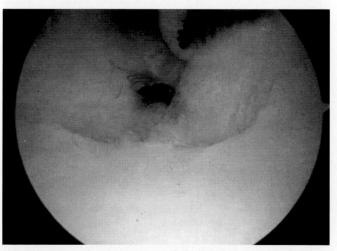

FIGURE 7.7. Arthroscopic view of the braided permanent suture securing the radial articular disk tear back to the sigmoid notch of the radius.

wire again inserted into the 6-U portal. A very small incision is then made over the radial side of the wrist, where the Kirschner wire has exited. Dissection is carried bluntly down to the bone where the Kirschner wire is seen exiting. An inserting device is then placed through the drill hole of the radius and out the sigmoid notch of the radius (Figure 7.8). A grasper is inserted through the 6-R portal to invert the edge of the articular disk. The inserter needle is then passed through the articular disk under direct observation with the arthroscope in the 3-4 portal (Figure 7.9). The absorbable PLA backstop is then deployed through the inserter needle across the radial-sided tear of the articular disk. The PLA TopHat is then slid down, with a pretied slipknot, the attached 2/0 ETHIBOND® (ETHICON, Inc., Somerville, NJ) securing the TopHat against the bone of the distal radius. This greatly simplifies the radial-sided repair of the articular disk. One or two devices are placed utilizing this technique. This new technique appears quite promising, particularly for its simplicity; however, continued clinical evaluation will need to be performed to evaluate its effectiveness. Ulnar repairs may also be performed with appropriate modifications to the technique and inserter.

RESULTS

Open and arthroscopic repair of radial-sided tears of the triangular fibrocartilage complex have been reported with acceptable results in the literature. Cooney et al reported on the results of open radial-sided triangular fibrocartilage repairs in 23 patients.[5] Eleven patients had concomitant shortening of the ulna. In their series, 18 patients had good or excellent results, 4 had fair results, and 1 patient had a poor re-

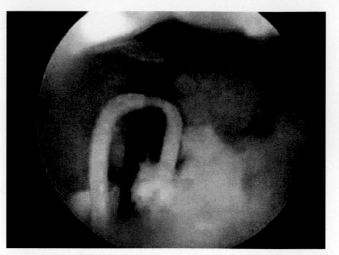

FIGURE 7.9. Arthroscopic view of the needle passed through the radius and articular disk before the backstop is inserted through the radial TFCC tear.

sult. Of the patients with an unsatisfactory result, 2 had experienced reinjury and 1 had experienced postoperative pain syndrome. As noted earlier, 5 patients in the study underwent MRI imaging after more than 2 years post repair. MRI documented healing in 4 of the 5 patients. The authors concluded that repair of radial-sided tears of the triangular fibrocartilage complex is warranted, given the important biomechanical function to the wrist.

Sagerman and Short reported their results of arthroscopic repair of peripheral radial-sided tears of the TFCC in 12 patients.[7] They reported good or excellent results in 8 of 12 patients. Five patients underwent postoperative arthrogram evaluation. There was no leak found in 3 of 5 patients who underwent a postoperative arthrogram evaluation. Trumble reported on 13 patients with isolated Palmer Type 1D triangular fibrocartilage complex tears with an average follow-up of 34 months.[4] In his study, patients regained 87% of their total range of motion and 89% of their strength, compared with the contralateral wrist. This compares favorably with reports of ulnar-sided TFCC repairs. The authors also addressed the fate of radial-sided repairs in 10 of the 13 patients. The triangular fibrocartilage complex was found to be intact in 4 of 5 patients who underwent postoperative arthrograms, in 3 of 3 patients who underwent postoperative MRI imaging studies, and in both of 2 patients who were followed up by arthroscopy.

Traumatic radial-sided tears of the triangular fibrocartilage complex are much less common than central perforations or ulnar-sided tears. However, radial-sided tears of the TFCC are an important potential cause of ulnar-sided wrist pain, particularly when involvement of the volar and/or dorsal radioulnar ligaments leads to potential chronic pain and instability of the distal radioulnar joint.

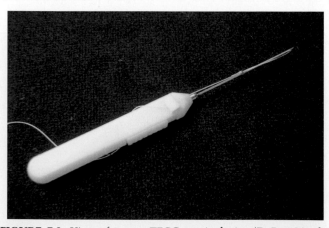

FIGURE 7.8. View of a new TFCC repair device (DePuy Mitek, Norwood, MA) to fix both radial and ulnar-sided peripheral tears of the articular disk. The needle perforates the articulate disk and the backstop is inserted through the disk. The TopHat is then slid down with a pre-tied slip knot to secure the tear against the radius (radial TFCC tear) or the tendon sheath of the extensor carpi ulnaris (ulnar TFCC tear).

CONCLUSION

Wrist arthroscopy is a sensitive modality to evaluate for tears of the triangular fibrocartilage complex. It allows precise identification of the tear pattern as well as the severity of the tear. Wrist arthroscopy allows evaluation of the integrity of the articular disk through palpation with a probe and documents when the tear extends to involve radioulnar ligaments. When a radial-sided tear of the articular disk includes the volar and/or dorsal radioulnar ligaments, arthroscopic repair of the TFCC should be considered. Although anatomic studies have shown decreased vascularity on the radial side of the triangular fibrocartilage complex, several studies have shown successful repair of the articular disk, both clinically and by objective imaging with arthrograms and MRI.

Arthroscopic repair of radial-sided tears of the TFCC is safe and effective. Several surgical techniques have been described in the literature. Arthroscopic techniques have less morbidity and potentially accelerated rehabilitation for patients compared to open repair. New techniques continue to be developed to further simplify the procedure.

References

1. Chidgey LK, Dell PC, Bittar ES, et al. Histologic anatomy of the triangular fibrocartilage. *J Hand Surg* 1991;16:1084–1100.
2. Thiru RG, Ferlic DC, Clayton MI, et al. Arterial anatomy of the triangular fibrocartilage of the wrist and its surgical significance. *J Hand Surg* 1986;11:258–263.
3. Bednar MS, Arnoczky SP, Weiland AJ. The microvasculature of the triangular fibrocartilage complex: its clinical significance. *J Hand Surg* 1991;16:1101–1105.
4. Trumble TE, Gilbert M, Vedder N. Isolated tears of the triangular fibrocartilage: management by early arthroscopic repair. *J Hand Surg* 1997;22:57–65.
5. Cooney WP, Linscheid RL, Dobyns JH. Triangular fibrocartilage tears. *J Hand Surg* 1994;19:143–154.
6. Fellinger M, Peicha G, Seibert FJ, et al. Radial avulsion of the triangular fibrocartilage complex in acute wrist trauma: a new technique for arthroscopic repair. *Arthroscopy* 1997;13:370–374.
7. Sagerman SD, Short W. Arthroscopic repair of radial-sided triangular fibrocartilage complex tears. *Arthroscopy* 1996;12:339–342.
8. Herrmannsdorfer JD, Kleinman WB. Management of chronic peripheral tears of the triangular fibrocartilage complex. *J Hand Surg* 1991;16:340–346.
9. Jantea CL. Radial TFCC repairs. *Hand Clin* 1995;11:31–38.
10. Jantea CL, Baltzer A, Ruther W. Arthroscopic repair of radial sided lesion of the triangular fibrocartilage complex. *Hand Clin* 1995;11:31–36.
11. Jones MD, Trumble TE. Arthroscopic repair of radial sided triangular fibrocartilage complex tears. *Atlas Hand Clin* 2001;6:221–239.
12. Plancher KD. Arthroscopic repair of radial TFCC tears. *Techn Hand Upper Ext* 1999;3:44–50.
13. Palmar AK. Triangular fibrocartilage complex lesions: a classification. *J Hand Surg* 1989;14:594–606.
14. Adams B. Partial excision of the triangular fibrocartilage complex articular disk, a biomechanical study. *J Hand Surg* 1993;184:334–340.
15. Levinsohn EM, Rosen ID, Palmer AK. Wrist arthrography: value of the three-compartment injection method. *Radiology* 1991;179:231–239.
16. Zinberg EM, Palmer AK, Coren AB, et al. The triple injection wrist arthrogram. *J Hand Surg* 1988;13:803–809.
17. Brown JA, Janzen DL, Adler BD, et al. Arthrography of the contralateral, asymptomatic wrist in patients with unilateral wrist pain. *Can Assoc Radiol J* 1994;45:292–296.
18. Minami A, Kaneda K, Itoga H. Hemiresection interposition arthroplasty of the distal radioulnar joint associated with repair of triangular fibrocartilage complex lesions. *J Hand Surg* 1991;16:1120–1125.
19. Geissler WB, Fernandez DL, Lamey DM. Distal radioulnar joint injuries associated with fractures of the distal radius. *Clin Orthop* 1996;327:135–146.

8

Management of Type C TFCC Tears

Matthew M. Tomaino

When a patient presents with ulnar-sided wrist pain, the history and physical exam may prompt conservative treatment initially, unless symptoms are chronic. Because the diagnostic accuracy of wrist arthroscopy exceeds that of either MR imaging or triple-phase arthrography,[1,2] many clinicians may justifiably recommend arthroscopy when a triangular fibrocartilage complex (TFCC) or intercarpal ligament tear is suspected, avoiding these studies completely. Indeed, wrist arthroscopy allows not only diagnosis but also minimally invasive treatment of internal derangement of the wrist.

Whether a TFCC tear is repaired or debrided, and whether concomitant ulnar shortening needs to be performed depends upon its location and blood supply, its chronicity, the ulnar variance, and the arthroscopic skills of the surgeon. This chapter will address these issues as they pertain to the diagnosis and management of Palmer Type C TFCC tears.[3] Palmer's classification of TFCC lesions divides tears into traumatic (Type I) and degenerative (Type II) tears, and each type is further subdivided based on the details of the anatomic lesion (Figure 8.1).

PREOPERATIVE PLANNING

Diagnosis

Traumatic and degenerative TFCC tears may be indistinguishable in terms of the symptoms they elicit. Both result in ulnar wrist pain, particularly with activities that load the wrist during pronation and supination. The pain may also be accompanied by a sensation of catching or snapping in the wrist. It would seem, therefore, that Palmer's classification highlights differences in the etiologies of these two types of tears, rather than differences in symptoms. Indeed, Type I lesions are more apt to follow a fall on an outstretched hand, or an abrupt load to the pronated and/or ulnarly deviated wrist. By contrast, the history for Type II lesions may be more insidious and chronic, without any history of a traumatic precipitant.

Physical examination is the most valuable method of evaluating a suspected TFCC tear. When a complaint of ulnar wrist pain exists, other causes should first be excluded, such as extensor carpi ulnaris tenosynovitis or subluxation, isolated lunotriquetral ligament strain or disruption, pisotriquetral arthritis, and ulnar styloid–carpal impaction. Exclusion of these potential diagnoses is relatively easy by means of a careful exam and the selective injection of lidocaine when necessary. The two most valuable and sensitive tests include Nakamura's ulnocarpal stress test[4] and Berger's fovea test. Nakamura's test is performed by passively pronating and supinating the wrist while it is axially loaded and ulnarly deviated. While it may not differentiate between a traumatic, degenerative TFCC tear, or an LT tear, this test is sufficiently sensitive to warrant further evaluation by arthroscopy if crepitus is palpated. The fovea test is performed by palpating the volar aspect of the TFCC between the flexor carpi ulnaris (FCU) tendon volarly, and the ulnar styloid process dorsally. The presence of tenderness suggests a lesion of the ulnocarpal ligaments.[5]

Radiographic assessment includes the use of neutral rotation[6] and pronated grip radiographs.[7,8] These will allow assessment of both static and dynamic ulnar variance. If physical examination suggests a TFCC lesion, MR imaging is not required preoperatively, since wrist arthroscopy is more sensitive and allows concomitant treatment as well. But, if one is concerned that the potential lesion is degenerative—consistent with ulnar impaction syndrome (a Type II tear)—an MRI may be helpful in showing marrow edema in the ulnar corner of the lunate.[9] In cases where a TFCC perforation is not present but exam and MR imaging suggest ulnar impaction (Type II A and B lesions), an ulnar recession procedure may be indicated nevertheless.[10–14] The availability and scope of MR imaging, when further preoperative workup is felt to be necessary, has significantly decreased the indications for either bone scintigraphy or wrist arthrography.

Biomechanical Considerations

Both traumatic and degenerative TFCC lesions develop because of similar biomechanical alterations. Indeed, an increase in ulnar variance results in an in-

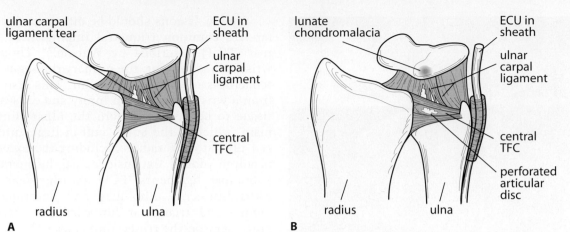

FIGURE 8.1. Illustration of a Type IC and IIC TFCC lesion. **A.** A Type IC lesion involves the volar ulnocarpal ligaments (ulnolunate and/or ulnotriquetral), which extend from the carpus to the volar rim (volar radioulnar ligament) of the articular disk of the TFCC. **B.** A Type IIC lesion involves a perforation of the articular disk of the TFCC with chondromalacia of the ulnar head or lunate.

crease in load transfer across the ulnocarpal joint.[15] Whether as a result of a fall or the impact, over time, of the combination of forearm pronation and forceful grip, the TFCC either acutely tears or gradually attenuates and perforates because of its role in load transfer. And even though Type II tears occur most commonly in ulnar-positive wrists,[10,11] "dynamic" increases in variance which accompany forceful grip[7,8,12] explain why ulnar impaction syndrome may also develop in wrists with neutral and negative ulnar variance,[13,14] and why pain relief following debridement alone for Type I tears is not always satisfactory.[16–19]

Incomplete pain relief has been reported following TFCC debridement alone in as many as 25% of wrists, regardless of whether the tear is posttraumatic or degenerative, but only recently have the potential implications of positive ulnar variance been considered.[8,16–19] In 1996, Minami et al. were the first to report that positive ulnar variance was associated with poor outcome following TFCC debridement alone.[19] They measured ulnar variance with the forearm in pronation to mimic the dynamic increases in ulnar variance that might accompany functional activity. Their suggestion that persistent pain was related to positive ulnar variance was consistent with two other reports that showed the efficacy of combining ulnar shortening with TFCC repair to improve pain relief.[20,21] Similarly, Hulsizer et al. reported that ulnar shortening provided successful treatment of persistent ulnar wrist pain following TFCC debridement,[22] and most recently, Minimi and Kato reported successful treatment of TFCC tears associated with positive ulnar variance using ulnar shortening osteotomy alone.[23]

TFCC debridement alone may not provide complete pain relief in wrists with positive ulnar variance, regardless of whether the etiology is "traumatic" or "degenerative."[24,25] Tomaino and Weiser prospectively evaluated the feasibility and efficacy of com-

bining arthroscopic TFCC debridement with an arthroscopic "wafer procedure" as treatment for wrists in which both TFCC disruption and positive ulnar variance coexisted.[26] Seven Type I and 5 Type II tears were treated, and all patients reported satisfactory resolution of preoperative pain.

Therefore, whether the a TFCC lesion is classified as Type I or Type II may have more to do with etiology than with management. The management of Type C lesions will be discussed in the following section.

SURGICAL MANAGEMENT

A standard arthroscopic setup is used, and 10 to 12 pounds of traction are administered via index and long finger traps. A 2.7 mm arthroscope is used. Initially the 3-4 and 6-R portals are made, and occasionally a 4-5 portal is added. An 18-gauge needle attached to plastic IV tubing is placed in the radial styloid–scaphoid joint for outflow. Debridement is typically performed using a combination of a motorized shaver and the Mini-VAPR device (Mitek, Westwood, MA). A 2 mm burr is used to perform a wafer resection of the ulnar head when indicated.

Type IC Lesions

It is unusual to see a frank avulsion of the ulnocarpal ligaments from the carpus. Rather, partial fraying is identified—often at the junction with the volar rim of the articular disk (Figure 8.2). Thus, debridement is performed to remove any unstable ligamentous flaps both to prevent impingement, a mechanical source of pain, and to remove a potential source of pain-mediating cytokines.

Although simple debridement is likely to be effective, particularly since the mechanical integrity of

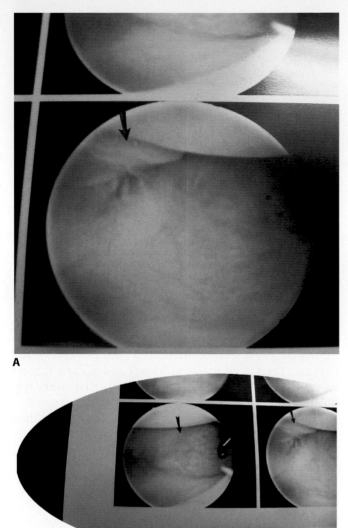

FIGURE 8.2. Type IC TFCC lesion. **A.** Type IC tear (ulnocarpal ligament fraying) is identified by the black arrow. **B.** The flap has been debrided.

the TFCC and its role in stabilizing the distal ulna is not typically compromised, repair of Type IC tears has also been described.[27] The authors emphasize the importance of identifying and protecting the ulnar nerve. It is worth noting that fraying of the ulnocarpal ligaments may reflect a chronic LT ligament disruption.[28] Zachee et al. found 10 Type IC tears in their series of 40 wrist arthroscopies, and complete LT disruption was confirmed on midcarpal arthroscopy in 9. They rightly acknowledge that the ulnocarpal ligaments are placed under tension following LT rupture and theorize that this portion of the TFCC may serve as a secondary restraint after LT injury. Indeed, the LT ligament should be assessed during the routine wrist arthroscopic exam when any lesion of the TFCC is suspected.

Type IC lesions should be differentiated from the far less common triquetral impingement ligament tear (TILT) described by Watson.[29] Though ulnar wrist pain is present, the primary finding is localized tenderness over the triquetrum. This lesion results from a wrist hyperflexion injury and causes a cuff of tissue to be displaced from the ulnar sling mechanism, which is the entire cuff of ligamentous collagen ulnar to the radius including the extensor retinaculum, dorsal extrinsic carpal ligaments, dorsal radioulnar ligaments, ECU sheath, volar extrinsic carpal ligaments, ulnolunate and ulnotriquetral ligaments, and triangular fibrocartilage. Chronic impingement on the triquetrum causes hyperemia, loss of articular cartilage, and softening of the bone. Surgical treatment consists of simply excising the impinging fibrous cuff.

Type IIC Lesions

Minami has emphasized that debridement of degenerative Type IIC tears alone may not provide satisfactory pain relief—presumably because of ulnar impaction. If either static or dynamic variance is positive, and a central perforation of the TFCC is identified, treatment should include either an ulnar shortening osteotomy,[10,11] an open wafer procedure,[14,30,31] or my current preference, a combined arthroscopic TFCC debridement and wafer procedure.[26]

I always excise enough of the articular disk to facilitate exposure but never violate the volar or dorsal radioulnar ligaments or the TFCC insertion at the base of the styloid (Figure 8.3). The Mini-VAPR device (Mitek, Westwood, MA) facilitates debridement, and cartilage of the ulnar head and subchondral bone are removed with a 2 mm bur. Knowing ahead of time that the diameter of the bur is 2 mm, I recess the radial portion of the ulnar head first to approximately the width of the bur beneath the top of the sigmoid notch. The bur is then moved more ulnarly toward the base of the styloid. Most of the resection can be performed with the scope in the 3-4 portal and the bur in the 6-R. With the hand maintained within the traction apparatus, passive forearm pronation provides exposure of that portion of the ulnar head that is most prominent during pronation. Completion of the wafer resection usually requires visualization through the 6-R portal to ensure that the ulnar recession is 2 mm beneath the cartilage of the lunate fossa with the wrist in neutral rotation all the way from dorsal to volar. Visualization through the 3-4 portal ensures adequate resection ulnarly to the base of the styloid. I use the tip of an arthroscopic probe, which measures 2 mm, to assess the extent of resection. Neither intraoperative X-ray nor fluoroscopy is used during the surgical procedure. Postoperatively, X-rays often seem to

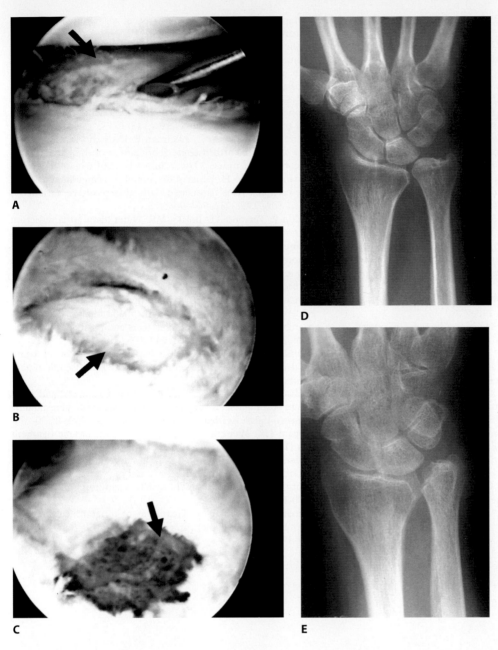

FIGURE 8.3. Type IIC TFCC lesion. **A.** Black arrow shows perforation of the articular disk. Above the needle, lunate chondromalacia is visible. **B.** TFCC articular disk has been debrided to expose the ulnar head. **C.** Recession of the ulnar head has been performed with the assistance of manual pronation and supination, using the end of the probe as a depth gauge relative to the level of the lunate fossa. **D.** Preoperative pronated grip X-ray. **E.** Postoperative pronated grip X-ray. The postoperative grip X-ray may exaggerate the magnitude of recession as compared to the intraoperative exam.

exaggerate the magnitude of the recession as compared to the intraoperative assessment (Figure 8.3).

CONCLUSION

Though the Palmer classification of TFCC tears has added tremendous value in terms of grouping lesions into traumatic and degenerative categories, it is important to remember that it is more useful in terms of differentiating etiology than in designating distinct treatment recommendations. Both Type I and Type II tears may reflect the biomechanical effects of increased ulnar variance, and both, in that light, may require more than simple debridement. Careful examination and the use of preoperative MR imaging and

fastidious diagnostic use of the arthroscope may reveal whether an element of ulnar impaction exists and, for that matter, whether other pathology, such as an LT tear, needs to be addressed.

For the most part, however, Type IC tears can be treated effectively with debridement alone and Type IIC tears by debridement and an arthroscopic wafer procedure.

References

1. Oneson SR, Timins ME, Scales LM, et al. MR imaging diagnosis of triangular fibrocartilage pathology with arthroscopic correlation. *Am J Roentgenol* 1997;168:1513–1518.
2. Cooney WP. Evaluation of chronic wrist pain by arthrography, arthroscopy, and arthrotomy. *J Hand Surg* 1993;18:815–822.

3. Palmer AK. Triangular fibrocartilage complex lesions: a classification. *J Hand Surg* 1989;14A:594–606

4. Nakamura R, Horii E, Imaeda T, et al. The ulnocarpal stress test in the diagnosis of ulnar-sided wrist pain. *J Hand Surg* 1997;22B:719–723.

5. Berger RA. Arthroscopic anatomy of the wrist and distal radioulnar joint. *Hand Clin* 1999;15:393–413.

6. Palmer AK, Glisson RR, Werner FW. Ulnar variance determination. *J Hand Surg* 1982;7:376–379.

7. Tomaino MM, Rubin DA. The value of the pronated grip view radiograph in assessing dynamic ulnar positive variance: a case report. *Am J Orthop* 1999;3:180–191.

8. Tomaino MM. The importance of the pronated grip x-ray view in evaluating ulnar variance. *J Hand Surg* 2000;25A:352–357.

9. Imaeda T, Nakamura R, Shionoya K, et al. Ulnar impaction syndrome: MR imaging findings. *Radiology* 1996;201:495–500.

10. Friedman SL, Palmer AK. The ulnar impaction syndrome. *Hand Clin* 1991;7:295–310.

11. Chun S, Palmer AK. The ulnar impaction syndrome: follow-up of ulnar shortening osteotomy. *J Hand Surg* 1993;18A: 46–53.

12. Friedman SL, Palmer AK, Short WH, et al. The change in ulnar variance with grip. 1993;18A:713–716.

13. Tomaino MM. Ulnar impaction syndrome in the ulnar negative and neutral wrist: diagnosis and pathoanatomy. *J Hand Surg* 1998;23B:754–757.

14. Tomaino MM. Results of the wafer procedure for ulnar impaction syndrome in the ulnar negative and neutral wrist. *J Hand Surg* 1999;24B:671–675.

15. Palmer AK, Werner FW. Biomechanics of the distal radioulnar joint. *Clin Orthop* 1984;187:26–35.

16. Bednar JM. Arthroscopic treatment of triangular fibrocartilage tears. *Hand Clin* 1999;15:479–488.

17. Osterman AL. Arthroscopic debridement of triangular fibrocartilage complex tears. *Arthroscopy* 1990;6:120–124.

18. Westkaemper JG, Mitsionis G, Giannakopoulos PN, et al. Wrist arthroscopy for the treatment of ligament and triangular fibrocartilage complex injuries. *Arthroscopy* 1998;14:479–483.

19. Minami A, Ishikawa J, Suenaga N, et al. Clinical results of treatment of triangular fibrocartilage complex tears by arthroscopic debridement. *J Hand Surg* 1996;21A:406–411.

20. Trumble TE, Gilbert M, Vedder N. Ulnar shortening combined with arthroscopic repairs in the delayed management of triangular fibrocartilage complex tears. *J Hand Surg* 1997;22A: 807–813.

21. Cooney WP, Linscheid RL, Dobyns JH. Triangular fibrocartilage tears. *J Hand Surg* 1994;19A:143–154.

22. Hulsizer D, Weiss APC, Akelman E. Ulna-shortening osteotomy after failed arthroscopic debridement of the triangular fibrocartilage complex. *J Hand Surg* 1997;22A:694–698.

23. Minami A, Kato H. Ulnar shortening for triangular fibrocartilage complex tears associated with ulnar positive variance. *J Hand Surg* 1998;23A:904–908.

24. Feldon P, Terrono AL, Belsky MR. Wafer distal ulna resection for triangular fibrocartilage tears and/or ulna impaction syndrome. *J Hand Surg* 1992;17A:731–737.

25. Wnorowski DC, Palmer AK, Werner FW, et al. Anatomic and biomechanical analysis of the arthroscopic wafer procedure. *Arthroscopy* 1992;8:204–212.

26. Tomaino MM, Weiser RW. Combined arthroscopic TFCC debridement and wafer resection of the distal ulna in wrists with triangular fibrocartilage complex tears and positive ulnar variance. *J Hand Surg* 2001;26A:1047–1052.

27. Trumble TE, Gilbert M, Vedder N. Isolated tears of the triangular fibrocartilage: management by early arthroscopic repair. *J Hand Surg* 1997;22A:57–65.

28. Zachee B, DeSmet L, Fabry G. Frayed ulno-triquetral and ulno-lunate ligaments as an arthroscopic sign of longstanding triquetro-lunate ligament rupture. *J Hand Surg* 1994;19B:570–571.

29. Watson HK, Weinzweig J. Triquetral impingement ligament tear (TILT). *J Hand Surg* 1999;24B:321–324.

30. Constantine KJ, Tomaino MM, Herndon JH, et al. Comparison of ulnar shortening osteotomy and the wafer resection procedure as treatment for ulnar impaction syndrome. *J Hand Surg* 2000;25A:55–60.

31. Tomaino MM, Shah M. Treatment of ulnar impaction syndrome with the wafer procedure. *Am J Orthop* 2001;30: 129–133.

9

Debridement of Central TFCC Tears

Gary R. Kuzma and David S. Ruch

The radiocarpal and midcarpal components of the wrist joint are capable of significant freedom of movement and act as a universal joint. The forearm architecture and distal radial ulnar joint (DRUJ) allow rotation through 180 degrees of pronation and supination to further enhance the arm's ability to position the hand in a vast array of functional positions. The triangular fibrocartilage complex (TFCC) extends the articular surface of the concave distal radius over the convex head of the distal ulna. The motion of each component of this multifaceted joint is extremely complex. Movements involve rotation, translation with shifting axis of movement, and changing points of load transmission. Further, because no muscle is attached to the carpal bones, they are loaded by the geometry of the distal radius and ulna. Stability is provided instead by the intrinsic and extrinsic ligaments, and motion is generated by the carpal bones being pushed or pulled into position. Wrist arthroscopy has made a significant contribution to the diagnosis and treatment of injury to the wrist. With minimal incision and no disruption to the major ligaments of the wrist, the arthroscope provides an unparalleled view of the interior of the wrist joint. Injury of the TFCC can affect the function of both radiocarpal and distal radial ulnar joints. Arthroscopy is especially useful in both the diagnosis and treatment of injury to the TFCC.

ANATOMY

The TFCC is a multifunctional structure comprised of ligamentous and cartilaginous components. Covering the head of the ulna, the complex is attached to the ulnar distal radius at the sigmoid notch and to the fovea of the distal ulna, just radial to the ulnar styloid process. As described by Gan and Richards, the components of the TFCC include the triangular fibrocartilage or articular disk, the meniscus homologue, the dorsal and palmar radial ulnar ligaments, and the extensor carpi ulnaris sheath.[1,2]

The dorsal and palmar radial ulnar ligaments are composed of both a superficial and deep component.

The deep portion of the dorsal and palmar component (subcuratum) inserts into the fovea of the ulna. The superficial portion surrounds the articular disk and unites at the periphery of the ulna. Between the united superficial ligaments and the joint capsule lies the meniscus homologue. The prestyloid recess may be a narrow slit, wide open, or not present at all and should not be confused with an injury to the TFCC. The ulnolunate ligament emerges from the palmar radial ulnar ligament, while the ulnotriquetral ligament inserts on the base of the ulnar styloid.[3] The vascular supply to the TFCC is fed by the dorsal and palmar branches of the anterior interosseous artery, the dorsal and palmar radiocarpal branches of the ulnar artery, and the interosseous branches from the foveal attachment of the TFCC at the ulnar head.[4–8] Vessels penetrate the periphery into approximately 15% to 20% of the dorsal and palmar radial ulnar ligaments of the articular disk. The central 80% to 85% of the articular disk is avascular and thus incapable of healing. The radial attachment of the articular disk contributes no blood supply[5–9] (Figure 9.1)

The histology of the TFCC contributes to the understanding of the function of various components. The radial attachment of the TFCC projects from the hyaline cartilage of the distal radius and is reinforced by thick collagen bundle within the fibrocartilage of the articular disk for approximately 1 to 2 mm.[4,9] The disk proper is composed of collagen fibers and fibrocartilage.[10,11] Arranged in an oblique pattern, collagen fibers coalesce into interwoven waves suited for both compressive and tension stresses.[2,4,9] Peripherally, these fibers band together to become the dorsal and palmar radial ulnar ligaments. The articular disk is comprised of chondrocytes in a collagen matrix, while the proximal portion is more fibrous. Loose connective tissue fills the disk between these two layers. The TFCC forms a hammock, which cradles the ulnar carpus, extending the distal radius articular surface over the dome of the ulnar head. The TFCC provides support for the carpus, a smooth gliding surface, a cushion and stability to the DRUJ.[5,10–12] The thickness of the TFCC is inversely proportional to the length of the ulna compared to the radius.[13] Injury of the tri-

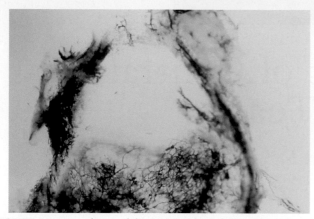

FIGURE 9.1. Vascularity of the TFCC. Ink studies indicate that the articular disk is relatively devoid of blood supply, while the periphery is well perfused. (Courtesy of Michael Bednar, MD).

angular fibrocartilage complex has been felt to be a cause of pain on the ulnar side of the wrist. The TFCC is innervated by branches of the posterior interosseous, ulnar, and dorsal sensory branch of the ulnar nerve.[14] In general, nerves follow blood vessels, and this principle of anatomy proves to be true with respect to the innervation of the TFCC. The paths of the nerves closely follow and parallel the vascular patterns described by Bednar, Chidgey, and Mikic.[4,7,8] The peripheral margins are well innervated, while the central and radial aspects of the TFCC are not innervated.[14]

BIOMECHANICS

There is no dispute that the dorsal and palmar coalescences are the primary stabilizers of the TFCC that provide stability to the DRUJ. The central two-thirds of the TFCC contributes little towards DRUJ stability and can be removed without adverse effects on wrist function.[15–17] However, many researchers disagree about which ligament stabilizes the DRUJ in pronation and supination. Several authors feel that during pronation the DRUJ is stabilized by the palmar component of the radial ulnar ligament in association with the dorsal rim of the sigmoid notch of the radius. These authors likewise feel that in supination it is the dorsal radial ulnar ligaments and palmar rim of the sigmoid notch of the distal radius that afford stability[18] (Figure 9.2). Conversely, others feel that the dorsal radial ulnar ligament is taut in pronation, and the palmar radial ulnar ligament is taut in supination.[19] Nakamura and Nagle found that the proximal portion of the dorsal and palmar condensations could be categorized into three types: fan shaped, V shaped, and funnel shaped, and represents the true radial ulnar ligaments. Nakamura also found that the dorsal portion was under tension from supination to pronation, while the palmar portion lengthened when the wrist moved

from pronation to supination. The fovea of the ulna is the axis of rotation of the wrist, while the ligament—either dorsal or palmar—attached nearest to the center of the fovea showed isometric lengthening. The change in length was greatest in those fibers attached at a distance from the fovea.[11,20]

The DRUJ is not a tight congruous joint. The radius of curvature of the ulnar head and sigmoid notch of the distal radius are significantly different (10 mm versus 15 mm, respectively) resulting in both rotation and sliding.[2] Moreover, the joint is stabilized not only by the dorsal and palmar radial ulnar ligaments of the TFCC and the bony architecture of the sigmoid notch, but also by the extensor carpi ulnaris and its subsheath, the interosseous membrane, pronator quadratus, and forearm muscles that cause the rotation of axis of the DRUJ.[2,21,22] The TFCC dorsal and palmar ligaments, however, are the primary stabilizers of the DRUJ except in full pronation or supination.[11,23,24]

Forced transmission of compressive loads across the wrist is determined by ulnar variance. Normally 82% of the compressed load is borne by the radius, and 18% is transmitted to the ulnar carpal articulation when there is neutral variance. When the ulna is 2.5 mm longer than the distal radius, the ulnocarpal load increases to 42%. If the ulna is 2.5 mm shorter than the radius, the load on the ulna decreases to 4.3%. Transmission of this load is obviously through the triangular fibrocartilage complex.[13,25] Ulnar variance is not static and changes with both grip and forearm rotation.[12,26] The ulna becomes functionally long in full pronation.

EVALUATION

History and physical examination should precede a routine and orderly investigation of the wrist. Range of motion, strength, and localization of pain should be

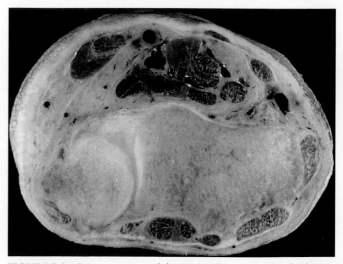

FIGURE 9.2. Gross anatomy of the DRUJ illustrating the thick confluence of fibers of the dorsal and palmar DRUJ ligaments.

examined. There are no pathognomic signs for injury of the TFCC. Instability of the DRUJ may be a subtle difference, when compared to the opposite wrist. North attempted to correlate the clinical examination to arthroscopic findings and found no association with ligament tear, chondromalacia, synovitis with mechanism of injury, duration of symptoms, click, or activity pain.[27]

The benefits and disadvantages of the vast array of available imaging studies have been weighed by many researchers. Imaging studies should include routine views of the wrist and standardized views to visualize the distal radial ulnar joint for ulnar variance.[28,29] Arthrography of the wrist with triple injection and digital subtraction, once the mainstay for the diagnosis of TFCC injury, is of questionable use.[30–35] Bone scans are of little use in diagnosing TFCC tears.[36] CT scans are useful for the diagnosis of DRUJ instability when comparing both sides in pronation, neutral rotation, and supination and may be enhanced by the addition of stress views.[37,38] Magnetic resonance imaging (MRI) provides accurate correlation to the TFCC abnormality.[18,39] Gadolinium arthrography, in addition to MRI scans, has been added to enhance sensitivity, but must be clinically correlated in light of normal degeneration and TFCC tears occurring as part of the natural aging process.[8,40–42]

Arthroscopic inspection of the radiocarpal joint is far superior to any imaging technique for the diagnosis of TFCC injuries.[18,43] In addition, therapeutic modalities can be instituted. Unfortunately, arthroscopic inspection of the DRUJ is technically difficult and has not enjoyed the same degree of acceptance as arthroscopy of the radiocarpal and midcarpal joints.[44–46]

CLASSIFICATION

Tears of the TFCC have been classified by Palmer into two general types: Type I, traumatic and Type II, degenerative. Traumatic tears are then subclassified depending on their location in the substance of the TFCC.[47,48]

There are four types of traumatic tears of the TFCC. Type 1A is a transverse tear 2 mm from the radial attachment of the TFCC that occurs at the termination of the collagen fibers of the TFCC. These are the fibers emanating from the sigmoid notch of the distal ulnar radius and proceeding into the triangular fibrocartilage radial side. This tear is in the articular disk's avascular portion. Type 1A tears can be debrided without altering the function of the TFCC if the dorsal and palmar condensations are not violated[15] (Figure 9.3).

Type 1B tears occur at the dorsal or peripheral margin attachment of the TFCC of the capsule or fovea of the ulna. These tears are in the vascular area of the triangular fibrocartilage and have the capacity to heal. They may require debridement of the synovial tissue

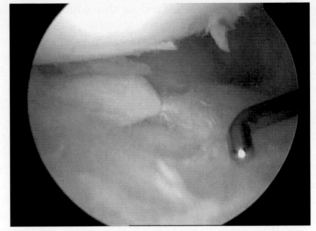

FIGURE 9.3. Traumatic central tear of the TFCC. Note the "loose" central fragment that acts effectively as a loose body.

that frequently heals and obscures the real TFCC tear. These tears should be repaired and not debrided. Type 1B tears have the potential for destabilizing the distal radial ulnar joint. Tears from the bone should be repaired back to the bone.[49]

Tears along the volar margin of the TFCC may include the attachment or involve the ulnotriquetral and/or ulnar lunate ligaments and can be repaired or, if partial, can be debrided. These are classified as type 1C tears.[50–52]

The TFCC may be pulled off from its origin on the distal radius. These tears also have the capacity to destabilize the DRUJ if they include the dorsal and/or palmar radial ulnar ligaments. The type 1D tears can be debrided and/or repaired if they do not include the ligament.[23,53–57]

If the dorsal or palmar ligament is detached from the distal radius, formal repair should be undertaken to stabilize the distal radial ulnar joint.[58]

Type II tears are degenerative in nature due to an ulnar-positive relationship to the radius. Degeneration begins on the proximal surface of the TFCC without perforation. With continued wear, chondromalacia of the ulnar head and the ulnar side of the lunate occurs. Type 2C injuries are evidenced by an ovoid perforation of the triangular fibrocartilage central disk with characteristic smooth margins. Type 2D injury includes the prior stages plus degeneration and tear of the lunotriquetral interosseous ligament. Continuation of the injury results in ulnocarpal arthritis with the addition of a defect occurring in the proximal ulnar aspect of the lunate, and is classified as a type 2E tear.[47,48]

TREATMENT

Arthroscopic Assessment

The technique of wrist arthroscopy is subject to some variability due to personal preferences. However, in general the patient is placed in the supine position with the arm abducted at the shoulder and with the surgeon and assistant sitting. The arm is supported on an arm board, and traction is applied by a simple traction apparatus or traction tower with the elbow flexed. A tourniquet may or may not be utilized.

Anatomical landmarks are defined prior to distending the joint. Portals are defined by the extensor tendon compartments and Lister's tubercle. Either tendon and bony landmarks are outlined, or portals are marked. The joint is inflated with a 22-gauge needle, introduced in the 3-4 portal. Flexing and extending the thumb assures the extensor pollicis longus (EPL) is not violated. The joint is distended with 10 cc of saline. An incision is made through the skin only with a #15 blade scalpel. The portal is deepened with a hemostat down to the capsule. The joint is gently entered with a blunt trocar and arthroscope sheath parallel to the articular surface, remembering that the radius has a 12-degree palmar tilt.

The arthroscope is introduced, and the joint undergoes an orderly inspection from radial to ulnar side. The articular surfaces and the extrinsic and intrinsic ligaments are evaluated. The outflow needle or catheter is introduced through the 6-U portal to obtain flow after introducing the scope, if visualization is poor. The 4-5 or 6-R portals are opened in a similar fashion to the 3-4 portal after localization with a 22-gauge needle. This is done while visualizing the dorsal ulnar capsule. The needle is used to assure that the portal position allows for adequate access to all positions of the joint with larger instruments.

To assess the integrity of the TFCC, a probe is introduced through the ulnar portal so that it can be probed and palpated. The trampoline effect is noted.[58] Significant synovitis is noted. If pressurized inflow is utilized, decreasing the pressure will allow the TFCC to assume a more normal position. To assess the integrity of the deep fibers, a Hook test may be performed. This is accomplished by inserting the probe under the peripheral rim of the TFCC and elevating the disk. If the deep fibers are intact, then only the peripheral rim is torn. In this case, repair of the TFCC to the subsheath is sufficient. If the entire TFCC is avulsed off the ulna, the entire disk needs to be reattached to the ulna. Subtle tears usually require insertion of the probe and elevation of the disk. Pronation and supination of the forearm allow visualization of the entire TFCC. The scope may need to be placed in the ulnar portal for visualization of the ulnar radius, TFCC, ulnar intercarpal, and ulnocarpal ligaments. This entire procedure is done with the wrist distracted with 10 pounds of traction.

Debridement

For debridement of the TFCC, midcarpal portals are not utilized. Debridement is performed with a suction punch, shaver, grafting forceps, scalpel, banana blade hook knife, radiofrequency probe, or laser. Selection is determined by the preference and training of the surgeon[20] (Figure 9.4A–E). A 377200# ophthalmic beaver blade has been useful for precise resections. The central portion of a type 1A or type 1D tear is amenable to debridement as treatment. The margin of the TFCC is smoothed and beveled following the central disk resection. With the scope in the 3-4 portal, the radial side of the TFCC articular disk may be resected using the ulnar-side portal. A banana blade is very useful in outlining and excising the torn fibers of the articular disk. They are then removed with a grasper. Next, the scope is placed in the ulnar-side portal, and the cutting instrument is inserted through the 3-4, and the ulnar side of the tear is resected. It is essential to the success of the procedure not to extend the resection into the peripheral margin of the TFCC and instead to resect only the articular disk (the central portion of the TFCC). Attention should then be directed at the lunotriquetral joint to assess for associated lunotriquetral ligament disruption, and to assess the quality of the articular cartilage of the lunate. If articular changes are noted, then debridement of loose flaps of articular cartilage or lunotriquetral ligaments should be considered as well.

Attritional tears of the TFCC are a consequence of the normal aging process. Mikic found an increasing incidence of degenerative tearing of the TFCC with progressing age. There were no tears in patients under the age of 20 years. Between 20 and 30 years of age, 7.6%; by 50 years of age, 18.1%; and over the age of 60 years, 53.1% of patients studied incurred tears of the TFCC. Veigas, on the other hand, found no patient under 45 years of age, and 27.5% of patients over 60 years old suffered degenerative tears of the TFCC.[41]

There has been controversy regarding the effect of partial excision of the TFCC.[16,59–61] While the mechanical stability of the DRUJ is provided primarily by the distal radial ulnar joint ligaments, there is concern that excision of the articular disk may result in instability. The effect of partial excision of the TFCC has been investigated in cadaver models. Palmer et al documented that resection of less than two-thirds of the horizontal portion of the articular disk caused no significant alteration to axial load transmission.[16] Similarly, Adams found no instability resulted from a partial central disk resection when compared to an intact specimen.[15] Consequently, partial resection of less than two-thirds of the horizontal portion of the TFCC can be performed without biomechanical alteration of the important functions of the TFCC.

RESULTS

Results of open debridement of the TFCC have met with limited success. There are few reports of open

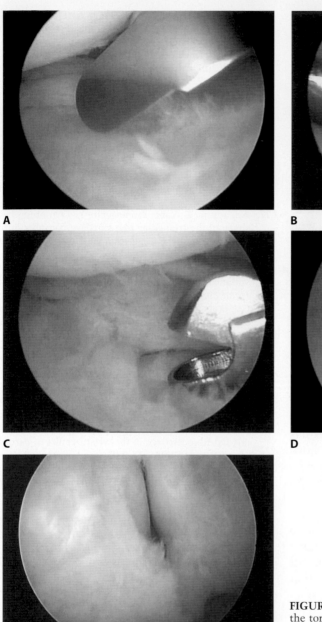

A

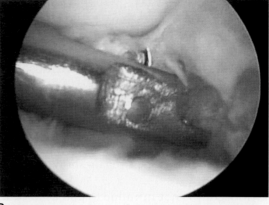

B

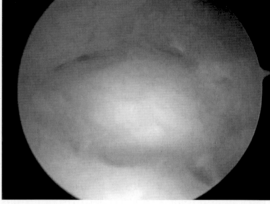

C

D

E

FIGURE 9.4. A. Demonstrates the use of a beaver blade to resect the torn margins of the TFCC radially and ulnarly. Suture forceps may then be placed **(B)** radially and **(C)** ulnarly to remove loose fragments of the disk. **D.** Appearance following resection of unstable margins. **E.** Inspection must be turned to the LT interval to identify potential interosseous ligament trauma.

excision of the TFCC, with the Darrach procedure being the treatment usually instituted for problems with the distal radial ulnar joint prior to the advent of wrist arthroscopy. Mennon et al reported their results in 16 patients who underwent partial excision of the TFCC. Sixty-nine percent had relief of symptoms, and the remaining 5% required Darrach procedures to relieve symptoms. They noted that all patients over 40 years of age did poorly. Failures were due to the presence of arthritic changes of the radiocarpal or distal radial ulnar joint. No mention was made of the type of TFCC tear found. All asymptomatic patients in follow up maintained stability of the distal radial ulnar joint without loss of motion or strength.[17]

Arthroscopic debridement of traumatic type 1A tears of the TFCC is now preferable to open debridement. These tears have no capacity to heal, due to the lack of blood supply. Removal of the central two-thirds portion with removal of any pads or flaps and with smoothing of the debrided margins will not destabilize the distal radial ulnar joint if 2 mm of rim is left intact.[15,62,63] There is no alteration in the biomechanics; therefore, immediate rehabilitation can be instituted.[16,64] There is actually no repair to heal, and postoperative immobilization is not necessary.

Earlier reports of "ectomy" by Roth and Osterman confirm the feasibility of arthroscopic debridement of the central portion of the TFCC as a standard arthroscopic procedure.[43,62] Thirty-four percent of Osterman's patients demonstrated a type 1A TFCC lesion, and 88% of 52 patients reported good or excellent results following arthroscopic treatment. Several reports subsequently confirm the advantage of arthroscopic debridement of the TFCC.[50,62,65–72]

Type 1D (radial) tears may also be amenable to simple debridement if the dorsal and palmar distal radial ulnar joint ligaments are intact.[1] If the dorsal and palmar condensation is involved, instability is present, and either arthroscopic or open repair should be performed.[56–58,73–75]

Wrist arthroscopy is not immune to potential complications.[76,77] The general complications are well known and described elsewhere in this book. Debridement of the TFCC is relatively free from complications specific to the procedure. However, care must be taken to avoid injury to the articular surface of the ulna or damage to the dorsal and palmar ligamentous condensations. Preoperatively, stability of the DRUJ must be present, the joint must be nonarthritic, and ulnar-positive variation must be addressed, or failure of simple debridement will result.[78,79] In the event that pain relief does not result from debridement, several investigations have reported favorable results with ulnar-shortening osteotomy.[79–82]

Our experience in over 778 wrist arthroscopies has paralleled the described experience of others for both 1A and 1D non-destabilizing tears. While a prospective series has not been performed, we have found no difference in results for patients with 1D tears either debrided or repaired using arthroscopic techniques. Type 1A tears debrided in the horizontal portion to maintain the distal radial ulnar joint ligaments have resulted in an 85% good or excellent outcome in our series. In conclusion, debridement of the TFCC tear in a stable wrist results in a high degree of satisfaction. Failures of the procedure are generally secondary to persistent occult instability of either the DRUJ or the lunotriquetral ligament.

References

1. Gan B, Richards R, Roth J. Arthroscopic treatment of triangular fibrocartilage tears. *Orthop Clin North Am* 1995;26:721–729.
2. Chidgey L. The distal radioulnar joint: problems and solutions. *J Am Acad Orthop Surg* 1995;3:95–109.
3. Ishii S, Palmer A, Werner F, et al. An anatomic study of the ligamentous structure of the triangular fibrocartilage complex. *J Hand Surg* 1998;23:977–985.
4. Chidgey LK. Histologic anatomy of the triangular fibrocartilage. *Hand Clin* 1991;7:249–262.
5. Cober S, Trumble T. Arthroscopic repair of triangular fibrocartilage complex injuries. *Orthop Clin North Am* 2001;30:279–294.
6. Thiru RG, Ferlic DC, Clayton ML, et al. Arterial anatomy of the triangular fibrocartilage of the wrist and its surgical significance. *J Hand Surg* 1986;11:258–263.
7. Bednar M, Arnoczky S, Weiland A. The microvasculature of the triangular fibrocartilage complex: its clinical significance. *J Hand Surg* 1991;16A:1101–1105.
8. Mikic Z. The blood supply of the human distal radioulnar joint and the microvasculature of its articular disk. *Clin Orthop Rel Res* 1992;275:19–28.
9. Mikic Z, Somer L, Somer T. Histologic structure of the articular disk of the human distal radioulnar joint. *Clin Orthop Rel Res* 1992;275:29–36.
10. Nakamura T, Makita A. The proximal ligamentous component of the triangular fibrocartilage complex. *J Hand Surg Br* 2000;25:479–486.
11. Nakamura T, Yabe Y. Histological anatomy of the triangular fibrocartilage complex of the human wrist. *Ann Anat* 2000;182:567–572.
12. Nakamura T, Yabe Y, Horiuchi Y. Dynamic changes in the shape of the triangular fibrocartilage complex during rotation demonstrated with high resolution magnetic resonance imaging. *J Hand Surg* 1999;24:338–341.
13. Palmer A, Glisson R, Werner F. Relationship between ulnar variance and triangular fibrocartilage complex thickness. *J Hand Surg* 1984;9A:681–683.
14. Gupta R, Nelson S, Baker J, et al. The innervation of the triangular fibrocartilage complex: nitric acid maceration rediscovered. *Plast Reconstr Surg* 2001;107:135–139.
15. Adams B. Partial excision of the triangular fibrocartilage complex articular disk: a biomechanical study. *J Hand Surg* 1993;18:334–340.
16. Palmer A, Werner F, Glisson R, et al. Partial excision of the triangular fibrocartilage complex. *J Hand Surg* 1998;13A:391–394.
17. Menon J, Wood V, Schoene H, et al. Isolated tears of the triangular fibrocartilage of the wrist: results of partial excision. *J Hand Surg* 1984;9A:527–530.
18. Pederzini L, Luchetti R, Soragni O, et al. Evaluation of the triangular fibrocartilage complex tears by arthroscopy, arthrography, and magnetic resonance imaging. *Arthroscopy* 1992;8:191–197.
19. Schuind F, An KN, Berglund L, et al. The distal radioulnar ligaments: a biomechanical study. *J Hand Surg* 1991;16:1106–1114.
20. Nagle D. Laser-assisted wrist arthroscopy. *Hand Clin* 1999;15:495–499.
21. Stuart P, Berger RA, Linscheid RL, et al. Dorsopalmer stability of the distal radioulnar joint. *J Hand Surg Am* 2000;25A:689–699.
22. Tang B, Ryu J, Kish V. The triangular fibrocartilage complex: an important component of the pulley for the ulnar wrist extensor. *J Hand Surg* 1998;23:986–991.
23. Bednar JM, Osterman AL. The role of arthroscopy in the treatment of traumatic triangular fibrocartilage injuries. *Hand Clin* 1994;10:605–614.
24. Gupta R, Bozentka DJ, Osterman AL. Wrist arthroscopy: principles and clinical applications. *J Am Acad Orthop Surg* 2001;9:200–209.
25. Werner F, Palmer A, Fortino M, et al. Force transmission through the distal ulna: effect of ulnar variance, lunate fossa angulation, and radial and palmar tilt of the distal radius. *J Hand Surg* 1992;17A:423–428.
26. Friedman SL, Palmer AK, Short WH, et al. The change in ulnar variance with grip. *J Hand Surg* 1993;18:713–716.
27. North ER, Meyers S. Wrist injuries: correlation of clinical and arthroscopic findings. *J Hand Surg* 1990;15(A):915–920.
28. Hardy DC, Totty WG, Gilula LA. Posteranterior wrist radiography: importance of arm positioning. *J Hand Surg* 1987;12:504–508.
29. Epner RA, Bowers WH, Guilford WB. Ulnar variance—the effect of wrist positioning and roentgen filming technique. *J Hand Surg* 1982;7:298–305.

30. Zinberg EM, Palmer AK, Coren AB, et al. The triple-injection wrist arthrogram. *J Hand Surg* 1988;13A:803–809.

31. Levinsohn EM, Palmer AK, Palmer AK. Wrist arthrography: value of the three-compartment injection method. *Radiology* 1991;179:231–239.

32. Pfirrmann C, Theumann N, Chung C, et al. What happens to the triangular fibrocartilage complex during pronation and supination of the forearm? Analysis of its morphology and diagnostic assessment with MR arthrography. *Skeletal Radiol* 2001;30:677–685.

33. Manaster BJ, Mann RJ, Ruby LK. Wrist pain: correlation of clinical and plain film findings with arthrographic results. *J Hand Surg* 1989;14:466–473.

34. Pittman CC, Quinn SF, Belsole R, et al. Digital subtraction wrist arthrography: use of double contrast technique as a supplement to single contrast arthrography. *Skeletal Radiol* 1988;17:119–122.

35. Yin Y, Wilson AJ, Gilula LA. Three-compartment wrist arthrography: direct comparison of digital subtraction with nonsubtraction images. *Radiology* 1995;197:287–290.

36. Pin PG, Semenkovich JW, Young VL, et al. Role of radionuclide imaging in the evaluation of wrist pain. *J Hand Surg* 1988;13A:810–814.

37. Wechsler RJ, Wehbe MA, Rifkin MD, et al. Computed tomography diagnosis of distal radioulnar subluxation. *Skeletal Radiol* 1987;16:1–5.

38. Pirela-Cruz MA, Goll SR, Klug M, et al. Stress computed tomography analysis of the distal radioulnar joint: a diagnostic tool for determining translational motion. *J Hand Surg* 1991; 16:75–82.

39. Skahen JR 3rd, Palmer AK, Levinsohn EM, et al. Magnetic resonance imaging of the triangular fibrocartilage complex. *J Hand Surg* 1990;15A:552–557.

40. Peh WCG, Patterson RM, Viegas S, et al. Radiographic-anatomic correlation at different wrist articulations. *J Hand Surg* 1999;24A:777–780.

41. Viegas SF, Patterson RM, Hokanson JA, et al. Wrist anatomy: incidence, distribution, and correlation of anatomic variations, tears, and arthrosis. *J Hand Surg* 1993;18A:463–475.

42. Kinninmonth AWG, Chan KM. A study of age-related changes of the articular disc of the wrist in Hong Kong Chinese. *J Hand Surg* 1990;15B:358–361.

43. Roth JH, Poehling GG. Arthroscopic "-ectomy" surgery of the wrist. *Arthroscopy* 1990;6:141–147.

44. Verheyden JR, Short WH. Arthroscopic wafer procedure. *Atlas of the Hand Clinics* 2001;6:241–252.

45. Leibovic SJ, Bowers WH. Arthroscopy of the distal radioulnar joint. *Orthop Clin North Am* 1995;26:755–757.

46. Zelouf DS, Bowers WH. Arthroscopy of the distal radioulnar joint. *Hand Clin* 1999;15:475–477.

47. Palmer AK. Triangular fibrocartilage complex lesions: a classification. *J Hand Surg* 1989;14A:594–606.

48. Palmer AK. Triangular fibrocartilage disorders: injury patterns and treatment. *Arthroscopy* 1990;6:125–132.

49. Hauck RM, Skahen JI, Palmer AK. Classification and treatment of ulnar styloid nonunion. *J Hand Surg* 1996;21A:418–422.

50. Trumble T, Gilbert M, Vedder N. Arthroscopic repair of the triangular fibrocartilage complex. *Arthroscopy* 1996;12:588–597.

51. Trumble T, Gilbert M, Vedder N. Isolated tears of the triangular fibrocartilage: management by early arthroscopic repair. *J Hand Surg* 1997;22:57–65.

52. Ruch DS, Poehling GG. Arthroscopic management of partial scapholunate and lunotriquetral injuries of the wrist. *J Hand Surg* 1996;21A:412–417.

53. Melone C, Nathan R. Traumatic disruption of the triangular fibrocartilage complex. *Clin Orthop Rel Res* 1992;275:65–73.

54. Sagerman SD, Short W. Arthroscopic repair of radial-sided triangular fibrocartilage complex tears. *Arthroscopy* 1996;12:339–342.

55. Cooney WP, Linscheid RL, Dobyns JH. Triangular fibrocartilage tears. *J Hand Surg* 1994;19:143–154.

56. Bednar J. Arthroscopic treatment of triangular fibrocartilage tears. *Hand Clin* 1999;15:479–488.

57. Jantea CL, Baltzer A, Ruther W. Arthroscopic repair of radial-sided lesions of the fibrocartilage complex. *Hand Clin* 1995;11: 31–36.

58. Hermansdorfer JD, Kleinman WB. Management of chronic peripheral tears of the triangular fibrocartilage complex. *J Hand Surg* 1991;16A:340–346.

59. Darrach W. Partial excision of lower shaft of ulnar for deformity following Colles's fracture. *Clin Orthop* 1992;275:3–4.

60. Kleinman WB, Greenberg JA. Salvage of the failed darrach procedure. *J Hand Surg* 1995;20A:951–958.

61. McKee MD, Richards RR. Dynamic radio-ulnar convergence after the Darrach procedure. *J Bone Joint Surg Br* 1996;78:413–418.

62. Osterman AL. Arthroscopic debridement of triangular fibrocartilage complex tears. *Arthroscopy* 1990;6:120–124.

63. Coleman H. Injuries of the articular disc at the wrist. *J Bone Joint Surg* 1960;42B:522–529.

64. Palmer AK. Partial excision of the triangular fibrocartilage complex. In: Gelberman RH (ed). *Master Techniques in Orthopaedic Surgery: The Wrist.* New York: Raven Press, 1994, pp. 207–218.

65. Nagle D, Benson L. Wrist arthroscopy: indications and results. *Arthroscopy* 1992;8:198–203.

66. Minami A, Ishikawa J, Suenaga N, et al. Clinical results of treatment of triangular fibrocartilage complex tears by arthroscopic debridement. *J Hand Surg* 1996;21A:406–411.

67. De Smet L, De Ferm A, Steenwerckx A, et al. Arthroscopic treatment of triangular fibrocartilage complex lesions of the wrist. *Acta Orthop Belg* 1996;62:8–13.

68. Westkaemper JG, Mitsionis G, Giannakopoulos PN, et al. Wrist arthroscopy for the treatment of ligament and triangular fibrocartilage complex injuries. *Arthroscopy* 1998;14:479–483.

69. Dailey S, Palmer A. The role of arthroscopy in the evaluation and treatment of triangular fibrocartilage complex injuries in athletes. *Hand Clin* 2000;16:461–476.

70. van der Linden A. Disk lesion of the wrist joint. *J Hand Surg* 1986;11A:491–497.

71. Husby T, Haugstvedt J. Long-term results after arthroscopic resection of lesions of the triangular fibrocartilage complex. *Scand J Plast Reconstr Surg Hand Surg* 2001;35:79–83.

72. Sotereanos DG, Giannakopoulos PN, Mitsionis GJ. Arthroscopic debridement for the treatment of wrist ligament tears and TFCC tears: results in 62 patients. *Arthroscopy* 1996;12:362.

73. Jones MD, Trumble TE. Arthroscopic repair of radial-sided triangular fibrocartilage complex tears. *Atlas of the Hand Clinics* 2001;6:221–239.

74. Mikic Z, Sad N. Treatment of acute injuries of the triangular fibrocartilage complex associated with distal radioulnar joint instability. *J Hand Surg* 1995;20A:319–323.

75. Whipple T, Geissler W. Arthroscopic management of wrist triangular fibrocartilage complex injuries in the athlete. *Orthopedics* 1992;16:1061–1067.

76. Culp RW. Complications of wrist arthroscopy. *Hand Clin* 1999;15:529–535.

77. del Pinal F, Herrero F, Cruz-Camara A, et al. Complete avulsion of the distal posterior interosseous nerve during wrist arthroscopy: a possible cause of persistent pain after arthroscopy. *J Hand Surg* 1999;24A:240–242.

78. Tomaino M, Weiser R. Combined arthroscopic TFCC debridement and wafer resection of the distal ulna in wrists with triangular fibrocartilage complex tears and positive ulnar variance. *J Hand Surg* 2001;26:1047–1052.

79. Fricker R, Pfeiffer K, Troeger H. Ulnar shortening osteotomy in posttraumatic ulnar impaction syndrome. *Arch Orthop Trauma Surg* 1996;115:158–161.

80. Hulsizer D, Weiss A, Akelman E. Ulna-shortening osteotomy after failed arthroscopic debridement of the triangular fibrocartilage complex. *J Hand Surg* 1997;22A:694–698.

81. Van Sanden S, De Smet L. Ulnar shortening after failed arthroscopic treatment of triangular fibrocartilage complex tears. *Chir Main* 2001;20:332–336.

82. Boulas HJ, Milek MA. Ulnar shortening for tears of the triangular fibrocartilaginous complex. *J Hand Surg* 1990;15A:415–420.

10

Arthroscopic Management of Ulnar Impaction Syndrome

Gregory J. Hanker

During the last 20 years, the orthopaedic community has become much more aware of ulnar-sided wrist problems in general, and ulnar impaction syndrome in particular.[1] Ulnar impaction syndrome (UIS) is a degenerative condition involving the ulnar column of the wrist joint. The chronic impaction or abutment of the dome of the ulnar head against the triangular fibrocartilage complex (TFCC) and the ulnar portion of the carpus results in an increased load across the ulnocarpal articulation and the subsequent progressive degeneration of the tissues with the development of ulnar-sided wrist pain.

PATHOPHYSIOLOGY

The increased load-bearing across the ulnar side of the wrist, associated with the repetitive impaction of the dome of the ulna into the TFCC and ulnar carpus, has been shown to cause progressive tissue degeneration.[2] In most instances, the excessive ulnar column load is associated with a static increase in ulnar variance (UV). Positive UV can be congenital or acquired. Most acquired varieties are the result of wrist trauma. Excessive ulnar load can also occur in a dynamic fashion as a direct result of forearm pronation, ulnar deviation, and power grip, which lead to a relative increase in UV.[3-5] Over time, chronic ulnar load-bearing from a static positive UV, or from a dynamic increase in ulnocarpal load, will produce tissue degeneration with wear and tear of the TFCC; chondromalacia of the lunate, triquetrum, and ulnar head; tearing of the lunotriquetral ligament (LTL); carpal instability; and joint arthrosis.[6]

CLASSIFICATION

This sequence of tissue degeneration has been described by Palmer in his classification scheme of TFCC abnormalities.[7] Palmer's class II degenerative lesions follow a progressive pattern of destructive tissue injury due to the ulnar abutment. In stage IIA, there is wearing of the TFCC, and in stage IIB there is associated lunate or ulnar dome chondromalacia. In stage IIC there is a central tear of the TFCC. Tearing of the LTL and the TFCC, with ulnar-sided chondromalacia, categorizes stage IID. Finally, in stage IIE there is associated ulnocarpal arthritis. Occasionally, the stages will overlap. As we will see, the classification of TFCC degeneration aids us in choosing appropriate treatment for UIS.[8-10]

CLINICAL EVALUATION

Patients with UIS typically present with ulnar-sided wrist pain, aggravated by activities that require forceful or repetitive gripping. Physical examination reveals pain with palpation over the ulnar carpus, TFCC, and lunotriquetral joint (LTJ) regions. Wrist motion is somewhat stiff and painful. Grip strength is diminished.[11] In my practice, UIS is one of the most overlooked work-related musculoskeletal disorders in patients whose careers involve repetitive hand manipulative tasks, such as packers, pickers, sorters, and so on.

Plain radiographs typically show a neutral or positive ulnar variance on the posteroanterior view. The dome of the ulnar head impinges upon the lunate, creating a cysticlike degeneration in the inferoulnar aspect of the lunate and sometimes on the inferoradial aspect of the triquetrum; and subchondral sclerosis of the ulnar head.[12] Infrequently, arthrosis about the ulnar aspect of the carpus or LTJ diastasis is present. Magnetic resonance imaging (MRI) is the most helpful diagnostic tool because it is able to detect subtle degenerative changes in the lunate early on, even before plain films reveal any abnormality.[13] In addition, MRI provides information on the extent of TFCC degeneration, integrity of the LTL and LTJ alignment, distal radioulnar joint (DRUJ) alignment, and ulnar-sided carpal arthrosis (Figure 10.1). MRI can also aid the treating physician to more accurately stage the extent of Palmer class II degeneration.

Diagnostic wrist arthroscopy is the most accurate tool for evaluation of UIS. Direct visualization of the ulnar aspect of the carpus enables the arthroscopist to

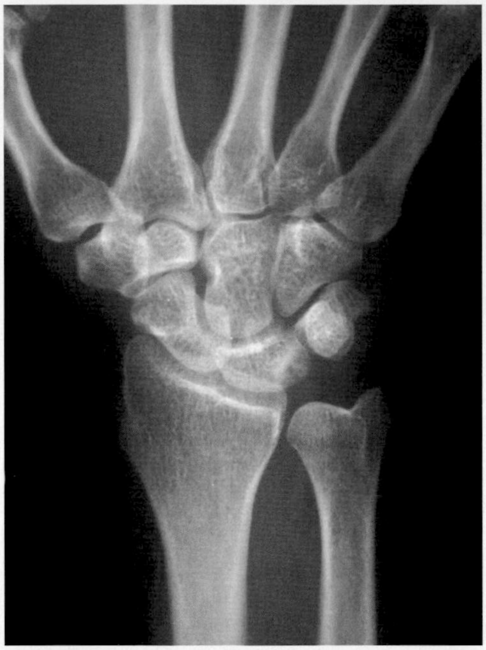

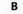

FIGURE 10.1. A. Plain X-ray of a 56-year old female patient with chronic ulnar-sided wrist pain attributable to work-related activities as a carrot sorter. **B.** MRI of the same patient. Note the signal abnormality in the inferoulnar aspect of the lunate.

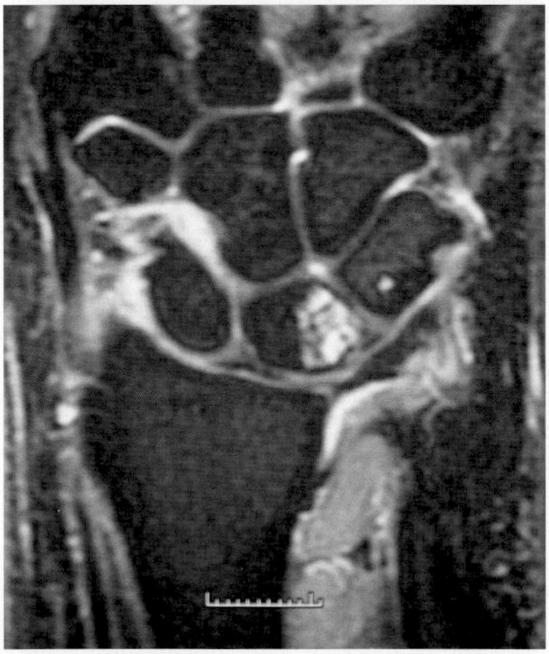

fully classify the extent of the tissue degeneration (Figure 10.2).[9,10,14–18]

TREATMENT

Initial management of UIS is conservative, with a recommendation for activity modification, antiinflam-matory medications, wrist splinting, cold application, and occupational therapy. Some patients respond to a cortisone injection administered about the ulnar aspect of the joint. Patients with neutral or negative ulnar variance and no significant ulnar-sided wrist pathology have the best chance to respond to this conservative care plan. Patients with positive ulnar variance and advanced TFCC degeneration—Palmer class IIC, IID, IIE—and those who cannot modify their work or avocational activities will often require surgery.[1,2,16]

The goal of surgical treatment for UIS is to unload the ulnar column of the wrist, i.e., the ulnocarpal articulation. Even small changes in the relative length of the ulna will lead to a marked decrease in axial load transmission through the TFCC.[19] Traditionally, this was accomplished with an ulnar shortening osteotomy and subsequently with an excision of the ulnar dome (open wafer procedure). With advances in wrist arthroscopy, it is now possible to shorten the ulna via an arthroscopic wafer procedure and debride the degenerative TFCC, chondromalacia, ligament tearing, capsular scar, and synovitis.

HISTORICAL PERSPECTIVE

In 1941, Milch treated malunited Colles' fractures by performing a cuff resection of the ulna, removing a segment of the ulnar shaft, and providing fixation with wire loops.[20] In 1985, Darrow et al. reported their results of distal ulna recession for a variety of DRUJ disorders. Darrow modified Milch's procedure by using a dynamic compression plate. By shortening the long ulna approximately 4 mm, they obtained very good results.[21] In 1990, Boulas and Milek reported good success with open ulnar osteotomy, shortening, and plate fixation for treatment of arthrographically proven TFCC tears.[22] In 1991 and 1993, Chun and Palmer used an oblique ulnar shortening osteotomy to treat patients with UIS, reporting overall very good results.[23] A variety of osteotomy techniques evolved in an attempt to facilitate the osteotomy procedure, improve healing time of the osteotomy, and lessen the need for later plate removal.[24–26] Recently, Constantine et al. have shown that either head or shaft shortening to treat UIS produces equivalent results.[27]

Feldon et al devised an open surgical technique in which a 2 to 4 mm segment of the distal ulna was removed as a "wafer." In 1987 and 1992, Feldon et al. reported their results of the open wafer procedure.[28] Similar good results with this technique were reported by Bilos and Cumberland in 1991.[29] These studies clearly showed that open excision of a 2 to 4 mm wafer of the dome of the ulnar head could decompress the load across the ulnocarpal articulation and lead to good results in the treatment of UIS.

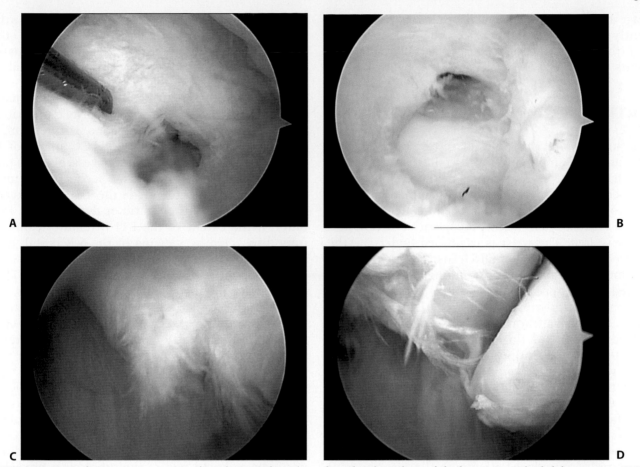

FIGURE 10.2. A. Arthroscopic appearance of a Palmer IIC lesion revealing chondromalacia of the lunate. **B.** Debrided degenerative TFCC tear with ulnar-sided chondromalacia. **C.** Extensive fraying and partial substance tearing of the LTL is characteristic of a Palmer IID injury. **D.** LTL tear with LTJ instability, and osteoarthritis of the triquetrum and lunate is typical of end-stage UIS seen in Palmer IIE lesions.

IMPORTANCE OF WRIST ARTHROSCOPY

Wrist arthroscopy is a minimally invasive procedure with low morbidity, high patient acceptance, and rapid recovery.[30] During the late 1980s and continuing into the 1990s, the technique of wrist arthroscopy greatly advanced. Operative wrist arthroscopy became the treatment of choice for most ulnar-sided wrist pathology, especially injuries of the TFCC, as classified by Palmer.[31–34] Credibility for the technique of arthroscopic debridement of acute traumatic and chronic degenerative TFCC tears arose from a biomechanical study done by Palmer et al. in 1988.[35] They showed that removal of the central avascular portion of the TFCC, leaving intact the peripheral rim, did not significantly alter load-bearing or stabilization of the DRUJ or the ulnar column of the wrist. Numerous clinical reports followed, recommending the technique of operative wrist arthroscopy to debride TFCC lesions. However, in 1995, Chidgey reported poor results with TFCC debridement in patients with posi-

tive ulnar variance when compared with favorable results in cases of neutral or negative ulnar variance.[36] In 1996, Minami et al. reported that arthroscopic debridement alone in patients with positive ulnar variance or degenerative lesions did not do well; but if an ulnar shortening osteotomy was included with a TFCC excision, the results were satisfactory.[31] Several other investigators, such as Hulsizer et al.[37] and Westkaemper et al.[18] indicated that positive ulnar variance or TFCC degeneration because of UIS played a key role in the poor results obtained from arthroscopic debridement alone.

Arthroscopy can also be employed to debride the ulnar dome, thus decompressing the ulnar aspect of the carpus. In 1990, the arthroscopic wafer procedure was used by Osterman in his debridement of TFCC tears.[38] Wnorowski et al. used a cadaver model to demonstrate that the arthroscopic wafer procedure significantly decreased ulnar load.[39] In 1992, Buterbaugh described the arthroscopic wafer technique for treatment of UIS.[40] Palmer then went on to report favorable results in his clinical study performed on patients with stage IIC pathology.[41] Several other reports have recently been presented indicating the effectiveness of an arthroscopic wafer procedure in select groups of patients with UIS.[42–47]

ARTHROSCOPIC WAFER PROCEDURE

The fundamental principles of setting up a large operating room, employing a well-trained surgical team, and having proper surgical instrumentation and arthroscopic equipment readily available are all necessary to carry out a successful procedure. Regional anesthesia is most often used. A preoperative antibiotic is administered. The wrist is examined under anesthesia to assess for carpal or DRUJ instability, limitation of motion, and crepitus or clunking. A tourniquet is placed on the upper arm, but it is used only if needed to control intra-articular bleeding that hampers arthroscopic visualization of the joint. The hand is placed in standard finger traps—usually the index, middle, and ring fingers—and then suspended vertically via attachment to a standard shoulder boom affixed to the opposite side of the operating table with 5 to 10 pounds of traction weight.

The radiocarpal joint (RCJ) is infused with sterile saline. A 3-4 dorsoradial portal is established, and the arthroscopic sheath (rotatable cannula and conical tip obturator) is introduced atraumatically into the joint. Inflow is established through this cannula. A fluid management system, such as the Dyonics InteliJet Fluid Management System (Smith & Nephew Inc, Andover, MA), is very helpful to control a smooth flow of fluid, especially when powered, suction surgical instrumentation is used during the procedure. The Dyonics 2.7 mm × 30-degree video arthroscope is seated into the cannula, and a systematic examination of the RCJ is begun. The arthroscopic examination is facilitated by obtaining through-and-through flow of the irrigation fluid. To do this, insert a 19-gauge needle into the vicinity of the 6-R or dorsoulnar portal, or proceed to establish the portal directly. The diagnostic arthroscopy is further facilitated by placing a 2.9 mm full-radius shaver (Dyonics disposable blade, Smith & Nephew, Inc, Andover, MA) into a second cannula positioned in the 6-R dorsoulnar portal. More often than not, you will encounter a significant amount of degenerated capsular tissue and posterior capsular scar that blocks arthroscopic view of the ulnar aspect of the carpus. The shaver can be used to tediously debride this tissue and any inflamed synovium. Having done this capsular debridement, it is now possible to pass the arthroscope ulnarly and to fully view the dorsal lunate and the TFCC.

Next, switch the arthroscope to the 6-R dorsoulnar portal to complete the examination of the ulnar portion of the RCJ. If excessive scarified and degenerated capsular tissue is still present in the dorsoulnar

wrist region, it may not be possible to view arthroscopically the LTL and LTJ, the inferior pole of the triquetrum, and the ulnarmost aspect of the lunate. If necessary, switch the scope back to the 3-4 portal, and redebride through the 6-R portal.

It is imperative that the full extent of the ulnar aspect of the RCJ be seen, or a proper classification of TFCC degeneration cannot be done. Furthermore, arthroscopic management of the TFCC injury or UIS will be hampered by inadequate access. Use of a probe is encouraged to feel out lesions such as sloughing of the lunate cartilage, tearing of the TFCC, and tearing of the LTL with either static or dynamic LTJ instability. If the extent of the LTJ instability cannot be fully discovered by viewing in the 6-R portal, establish a 6-U portal. The 6-U portal affords a unique vantage of the entire ulnar region, especially the LTJ and the dome of the distal ulna. In most instances, midcarpal arthroscopy is also performed to assess for injury in the midcarpal region of the wrist. Subtle carpal instabilities, especially of the LTJ, can be better appreciated. Rarely is a DRUJ portal necessary for treatment of TFCC degeneration or UIS.

The arthroscopic wafer procedure can be successfully undertaken only through a central disruption of the TFCC. Access to the dome of the distal ulna is only possible through a central tear of the TFCC. Absent such a tear, the arthroscopic wafer procedure is not indicated, and one of the other open procedures should be chosen instead.

To facilitate the arthroscopic wafer procedure, I introduce a third cannula through the 6-U portal. The 6-U portal becomes the workhorse for the entire procedure. The arthroscopic wafer procedure is begun by first debriding the entire central portion of the torn and degenerated TFCC, leaving behind a stout peripheral rim of tissue. In this way, the central opening through the TFCC provides a pathway to access the dome of the distal ulna, and the volar and dorsal radioulnar ligaments are preserved. The 2.9 mm full-radius shaver is utilized for this debridement. This same shaver is then introduced through the central defect of the TFCC, and excision of the radial one-half to two-thirds of the degenerated ulnar dome is begun (Figure 10.3). The shaver is swept dorsal to volar, removing a 2 to 3 mm depth of distal ulna. To ensure that the wafer excision is kept uniformly smooth, the forearm must be rotated into pronation and then supination. The depth of the debridement can be judged by comparing the diameter of the shaver, (i.e., approximately 3 mm) to the defect created in the ulna (Figure 10.4). Rarely is it necessary to remove more than 4 mm of the ulnar dome.

The radialmost aspect of the ulnar dome is difficult to excise, as it lies directly adjacent to the sigmoid notch. To facilitate excision of this portion of the distal ulna, a small 0.25" osteotome or a Freer instrument can be inserted through the 6-U portal and

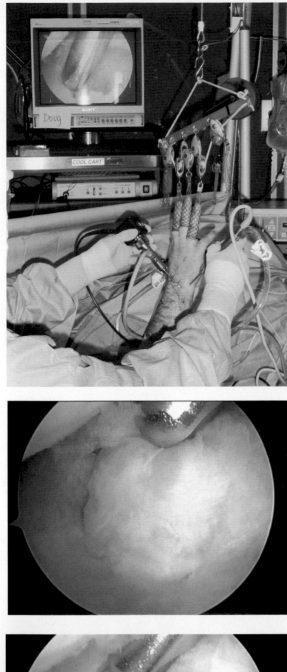

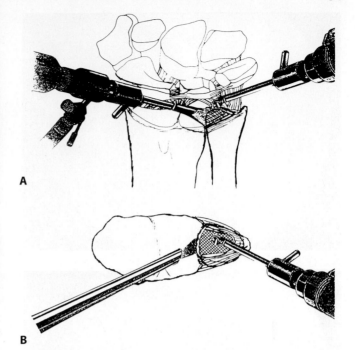

FIGURE 10.4. A. The dome of the distal ulna is systematically excised, represented by darkened area. **B.** Transverse schematic view depicting the position of distal ulna resection (darkened area).

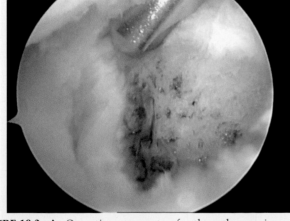

FIGURE 10.3. A. Operating room setup for the arthroscopic wafer procedure. Shaver is in the 6-U portal. **B.** The degenerated TFCC tear is debrided, revealing the protruding dome of the ulnar head. **C.** Resection of the ulnar head is begun through the central opening of the TFCC.

used to pry off the radial rim of tissue. In this way, a smooth declining osteotomy is made through the ulnar dome, decompressing the ulnocarpal articulation (Figure 10.5). To ensure that a satisfactory wafer excision has been accomplished, view the osteotomy site completely with the wrist rotated into full supination to pronation. Then use the small portable fluoroscope to view the DRUJ and ulnar column of the wrist (Figure 10.6). A negative ulnar variance of 1 to 3 mm should be observed, and the declivity of the wafer osteotomy should be smooth (Figure 10.7).

Note that viewing of the arthroscopic wafer procedure is done with the scope in the 3-4 portal. Also, view through the 4-5 or 6-R portals to get another perspective on the extent of the ulnar dome excision. Debriding with the shaver in the 4-5 or 6-R portal may help in excising the ulnar aspect of the distal ulnar head. Some authors have even recommended carrying out the wafer procedure through a DRUJ portal.[9]

I prefer to use the 2.9 mm full-radius shaver for the entire bony excision of the distal ulna. In younger patients with larger and harder bones, the Dyonics 3.5 mm Incisor or Razorcut full-radius shaver is more aggressive and will speed up the procedure. As an alternative, the Dyonics 2.9 mm Abrader or Barrel Abrader bur can be used. An electrosurgery probe (2.3 mm VAPR [short]; Mitek, Westwood, MA) can also accomplish the job with an effective excision of both the degenerated TFCC and the ulnar dome.

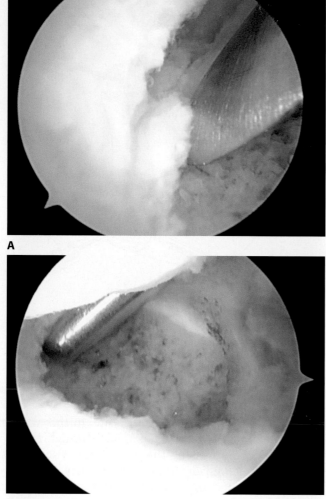

A

B

FIGURE 10.5. **A.** A Freer dissecting instrument is used to excise the difficult-to-reach distal ulnar rim adjacent to the sigmoid notch. **B.** The excision is completed by removing a depth of cartilage and bone about equal to the width of the shaver.

INDICATIONS FOR AN ARTHROSCOPIC WAFER PROCEDURE

The main indication for an arthroscopic wafer procedure is to treat chronic cases of UIS with a Palmer IIC lesion, a positive ulnar variance of 2 to 4 mm, and no arthroscopic evidence of LTJ instability. In those few instances where LTJ instability is detected as part of the arthroscopic wrist examination, these lesions are then upgraded to either a Palmer IID or IIE classification. It is then recommended to do a formal ulnar shortening osteotomy, since this partially stabilizes the ulnar aspect of the wrist joint through increased tension in the ulnocarpal ligament complex.[48] It may also be necessary to formally treat the LTJ instability. Surgical options include reconstruction, arthrodesis, and ulnocarpal plication.[49,50]

The arthroscopic wafer procedure is also the operation of first choice in Palmer IID lesions associated with UIS, as long as the injury to the LTL does not

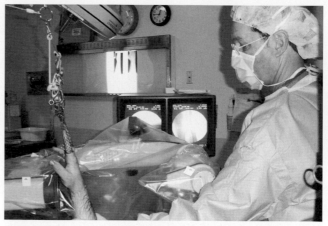

FIGURE 10.6. During the wafer excision, intraoperative portable fluoroscopic imaging confirms the amount of distal ulna resection.

result in LTJ instability. This determination is best made at the time of wrist arthroscopy.[51] For a partial LTL injury, the arthroscopic procedure can be used to debride the frayed portion of the ligament. This debridement is best accomplished by placing the shaver or suction punch in the 6-U portal and the scope in the 4-5 or 6-R portal.

In those patients with symptomatic UIS, but a neutral or negative ulnar variance, it is possible to proceed with a TFCC debridement of the central two-thirds of the degenerated disk. However, if there is any arthroscopic evidence of ulnar dome, lunate, or triquetral chondromalacia, it is recommended to include the arthroscopic wafer excision.

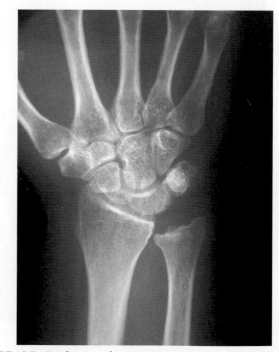

FIGURE 10.7. Final X-ray of patient in Figure 10.1. Approximately 4 to 5 mm of the ulnar dome has been removed, adequately decompressing the ulnocarpal impaction.

The arthroscopic wafer procedure is not appropriate for Palmer class IIA or IIB lesions associated with UIS because the TFCC typically remains intact, blocking arthroscopic access to the dome of the distal ulna. In these two instances, either an open wafer (Feldon) procedure for shortening less than 4 mm of distal ulna, or an open shortening ulnar osteotomy are better choices. In my experience, the Palmer IIE lesion is frequently discovered at the time of wrist arthroscopy. Often, the lunate chondromalacia, and sometimes the triquetral chondromalacia, is of a type 4 cartilage injury, i.e., full-substance loss of cartilage consistent with arthrosis. When arthritis has developed, even in the presence of a class IIA, IIB, or IIC lesion associated with UIS, it is best to proceed to an ulnar shortening osteotomy and debride the cartilage injury or perform a chondroplasty (Figure 10.8).

The arthroscopic wafer procedure offers several distinct advantages over an open wafer procedure (Feldon procedure) or an open ulnar osteotomy in the treatment of UIS. The arthroscopic operation avoids open surgery and either a long, unsightly forearm scar or an ulnar-sided wrist scar, and possible surgical alterations of the DRUJ anatomy. It avoids the risk of ulnar nonunion, the pain associated with postoperative forearm tendinitis, subsequent surgery for plate removal, risk of pathologic fracture, and prolonged postoperative immobilization to effect ulnar osteotomy union.

REHABILITATION

All patients are sent to occupational therapy (OT) preoperatively so they can be instructed in digital flexibility exercises and extremity elevation techniques. Doing this before surgery enables the patient to more fully comprehend their preoperative education. At surgery, an axillary block is administered for anesthesia. This type of regional block allows the patient an additional 12 to 18 hours of pain relief. In most cases, a "pain pump" is used to provide an additional 24 to 48 hours of relief. At the termination of the arthroscopic wafer procedure, the arm is immobilized in a modified long-arm, sugar-tongs splint. This blocks forearm rotation, which is usually quite painful.

One week later, the surgical dressings are removed, a supportive wrist splint is used, and a formal OT program is initiated, concentrating on active and passive wrist range of motion exercises, edema control, and scar modification. Approximately 3 weeks postoperatively, gentle resistance exercises are added. Most patients take approximately 3 months after surgery to return to their normal activities. Many patients will have mild to slight residual pain with activities, due to the chondromalacia or degenerative joint disease associated with UIS.

CONCLUSION

Arthroscopic wafer resection of the distal ulna has several distinct advantages that make it the surgical procedure of choice for the treatment of UIS with symptomatic Palmer IIC and select IID tears. Contraindications to the use of the arthroscopic wafer procedure include: LTJ instability typical of a Palmer IIE degenerative pattern, DRUJ instability or arthrosis, and excision of the ulnar dome in excess of 4 mm.

Recent clinical reviews of the arthroscopic wafer procedure indicate very good results; minimal complications when compared to open surgical procedures; minimal need for subsequent repeat surgery, such as plate removal, following osteotomy; and the ability to thoroughly evaluate the wrist joint for any

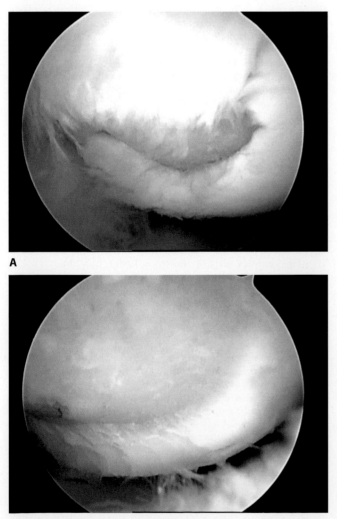

A

B

FIGURE 10.8. A. Complete loss of cartilage from the inferior aspect of the lunate, typical of a Palmer IIE lesion. **B.** Chondroplasty of the lunate arthritic lesion leaves behind a smooth rim of cartilage and encourages fibrocartilage growth.

associated intra-articular injuries. There is greater patient acceptance of the arthroscopic procedure over competing open surgical procedures. The rehabilitation following arthroscopy is relatively quick and better tolerated by patients.

References

1. Bowers W. The distal radioulnar joint. In: Green D, Hotchkiss R, Pederson W, (eds). *Green's Operative Hand Surgery*, 4th ed. Philadelphia: Churchill Livingstone, 1999, pp. 986–1032.

2. Moy O, Palmer A. Ulnocarpal abutment. In: Cooney W, Linscheid R, Dobyns J, (eds). *The Wrist—Diagnosis and Operative Treatment*. St. Louis: Mosby, 1998, pp. 773–787.

3. Palmer A, Glisson R, Werner F. Ulnar variance determination. *J Hand Surg* 1982;7:376–379.

4. Af Ekenstam F, Palmer A, Glisson R. The load on the radius and ulna in different positions of the wrist and forearm. *Acta Orthop Scand* 1984;55:363–365.

5. Friedman S, Palmer A, Short W, et al. The change in ulnar variance with grip. *J Hand Surg* 1993;18:713–716.

6. Friedman S, Palmer A. The ulnar impaction syndrome. In: Schneider L, (ed). *Hand Clinics 7:2*. Philadelphia: WB Saunders Co., 1991, pp. 295–310.

7. Palmer A. Triangular fibrocartilage complex lesions: a classification. *J Hand Surg* 1989;14:594–606.

8. Fulcher S, Poehling G. The role of operative arthroscopy for the diagnosis and treatment of lesions about the distal ulna. In: Graham T, (ed). *Hand Clinics 14:2*. Philadelphia: WB Saunders Co., 1998, pp. 285–296.

9. Verheyden J, Short W. Arthroscopic wafer procedure. In: Geissler W, (ed). *Atlas of the Hand Clinics 6:2*. Philadelphia: WB Saunders Co., 2001, pp. 241–252.

10. Pomerance J. Arthroscopic debridement and/or ulnar shortening osteotomy for TFCC tears. *J Am Soc Hand Surg* 2002;2:95–101.

11. Deitch M, Stern P. Ulnocarpal abutment—treatment options. In Graham T, (ed). *Hand Clinics 14:2*. Philadelphia: WB Saunders Co., 2001, pp. 251–263.

12. Pope T, Poehling G, Siegel D, et al. Imaging of the wrist. In: McGinty J, (ed). *Operative Arthroscopy*, 2nd ed. Philadelphia: Lippincott-Raven Publishers, 1996, pp. 937–974.

13. Imaeda T, Nakamura R, Shionoya K, et al. Ulnar impaction syndrome: MR imaging findings. *Radiology* 1996;201:495–500.

14. Pederzini L, Luchetti R, Soragni O, et al. Evaluation of TFCC tears by arthroscopy, arthrography, and MRI. *Arthroscopy* 1992;8:191–197.

15. Cooney W. Evaluation of chronic wrist pain by arthrography, arthroscopy and arthrotomy. *J Hand Surg* 1993;18A:815–822.

16. Palmer A, Harris P. Classification and arthroscopic treatment of TFCC lesions. In: McGinty J, (ed). *Operative Arthroscopy*, 2nd ed. Philadelphia: Lippincott-Raven Publishers, 1996, pp. 1015–1022.

17. Hanker G, Hanker K. Role of arthroscopy in the management of TFCC injuries and wrist fractures. In: Parisien J, (ed). *Current Techniques in Arthroscopy*, 3rd ed. New York: Thieme, 1998, pp. 137–147.

18. Westkaemper J, Mitsionis G, Giannakopoulos P, et al. Wrist arthroscopy for the treatment of triangular fibrocartilage complex injuries. *Arthroscopy* 1998;14:479–483.

19. Palmer A, Werner F. Biomechanics of the distal radioulnar joint. *Clin Orthop* 1984;187:26–35.

20. Milch H. Cuff resection of the ulna for malunited Colles' fracture. *J Bone Joint Surg* 1941;39:311–313.

21. Darrow J Jr, Linscheid R, Dobyns J, et al. Distal ulna recession for disorders of the distal radioulnar joint. *J Hand Surg* 1985; 10:482–491.

22. Boulas H, Milek M. Ulnar shortening for tears of the triangular fibrocartilaginous complex. *J Hand Surg* 1990;15:415–420.

23. Chun S, Palmer A. The ulnar impaction syndrome: follow-up of ulnar shortening osteotomy. *J Hand Surg* 1993;18:46–53.

24. Rayhack J, Gasser S, Latta L, et al. Precision oblique osteotomy for shortening of the ulna. *J Hand Surg* 1993;18:908–918.

25. Labosky D, Waggy C. Oblique ulnar shortening by a single saw cut. *J Hand Surg* 1996;21:48–59.

26. Mizuseki T, Tsuge K, Ikuta Y. Precise ulna-shortening osteotomy with a new device. *J Hand Surg* 2001;26:931–939.

27. Constantine K, Tomaino M, Herndon J, et al. Comparison of ulnar shortening osteotomy and the wafer resection procedure as treatment for ulnar impaction syndrome. *J Hand Surg* 2000; 25:55–60.

28. Feldon P, Terrono A, Belsky M. Wafer distal ulna resection for triangular fibrocartilage tears and/or ulnar impaction syndrome. *J Hand Surg* 1992;17:731–737.

29. Bilos Z, Cumberland D. Distal ulnar head shortening for treatment of triangular fibrocartilage complex tears with ulna positive variance. *J Hand Surg* 1991;16:1115–1119.

30. Whipple T. *Arthroscopic Surgery: The Wrist*. Philadelphia: J.B. Lippincott, 1992.

31. Minami A, Ishikawa J, Suenaga N, et al. Clinical results of treatment of triangular fibrocartilage complex tears by arthroscopic debridement. *J Hand Surg* 1996;21:406–411.

32. Schneider L, ed. *Hand Clinics—Problems of the DRUJ*; 7(2). Philadelphia: WB Saunders Co., 1991.

33. Bednar J, Osterman A. The role of arthroscopy in the treatment of traumatic triangular fibrocartilage complex injuries. *Hand Clin* 1994;10:605–614.

34. Graham J (ed). *Hand Clinics—Problems About the Distal End of the Ulna*; 14(2). Philadelphia: WB Saunders Co., 1998.

35. Palmer A, Werner F, Glisson R, et al. Partial excision of the triangular fibrocartilage complex: an experimental study. *J Hand Surg* 1988;13:391–394.

36. Chidgey L. The distal radioulnar joint: problems and solutions. *J Am Acad Orthop Surg* 1995;3:95–109.

37. Hulsizer D, Weiss A, Akelman E. Ulna-shortening osteotomy after failed arthroscopic debridement of the triangular fibrocartilage complex. *J Hand Surg* 1997;22:694–698.

38. Osterman A. Arthroscopic debridement of triangular fibrocartilage complex tears. *Arthroscopy* 1990;6:120–124.

39. Wnorowski D, Palmer A, Werner F, et al. Anatomy and biomechanical analysis of the arthroscopic wafer procedure. *Arthroscopy* 1992;8:204–212.

40. Buterbaugh G. Ulnar impaction syndrome: treatment by arthroscopic removal of the distal ulna. *Tech Orthop* 1992;7:66–71.

41. Wrobeleski A, Palmer A, Short W, et al. *Arthroscopic Wafer for Ulnar Impaction*. Presented at the American Society for Surgery of the Hand Annual Meeting, Denver, Colorado, 1997.

42. Osterman A, Bednar J, Gambin K, et al. *The Natural History of Untreated Symptomatic Tears in the TFCC*. Presented at the American Society for Surgery of the Hand Annual Meeting, Nashville, Tennessee, 1996.

43. Trumble T, Gilbert M, Vedder N. Ulnar shortening combined with arthroscopic repairs in the delayed management of triangular fibrocartilage complex tears. *J Hand Surg* 1997;22:807–813.

44. Minami A, Kato H. Ulnar shortening for triangular fibrocartilage complex tears associated with ulnar positive variance. *J Hand Surg* 1998;23:904–908.

45. Nakamura T, Yabe Y, Horiuchi Y, et al. Ulnar shortening procedure for the ulnocarpal and DRUJ's. *J Jpn Soc Surg Hand* 1998;15:119–126.

46. Tomaino M, Weiser R. Combined arthroscopic TFCC debridement and wafer resection of the distal ulna in wrists with triangular fibrocartilage complex tears and positive ulnar variance. *J Hand Surg* 2001:26;1047–1052.

47. Nagle D, Geissler W. Laser-assisted wrist arthroscopy. In: Geissler W, (ed). *Atlas of Hand Clinics—New Techniques in Wrist Arthroscopy; 6(2)*. Philadelphia: WB Saunders Co., 2001, pp. 189–201.

48. Smith B, Short W, Werner F, et al. The effect of ulnar shortening on lunotriquetral motion and instability: a biomechanical study. Presented at the American Society for Surgery of the Hand, Annual Fellows and Residents Meeting, 1994.

49. Bishop A, Reagan D. Lunotriquetral sprains. In: Cooney W, Linscheid R, Dobyns J, (eds). *The Wrist—Diagnosis and Operative Treatment*. St. Louis: Mosby, 1998, pp. 527–549.

50. Tolan W, Savoie III F, Field L. Arthroscopic management of lunotriquetral instability. In: Geissler W, (ed). *Atlas of the Hand Clinics; 6(2)*. Philadelphia: WB Saunders Co., 2001, pp. 275–283.

51. Ritter M, Chang D, Rush D. The role of arthroscopy in the treatment of lunotriquetral ligament injuries. In: Culp R, (ed). *Hand Clinics—Wrist and Hand Arthroscopy; 15(3)*. Philadelphia: WB Saunders Co., 1999, pp. 445–454.

11

Kinematics and Pathophysiology of Carpal Instability

Alan E. Freeland and William B. Geissler

The wrist is the subject of continuing anatomic and functional analysis. A precise understanding of normal and pathophysiologic wrist kinematics remains a challenge. Although much is known, more has yet to be discovered. Arthroscopy has been, and will continue to be, instrumental in unlocking the secrets of carpal pathophysiology by identifying the scope and extent of wrist ligament injuries, especially those of the scapholunate and lunotriquetral ligaments.

Although the wrist is commonly thought to move in the flexion-extension and radioulnar planes, it is actually a universal joint that is capable of multidirectional motion. While full motion may allow peak performance, most important daily functions are performed in the midrange.[1-3] Reciprocal synchronization occurs between wrist and digital function. Grip strength increases with wrist extension until it maximizes at 37 degrees.[4] Finger extension strength increases with progressive wrist flexion.[5]

The wrist is comprised of 8 carpal bones, 7 of which act synchronously and synergistically to allow normal wrist motion.[6] The pisiform articulates with the palmar surface of the triquetrum but acts primarily as a fulcrum to enhance flexor carpi ulnaris strength and power, rather than to influence wrist kinematics or stability. The carpal bones are guided and constrained by a complex system of intrinsic and extrinsic ligaments. A total of 24 muscles cross or insert on the carpal bones.

HISTORICAL PERSPECTIVE

Early investigations applied planar concepts that correlated carpal structure and function. Johnston reported in 1907 that carpal motion was always initiated at the midcarpal joint and occurred largely between two immobile carpal rows.[7] In 1943, Guilford et al described the scaphoid as a rod linking the carpal rows.[8] In 1972, Linscheid et al. refined the "link" concept of carpal motion to propose the "slider crank" analogy, in which the scaphoid acts as a mobile bridge between the two carpal rows, much as the

slider crank controls motion between a piston and a drive shaft (Figure 11.1).[9] In 1977, Sarrafian et al. noted that radiocarpal motion comprised 40% and midcarpal motion 60% of maximum wrist flexion, while motion was 66.5% radiocarpal and 33.5% midcarpal during maximum extension. These researchers theorized that the scaphoid functioned with the proximal row during flexion and with the distal row during extension.[10]

Although Wright reported in 1935 that the center of rotation (COR) of the wrist joint resided in the head of the capitate during wrist flexion and shifted to the intercarpal joint during extension, most investigators long believed that the COR was confined solely within the head of the capitate.[11-18] However, Patterson et al. determined in 1998, through an instantaneous screw axis (ISA) calculated for the third metacarpal with respect to the radius, that normal carpal kinematics does not have an ISA fixed in or limited to the capitate during flexion and extension of the wrist.[19]

In 1921, Navarro conceptualized a columnar wrist model to better explain the sophisticated and multidimensional movements of the wrist.[20] His theory held that 3 interdependent columns correlated carpal anatomy with function. The lateral column (scaphoid, trapezium, and trapezoid) supported the thumb and transferred load between the two carpal rows. The central column (lunate, capitate, and hamate) flexed and extended the wrist. Rotation was controlled by the medial column (triquetrum and pisiform). In 1978, Taleisnik modified the column theory to exclude the pisiform, recognizing that it played no integral role in intercarpal motion. He also determined that the normal distal carpal row has very little intercarpal motion and acts as a unit. He therefore included the trapezium and trapezoid as part of the central column (Figure 11.2).[21]

Meanwhile, Weber took a slightly different view of the columnar theory. He divided the carpus into two columns: the load-bearing radial column, composed of the lunate, capitate, scaphoid, and trapezoid; and the ulnar control column, consisting of the triquetrum and hamate. He viewed the helicoid triquetrohamate joint as the key to wrist position during load changes.[22]

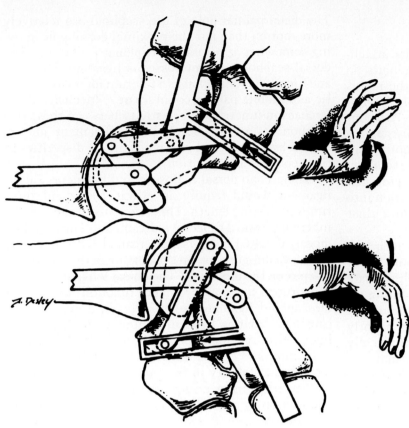

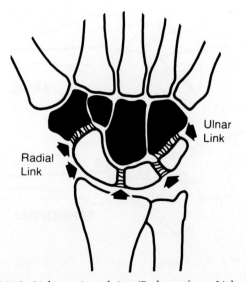

FIGURE 11.1. The "slider crank" concept of wrist flexion and extension. (Reprinted from: Linscheid RL, Dobyns JH, Beabout JW, Bryan RS: Traumatic instability of the wrist. *J Bone Joint Surg.* © 1972;54A: p. 1631 by permission of the Journal of Bone and Joint Surgery.)

Lichtman et al. formulated the next step toward a better understanding of 3-dimensional wrist motion with their "oval-ring" theory (Figure 11.3).[23] This theory conceives the wrist as four interdependent segments: the distal carpal row, scaphoid, lunate, and triquetrum. Ligamentous links connect each segment to its two adjacent elements. Continuity of the ligaments assures synchronous synergistic wrist motion. Disruption of any link(s) results in dysfunction. Craigen and Stanley pointed out that certain elements of both the column and the oval-ring theories, although sometimes contradictory, are useful in our understanding of the multidimensionality of wrist motion.[24]

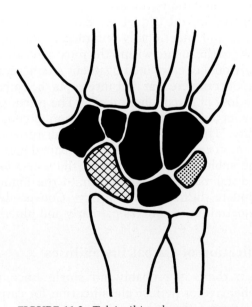

FIGURE 11.2. Taleisnik's columnar concept.

FIGURE 11.3. Lichtman's oval ring. (Redrawn from: Lichtman DM, Schneider R, Swafford AR, Mack GR. Ulnar midcarpal instability: Clinical and laboratory analysis. *J Hand Surg* 1981;6: p. 522.)

CARPAL KINEMATICS

The proximal carpal row has no tendinous attachments, except for that of the flexor carpi ulnaris on the pisiform, and is intercalated between the radius and ulna proximally and the distal carpal row.[6] Wrist motion begins in the distal carpal row.[25–27] At about the midpoint of wrist motion, the proximal carpal row accommodates the remaining extremes of motion, integrating ulnar deviation with flexion, and radial deviation with extension.[28–32] Similarly, the proximal carpal row incorporates extension and supination into radial deviation, and flexion and pronation into ulnar deviation of the wrist.

The lunate is an intercalated segment within the proximal row.[6] Lunate flexion and extension occur with the wrist during normal motion. The lunate flexes during radial deviation and extends during ulnar deviation. Within the proximal row, it is normally balanced between the scaphoid, which independently tends to flex, and the triquetrum, which intrinsically tends to extend. Although the normal proximal row moves synchronously in all directions, flexibility increases from the triquetrum across the lunate and to the scaphoid, and from dorsal to palmar at the scapholunate joint.[10,33–36]

The axial and tangential methods are equally accurate in assessing carpal angles (Figure 11.4).[37] The scapholunate angle on lateral X-ray views increases from an average of 35 degrees in full wrist extension to 76 degrees in full flexion. With the wrist in a neutral position, the scaphoid is flexed at about 47 degrees. The scaphoid rotates slightly, pronating during flexion and supinating during extension, while pivoting over the radioscaphocapitate ligament at its waist.

The distal palmar pole of the scaphoid has relatively more motion than has the proximal dorsal pole, moving somewhat as a rotating triplanar pendulum. The dorsal scapholunate interosseous ligament is stouter and functions somewhat as a fulcrum for its more elastic and mobile palmar counterpart.[38] Mechanical differences in function and elasticity between these two components of the scapholunate ligament are reflected by histological and biochemical disparities in their collagen composition.[39]

There is no dorsal radioscaphoid ligament. Such a ligament would require an elastic coefficient three times its resting length. This prerequisite exceeds the inherent physical capacity of ligaments. The dorsal radiocarpal (DRC) and dorsal intercarpal (DIC) ligaments form a V configuration on the dorsum of the wrist with its apex on the ulnar side. The dorsal V ligament (DVL) substitutes for some of the function that a radioscaphoid ligament might provide during normal carpal kinematics by maintaining an indirect stabilizing effect on the scaphoid throughout the range of wrist motion.[40,41] The transverse carpal ligament also lends some stability to the carpus.[42]

The triquetrum is the fulcrum for wrist rotation and motion in the radioulnar plane. The helicoid triquetrohamate joint is instrumental in accommodating this movement.[22,23] Although the palmar component of the lunotriquetral ligament is stronger, it is less flexible than its dorsal element.[30]

PATHOPHYSIOLOGY

Intrinsic Intercarpal Injuries

There are separate midcarpal joint ligamentous connections between the distal carpal row as a unit and the scaphoid and triquetrum in the proximal carpal row. The scaphoid and the triquetrum have anatomically independent and functionally interdependent ligamentous links to the lunate within the proximal carpal row. Any individual or combined ligament attenuation, partial tear, or complete tear that interrupts the carpal ring causes a loss of carpal alignment.[22] The proximal row assumes its lowest energy state position of collapse or instability. There are commensurate disturbances of wrist motion and joint loads.[6] The proximal pole of the scaphoid subluxes dorsoradially in the scaphoid fossa of the distal radius in proportion to the amount of scapholunate ligament diastasis.[43] Conversely, the lunotriquetral unit subluxes palmarly and ulnarly.

Classification of Carpal Instabilities

Although there is probably no single uncontested comprehensive or perfect classification for carpal instabilities, several parameters allow some measure of

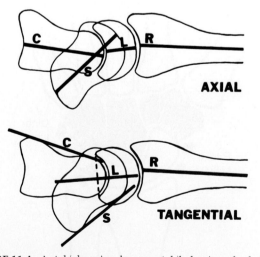

FIGURE 11.4. Axial (above) and tangential (below) methods of measuring carpal angles. C = capitate, S = scaphoid, L = lunate, R = radius. (Reprinted with permission from, Garcia-Elias M, An KN, Amadio PC, et al.: Reliability of carpal angle determinations. *J Hand Surg* 14A: Fig. 1, p 1018.)

quantification that is useful for analysis, comparison, communication, and management of these injuries.[44] These parameters include chronicity, constancy, ctiology, location, direction, and pattern.

CHRONICITY

The classification by chronicity relates to the time interval between injury and diagnosis. This categorization is based on the capacity for carpal reduction and especially upon the intrinsic capability for ligament healing after treatment. Acute carpal instabilities are those diagnosed within one week of injury. These instabilities are reducible and have the highest potential for ligament healing. Subacute tears are those diagnosed between 1 and 6 weeks after injury. Although they are reducible, the capacity for primary ligament healing is diminished. Injuries seen after longer than 6 weeks are considered chronic, have little capacity for ligament healing, and may occasionally be irreducible.

CONSTANCY

Carpal instability and symptoms may be apparent immediately in some cases; in others, they may take an initially indeterminate amount of time to appear. Ligaments that tear beyond the center of rotation of the two bones that they connect often have carpal malalignment that may be seen on standard wrist X-rays with the wrist at rest. This type of carpal collapse is termed *static carpal instability*.[45] This category may be further divided into reducible and irreducible injuries.

Patients with lesser ligament injuries often have normal standard X-rays, yet carpal malalignment and symptoms occur during motion and loading. This type of carpal collapse is termed *dynamic carpal instability*. The diagnosis of dynamic instability may require stress X-rays, such as an anteroposterior (AP) X-ray with digital traction; a 6-view AP (radial deviation, neutral, and ulnar deviation) and lateral (extension, neutral, and flexion) X-ray with a tightly gripped fist; cineradiography; or arthroscopic evaluation. Small ligament tears may propagate over a period of time, and carpal collapse and correlative symptoms may advance accordingly.[45–47]

ETIOLOGY

Trauma and synovitis are the principal causes of carpal ligament disruption. The former is more common. The healing capacity of traumatic ligament injuries is limited and unreliable, owing to a meager blood supply and technical difficulties in achieving successful repair by suturing. Synovitis erodes ligaments and renders them irreparable.

LOCATION

Location refers to the specific ligament or ligaments injured. Diagnosis and treatment of these injuries will be addressed in Chapter 12.

DIRECTION

The doubly intercalated lunate is a prime radiographic marker for both normal and pathophysiologic carpal kinematics.[6] The normal lunate is colinear with the capitate, as viewed on a lateral X-ray. Scapholunate, palmar radiocarpal, dorsal midcarpal ligament tears, or combinations of these injuries cause the lunate to dorsiflex and sublux under the head of the capitate. These injuries are termed *dorsal intercalary segment instability (DISI) patterns*.[9] Lunotriquetral, dorsal radiolunate, palmar scaphotrapezial, and palmar hamatolunate ligament tears or combinations of these injuries cause the lunate to volarflex and sublux over the head of the capitate. These injuries are termed *volar intercalary segment instability (VISI) patterns*.

PATTERN

Four intrinsic carpal instability patterns are recognized. When the ligaments restraining the scaphoid and triquetrum to the lunate are intact, the proximal row of carpals flexes and extends as a unit. Scapholunate or lunotriquetral ligament injuries cause disruption and reciprocally opposite rotation of the scaphoid and the triquetrum within the proximal carpal row. These injuries are therefore defined as *carpal instability dissociative (CID)*.[6,9] Displaced transtriquetral, and especially transscaphoid fractures may result in similar problems. When a fracture occurs proximal to the waist of the scaphoid, it is predisposed to displacement, owing to the opposing forces on the proximal and distal fragments.[48] Ligament injuries between the radius and/or ulna and the proximal carpal row (the radiocarpal and/or ulnocarpal joints) or between the proximal and distal carpal rows (the midcarpal joint) are labeled *carpal instability nondissociative (CIND)*.[6,9] Carpal instability adaptive (CIA) refers to carpal malalignment from a skeletal injury adjacent to, but not directly involving, the carpal bones and their connecting ligaments. Extra-articular distal radial fractures or malunions with loss of dorsal inclination and dorsal carpometacarpal dislocations may cause CIA.[49,50] If carpal instability adaptive is corrected with reduction of the causative skeletal deformity, the carpal bones usually realign in a normal or nearly normal posture. Coexisting CID and CIND are classified as *carpal instability combined (or complex) (CIC)*.

Axial carpal instability (ACI) refers to splits between metacarpal bases and bones in both carpal rows.[51,52] Axial wrist dislocations are not purely intrinsic carpal injuries, but may be further complicated by a variety of intrinsic carpal disturbances. Although isolated scaphoid dislocations are rare, they do occur.

MECHANISM AND PROGRESSION OF INJURY

Progressive perilunate instability (PPI) may result from sequential ligamentous injuries due to wrist extension, ulnar deviation, and supination during a fall on or injury to the outstretched hand (FOOSH).[53–55] These forces may also disrupt the wrist ligaments when they occur during other wrist injuries, especially intra-articular distal radial fractures.[56,57] Injuries to the scapholunate and lunotriquetral ligaments are classified as lesser arc injuries. Transscaphoid, transcapitate, and transtriquetral fractures are considered greater arc lesions (Figure 11.5). Combinations of wrist fractures and ligament injuries may occur. Concurrent transscaphoid fracture and scapholunate ligament (SLL) tear have been reported.[58–60] Fractures in these instances are more easily treated and heal more reliably than ligament injuries.

Ligament injury is one of degree and may be divided into attenuation injuries in which the elastic coefficient of the ligament is exceeded, partial tears, and complete tears.[57,61,62] Bone avulsion may occur in concert with complete ligament tears and sometimes helps to identify these injuries. Ligament lesions with a reparable avulsion fragment may have a better chance of healing than those confined within the substance of the ligament.

Progressive Perilunate Injury

Mayfield et al. have reported four progressive stages of perilunate injury (Figure 11.6).[53–55] The scapholunate ligament tear initiates distally in the volar extrinsic ligaments, progresses proximally, then attenuates the scapholunate ligament, later tearing it from volar to dorsal, and finally tears the dorsal radiolunate ligament.

Stage I injury is confined to attenuation or partial tear of the palmar radioscaphocapitate and scapholu-

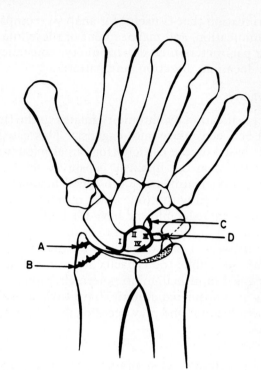

FIGURE 11.6. Mayfield's stages of progressive perilunate dislocation. (Reprinted with permission from: Mayfield JK, Johnson RP, Kilcoyne RK: Carpal dislocations: pathomechanics and progressive perilunate instability. *J Hand Surg* 1980;5A: p. 239.)

nate interosseous ligaments (Figure 11.6). The lesion starts distally and progresses proximally. This is a progressive scapholunate ligament disruption that may be further subdivided into three groups by combined radiocarpal and midcarpal diagnostic arthroscopy evaluation.[57] Progressive correlative scaphoid flexion, lunate (and triquetral) extension, and scapholunate gap widening may be seen on standard X-rays as the tear extends through the arthroscopic stages of classification.

The normal relationship of the scaphoid, lunate, and their related ligaments is illustrated in Figure 11.7. The normal scapholunate ligament has an inverted V appearance with the apex of the V distally, as visualized from the radiocarpal (3-4) arthroscopic portal. From the radial midcarpal portal, the normal scapholunate joint is congruently aligned and immobile (Figure 11.8). The scaphoid is flexed approximately 47 degrees relative to the lunate in the lateral X-ray view. The scapholunate joint space is congruent and does not exceed 2 mm on the AP X-ray.

Arthroscopic Grade I lesions are predynamic and have a tear of the volar extrinsic ligaments that may extend proximally to, but not beyond, the axis of rotation between the scaphoid and lunate (Figure 11.9). The interligamentous sulcus may be involved. The scapholunate ligament may be attenuated but is not torn. This attenuation is visualized from the radiocarpal (3-4) portal. From the radial midcarpal portal, the normal scapholunate joint remains congruently

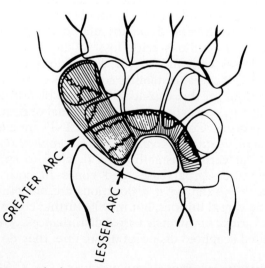

FIGURE 11.5. The lesser and greater carpal arcs. (Redrawn from: Blazar PE, Lawton JN. Diagnosis of carpal ligament injuries. In: Trumble TE (ed.): *Carpal Fracture-Dislocations.* Rosewood, IL: American Academy of Orthopaedic Surgery, 2002; p. 21.)

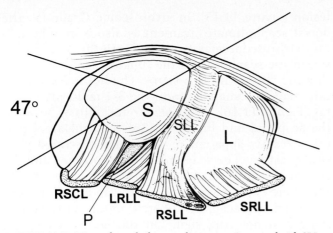

FIGURE 11.7. Normal scapholunate alignment. S = scaphoid, SLL = scapholunate ligament, L = lunate, RSCL = radioscaphocapitate ligament, P = interligamentous sulcus leading to the space of Portier, LRLL = long radiolunate ligament, RSLL = radioscapholunate ligament, SRLL = short radiolunate ligament.

ligament. They attenuate the midsubstance of the scapholunate ligament and cause dynamic instability (Figure 11.11). The scapholunate ligament may be partially torn at its volar corner, not extending past its midportion as seen from the radiocarpal (3-4) portal. From the radial midcarpal portal, scapholunate incongruity may be apparent, but a standard probe may not be introduced between the two bones (Figure 11.12). Slight multiplanar instability may be demonstrated by stressing either bone with the probe or by ballottement of the scaphoid tubercle. Usually, there is no discernible abnormality on standard X-rays.

In arthroscopic Grade III lesions, the tear extends through the substance of the scapholunate ligament, while the dorsal scapholunate component remains intact (Figure 11.13). The tear may be seen from both the 3-4 radiocarpal and the midcarpal portals, and a probe (but not the 2.7 mm arthroscope) may be introduced between the scaphoid and the lunate (Figure 11.14). Multiplanar instability is present and is easily demonstrated with the probe or by digital compression of the scaphoid tubercle. The dorsal portion of the scapholunate ligament remains intact. There is mild static instability. Slight scapholunate diastasis

aligned and immobile. No abnormality is seen on plain X-rays (Figure 11.10).

Grade II injuries continue proximally past the axis of rotation between the scaphoid and lunate and may involve the palmar portion of the scapholunate

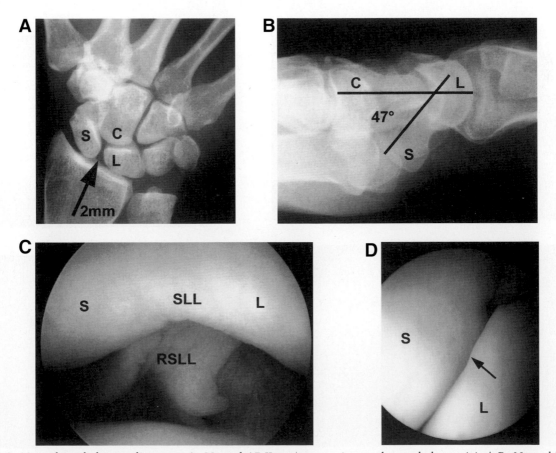

FIGURE 11.8. Normal scapholunate alignment. **A.** Normal AP X-ray (*arrow* points to the scapholunate joint). **B.** Normal lateral X-ray and scapholunate angle. **C.** Radiocarpal (3-4 portal) arthroscopic image demonstrating a normal SLL and RSLL. **D.** Midcarpal arthroscopic view with normal scapholunate alignment.

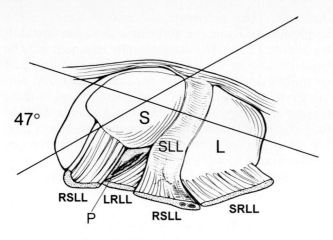

FIGURE 11.9. Grade I scapholunate ligament tear.

(3 to 4 mm) is seen on AP X-ray, and slight scaphoid flexion and lunate extension are seen on lateral X-ray.

In Stage II injury, there is dislocation of the capitolunate joint through the interligamentous sulcus into the space of Portier, indicating a complete scapholunate interosseous ligament tear (Figure 11.6). This correlates with an arthroscopic Grade IV

lesion (Figure 11.15). In arthroscopic Grade IV, the dorsal scapholunate ligament is also torn. The 2.7-mm arthroscope may be passed into the interval between the scaphoid and the lunate. Geissler termed this the "drive-through sign." The head of the capitate may be visualized from the 3-4 radiocarpal portal (Figure 11.16). Multiplanar instability between the scaphoid and lunate within the midcarpal portal is readily apparent or easily demonstrated with stress testing. The scaphoid is foreshortened and the carpus collapses, creating a SLAC wrist. On AP X-ray, there is a wide scapholunate gap (4 to 5 mm or more), and the scaphoid tubercle appears circular creating a signet ring sign. On the lateral view, the scaphoid is vertical, or nearly so, and the lunate is extended.

In Stage III, there is separation between the lunate and the triquetrum, indicating at least attenuation or partial tear of the lunotriquetral ligament (Figure 11.6). The dorsal wrist ligaments remain intact. In type IIIA, the head of the capitate remains contained, albeit sometimes dorsally subluxed, in the lunate concavity so as to create a DISI deformity. In type IIIB, the capitate is dorsally dislocated on top of the lunate (perilunate dislocation), indicating a complete tear of the lunotrique-

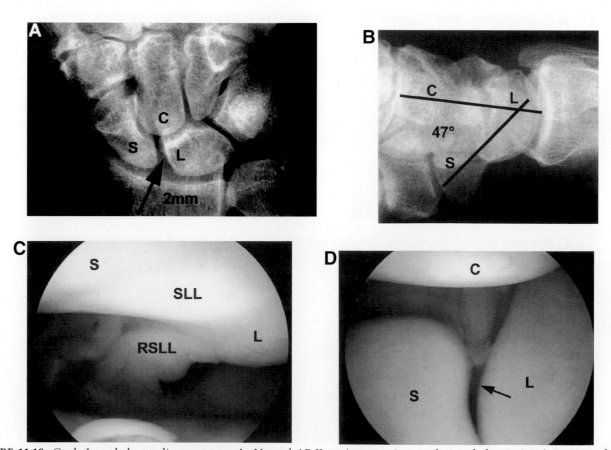

FIGURE 11.10. Grade I scapholunate ligament tear. **A.** Normal AP X-ray (*arrow* points to the scapholunate joint). **B.** Normal lateral X-ray and scapholunate angle. **C.** Radiocarpal (3-4 portal) arthroscopic image demonstrating attenuation of the SLL and RSLL. **D.** Midcarpal arthroscopic view with opening of the volar portion of the scapholunate interval.

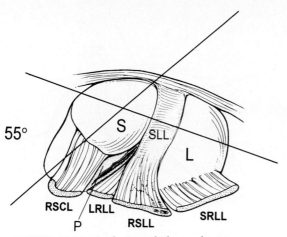

FIGURE 11.11. Grade II scapholunate ligament tear.

tral ligament. When both the scapholunate and lunotriquetral ligaments are torn, the lunate may appear neutral or be flexed or extended on lateral imaging, but the scaphoid will usually be abnormally flexed.

In Stage IV injury, the dorsal radiocarpal ligament is torn, producing a wide lunotriquetral gap (Figure 11.6).

Palmar rotatory dislocation of the lunate occurs through the space of Poirier (between the radioscaphocapitate and long radiolunate ligaments) and volar to the carpus.

Progressive Lunotriquetral Dissociation

Lunotriquetral dissociation has been less extensively studied and understood than its dissociative counterpart at the scapholunate joint. Because the triquetrohamate joint has a reciprocal relationship with the scaphotrapeziotrapezoid joint, it is currently believed that isolated injury to the lunotriquetral joint results from an injury that is the reverse of that described at the scapholunate joint. Lunotriquetral dissociation has been postulated to result from a fall or a force on the hypothenar eminence of the outstretched hand positioned in radial deviation with carpal pronation. The palmar aspect of the lunotriquetral ligament is stronger than its dorsal counterpart, while the midsubstance is of comparable strength to the midsubstance of the scapholunate ligament.[63,64] Isolated tears are believed to progress through a spectrum of sever-

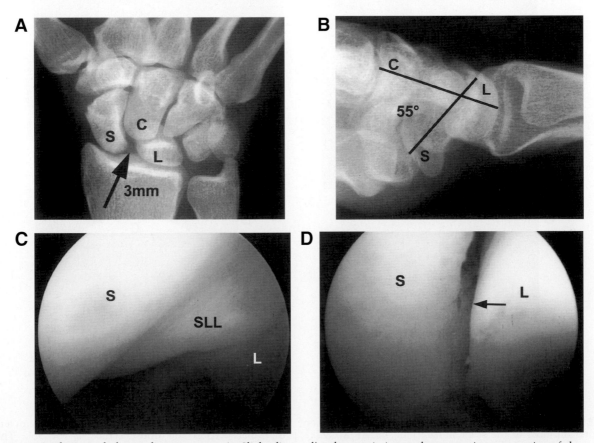

FIGURE 11.12. Grade II scapholunate ligament tear. **A.** Slight diastasis of the scapholunate joint on AP X-ray (*arrow* points to the scapholunate joint). **B.** Slight flexion of the scaphoid and increase of the scapholunate angle on lateral X-ray. **C.** Radiocarpal (3-4 por-

tal) arthroscopic image demonstrating attenuation of the SLL. **D.** Midcarpal arthroscopic view with a uniform opening (1.0 to 1.5 mm) of the scapholunate interval.

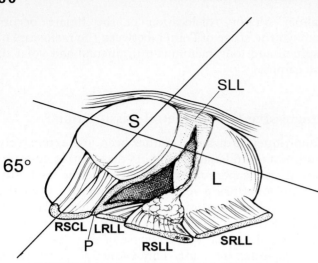

FIGURE 11.13. Grade III scapholunate ligament tear.

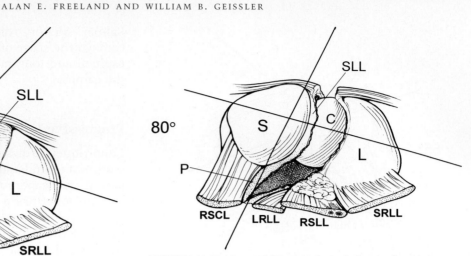

FIGURE 11.15. Stage II (Grade IV) scapholunate ligament tear.

ity similar to that of the scapholunate ligament but occurring in a dorsal to palmar direction (Figure 11.17).[30,65] The triquetrum extends in proportion to the injury[15] severity and becomes increasingly unsta-

ble. The lunotriquetral angle increases from a normal value of 14 degrees as lunotriquetral dissociation progresses (Figure 11.18).[66] Sectioning of the lunotrique-tral ligament alone does not produce a VISI defor-

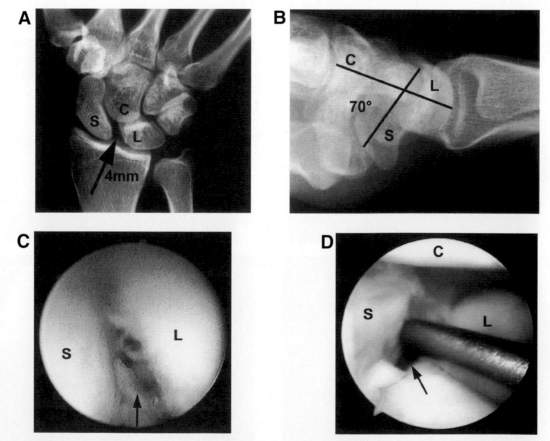

FIGURE 11.14. Grade III scapholunate ligament tear. **A.** Four-millimeter diastasis of the scapholunate joint on AP X-ray (*arrow* points to the scapholunate joint). **B.** Moderate flexion of the scaphoid and increase of the scapholunate angle to 70° on lateral X-ray. There is slight extension of the lunate in relation to the head of the capitate, a sign of early DISI pattern. **C.** Radiocarpal

(3-4 portal) arthroscopic image demonstrating a complete tear of the volar portion and midsubstance of the SLL. The dorsal scapholunate segment remains intact. **D.** Midcarpal arthroscopic view demonstrating increased widening and instability of the scapholunate joint sufficient to allow the introduction of a metallic probe.

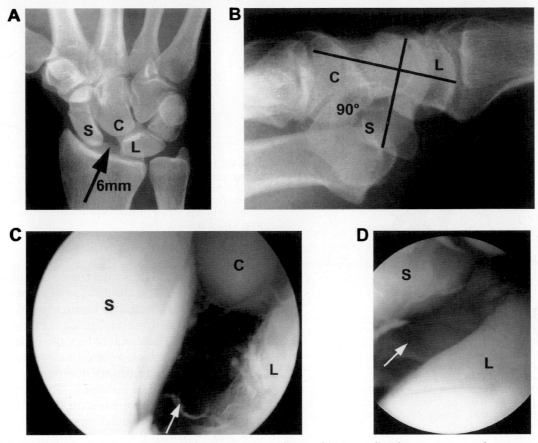

FIGURE 11.16. Stage II (Grade IV) scapholunate ligament tear. **A.** Six-millimeter diastasis of the scapholunate joint on AP X-ray (*arrow* points to the scapholunate joint). **B.** Severe flexion of the scaphoid and increase of the scapholunate angle to 90 degrees on lateral X-ray. The lunate is extended and subluxed in relation to the head of the capitate, a sign of an established DISI pattern. **C.** Ra-diocarpal (3-4 portal) arthroscopic image demonstrating a complete tear of the entire SLL. The head of the capitate can be visualized in the widened interval between the scaphoid and the lunate. **D.** A midcarpal arthroscopic view demonstrating severe widening and instability of the scapholunate joint sufficient to allow the introduction of the arthroscope.

mity.[67] Loss of integrity of the dorsal radio triquetral and dorsal scaphotriquetral ligaments further accentuates lunotriquetral instability. The scapholunate complex rotates into volar flexion and subluxes dorsally and radially in the scaphoid fossa of the distal radius. A VISI deformity then occurs, and the capitate tends to sublux palmarly.[30] The triquetrum supinates away from the lunate as lunotriquetral ligament integrity is lost.

Carpal Instability Nondissociative (Midcarpal Instability)

In nondissociative carpal instability (CIND), there is no dissociation of bones in the same row. Rather, there is dissociation between the carpal rows leading to dysfunction at both the radiocarpal and midcarpal joints (Figures 11.19 and 11.20). Midcarpal deformity is usually the more prevalent of the two.

Ulnar midcarpal instability is caused by injury to the triquetral-hamate-capitate ligaments.[23] A VISI deformity may occur. During ulnar deviation, the triquetrohamate joint undergoes an exaggerated shift or subluxation from palmar flexion to dorsiflexion that may be accompanied by a click or snap.

Radial midcarpal instability results from injury to the scaphoid-capitate-trapezoid-trapezium ligament complex.[68–70] A VISI pattern may result. Adaptive extrinsic midcarpal VISI deformity has been reported.[50]

The head of the capitate progressively subluxes dorsally on the lunate, especially during ulnar deviation in radiocapitate ligament injuries, creating a DISI deformity. This has been termed capitolunate instability pattern (CLIP).[71,72] Adaptive DISI CIND occurs with progressive loss of lateral inclination of the radius in distal radius fractures and malunions. In one study, all malunions of the distal radius with 30 degrees or more loss of lateral inclination had this type of collapse pattern.[49]

Other Intercarpal Disruptions

AXIAL DISLOCATIONS OF THE CARPUS

A longitudinal split of the carpus and metacarpal bases characterizes axial dislocations of the carpus (Figure

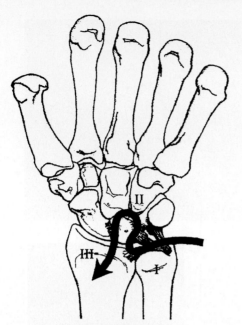

FIGURE 11.17. The direction, pattern, and stages of progressive lunotriquetral tear leading to perilunate involvement. A Stage I injury has disruption of the ulnolunate and ulnotriquetrial (ulnar leash) ligament complex. The lunotriquetral ligament is involved in a Stage II injury. In Stage III, the lesion progresses through the midcarpal joint and the scapholunate ligament is disrupted. (Reprinted with permission from: Shin AY, Murray PM. Biomechanical studies of wrist ligament injuries. In: Trumble TE (ed.): *Carpal Fracture-Dislocations.* Rosewood, IL: American Academy of Orthopaedic Surgery, 2002; p. 14.)

11.21). Both the proximal (carpal) and distal (metacarpal) transverse arches are disrupted. There are three types of axial wrist dislocations: radial, ulnar, and combined radioulnar.[51,52] In radial and ulnar dislocations, the carpus splits into two columns. In radial axial dislocations, the ulnar column maintains a normal

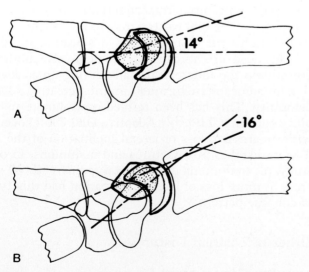

FIGURE 11.18. Normal lunotriquetral angle **A.** and the loss of this relationship with lunotriqetrial tear **B**. (Reprinted with permission from Reagan DS, Linscheid RL, Dobyns JH. Lunotriquetral sprains. *J Hand Surg* 1984; 9A: p. 506.)

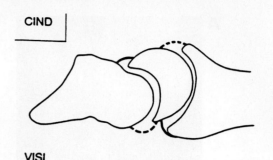

FIGURE 11.19. A VISI pattern of deformity occurs with CIND owing to attenuation or tear of the dorsal radiocarpal or volar midcarpal ligaments or of both. (Reprinted from: Amadio PC. Carpal kinematics and instability: A clinical and anatomic primer. *Clin Anat* 1991; 4: p. 7 by permission of Wiley-Liss, Inc., a subsidiary of John Wiley & Sons, Inc.)

and stable relationship with the distal radius and ulna, whereas the radial column displaces proximally and radially and may pronate. In ulnar axial dislocations, the radial column maintains a normal and stable relationship with the distal radius and ulna, whereas the ulnar column separates proximally and ulnarly and may supinate. In combined radioulnar axial dislocation, there are three columns. The central column, consisting of the lunate, capitate, and third metacarpal, maintains its normal relationship with the distal radius and ulna, while the radial and ulnar columns displace as detailed above. Axial dislocations may occur in combination with carpal ligament injuries and additional intercarpal deformities.

TRANSLATION INSTABILITY OF THE CARPUS

Siegal et al. demonstrated the importance of the integrity of the radioscaphocapitate and the radiolunate ligaments in preventing ulnar radiocarpal translocation.[73] There are two configurations of this lesion.[74,75] Type I involves ulnar translocation of the proximal carpal row as a unit owing to radioscaphocapitate and

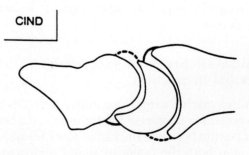

FIGURE 11.20. A DISI pattern of deformity occurs with CIND owing to attenuation or tear of the palmar radiocarpal or dorsal midcarpal ligaments or of both. (Reprinted from Amadio PC. Carpal kinematics and instability: a clinical and anatomic primer. *Clin Anat* 1991; 4: p. 6, by permission of Wiley-Liss, Inc., a subsidiary of John Wiley & Sons, Inc.)

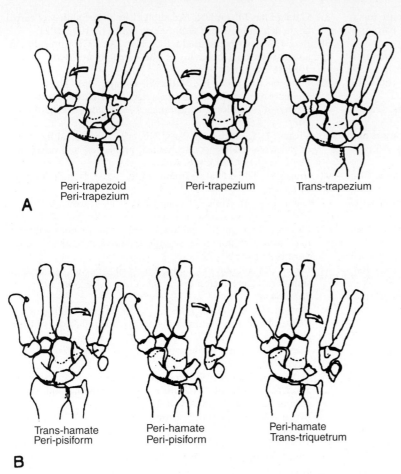

FIGURE 11.21. Some of the more common patterns of (**A**) axial-radial dislocation and (**B**) axial-ulnar dislocation patterns. (Reprinted with permission from: Garcia-Elias M, Dobyns JH, Cooney WP III, Linscheid RL: Traumatic axial dislocation of the carpus. *J Hand Surg* 1989; 14A: p. 449.)

radiolunate ligament injuries. Type II has an additional dissociative lesion of the scapholunate ligament. In Type II injuries, the radioscaphocapitate ligament may remain intact. Tear or avulsion of the ulnocarpal ligaments and attenuation or tear of the short radiolunate ligament form the basis for radial radiocarpal translation.[76] This constellation of injuries may present dynamic or static patterns and may be accompanied by dorsal or volar subluxation or dislocation. Static radiocarpal shifts of this nature may be identified on AP X-rays using standardized measurements of carpal position in relation to the longitudinal axis of the radius.[61,77]

Individual Carpal Dislocations

Although isolated carpal bone dislocations are rare, they may occur. Volar dislocation of the scaphoid is the most common. The scapholunate ligament is torn, followed by dislocation of the proximal pole of the scaphoid. Hyperpronation forces acting upon an extended and ulnarly deviated wrist, a direct dorsal to volar impact over the scaphoid with the distal radius stabilized, and occurrence during an effort to reduce a perilunate dislocation have each been reported. This is a type I or simple scaphoid dislocation.[78–80] Type II

or complex scaphoid dislocation is accompanied by axial disruption of the capitohamate joint. The lunotriquetral and scaphotrapeziotrapezoid joints are preserved in both types. CID often occurs. Lunate dislocations are the final stage (Stage IV) of progressive perilunate dislocation.

References

1. Amadio PC. Carpal kinematics and instability: a clinical and anatomic primer. *Clin Anat* 1991;4:1–12.
2. Brumfield RH, Champoux JA. A biomechanical study of normal functional wrist motion. *Clin Orthop* 1984;187:23–25.
3. Palmer AK, Werner FW, Murphy D, et al. Functional wrist motion: a biomechanical study. *J Hand Surg* 1985;10A:39–46.
4. Ryu JY, Cooney WP 3rd, Askew LJ, et al. Functional ranges of wrist joint motion. *J Hand Surg* 1991;16A:409–419.
5. O'Driscoll SW, Horii E, Ness R, et al. The relationship between wrist position, grasp size, and grip strength. *J Hand Surg* 1992;17A:169–177.
6. Zhao C, Amadio PC, Momose T. Effect of synergistic wrist motion on adhesion formation after repair of partial flexor digitorum profundus tendon lacerations in a canine model in vivo. *J Bone Joint Surg* 2002;84A:78–84.
7. Johnston HM. Varying positions of the carpal bones in the different movements at the wrist. Part I. Extension, ulnar, and radial flexion. *J Anat Physiol* 1907;41:109–122.
8. Guilford W, Boltan R, Lambrinudi C. The mechanism of the wrist joint. *Guy's Hosp Report* 1943;92:52–59.

9. Linscheid RL, Dobyns JH, Beabout JW, et al. Traumatic instability of the wrist: diagnosis, classification, and pathomechanics. *J Bone Joint Surg* 1972;54A:1612–1632.

10. Sarrafian SK, Malamed JL, Goshgarian GM. Study of wrist motion in flexion and extension. *Clin Orthop* 1977;126:153–159.

11. Wright DR. A detailed study of the movement of the wrist joint. *J Anat* 1935;70:137–143.

12. Fick R. *Anatomie und Meckanik der Gelenke.* Jena: Gustav Fisher, 1911, pp. 357.

13. MacConaill MA. The mechanical anatomy of the carpus and its bearings on some surgical problems. *J Anat* 1941;75:166–175.

14. Voltz RG. The development of a total wrist arthroplasty. *Clin Orthop* 1976;116:209–214.

15. Andrews JG, Youm YA. A biomechanical evaluation of wrist kinematics. *J Biomech* 1979;12:63–93.

16. Youm YA, Flatt AE. Kinematics of the wrist. *Clin Orthop* 1980;149:21–32.

17. Brumbaugh RB, Crowninshield RD, Blair WF, et al. An in-vivo study of normal wrist kinematics. *J Biomech Eng* 1982;104:176–181.

18. Jackson WT, Hefzy MS, Guo H. Determination of wrist kinematics using a magnetic tracking devise. *Med Eng Phys* 1994;16:123–133.

19. Patterson RM, Nicodemus CL, Viegas SF, et al. High speed, three-dimensional kinematic analysis of the normal wrist. *J Hand Surg* 1998;23A:446–453.

20. Navarro A. Luxaciones del carpo. *Anal Fac Med Montevideo* 1921;6:113–141.

21. Taleisnik J. Wrist anatomy, function, and injury. *AAOS Instr Course Lect.* St. Louis: Mosby, 1978, pp. 61–87.

22. Weber ER. Concepts governing the rotational shift of the intercalated segment of the carpus. *Orthop Clin North Am* 1984;15:193–207.

23. Lichtman DM, Schneider JR, Swafford AR, et al. Ulnar midcarpal instability. *J Hand Surg* 1981;6:515–523.

24. Craigen MA, Stanley JK. Wrist kinematics. Row, column or both? *J Hand Surg* 1995;20B:165–170.

25. Bradley KC, Sunderland S. The range of movement at the wrist joint. *Anat Rec* 1953;116:139–145.

26. Ruby LK, Cooney WP 3rd, An KN, et al. Relative motion of selected carpal bones: a kinematic analysis of the normal wrist. *J Hand Surg* 1988;13A:1–10.

27. Youm Y, McMurtry RY, Flatt AE, et al. Kinematics of the wrist. I. An experimental study of radial-ulnar deviation and flexion-extension. *J Bone Joint Surg* 1978;60A:423–431.

28. Kauer JMG. The interdependence of carpal articulation chains. *Acta Anat* 1974;88:481–501.

29. Kauer JMG. The mechanism of the carpal joint. *Clin Orthop* 1986;202:16–26.

30. Horii E, Garcia-Elias M, An KN, et al. A kinematic study of luno-triquetral dissociations. *J Hand Surg* 1991;16A:355–362.

31. Savelberg HH, Kooloos JG, DeLange A, et al. Human carpal ligament recruitment and three-dimensional carpal motion. *J Orthop Res* 1991;9:693–704.

32. Weaver L, Tencer AF, Trumble TE. Tensions in the palmar ligaments of the wrist. I. The normal wrist. *J Hand Surg* 1994;19A:464–474.

33. Schuind FA, Leroy B, Comtet J-J. Biodynamics of the wrist: radiologic approach to scapholunate instability. *J Hand Surg* 1985;10A:1006–1008.

34. Nakamura R, Hori M, Imamura T, et al. Method for measurement and evaluation of carpal bone angles. *J Hand Surg* 1989;14A:412–416.

35. Berger RA. The gross and histologic anatomy of the scapholunate ligament. *J Hand Surg* 1996;21A:170–178.

36. Berger RA, Imeada T, Bergland L, et al. Constraint and material properties of the subregions of the scapholunate interosseous ligament. *J Hand Surg* 1999;24A:953–962.

37. Garcia-Elias M, An KN, Amadio PC, et al. Reliability of carpal angle determination. *J Hand Surg* 1989;14A:1017–1021.

38. Berger RA, Crowninshield RD, Flatt AE. The three-dimensional rotational behavior of the carpal bones. *Clin Orthop* 1982;167:303–310.

39. Johnston RB, Seiler JG, Miller EJ, Drvaric DM. The intrinsic and extrinsic ligaments of the wrist. A correlation of collagen typing and histologic appearance. *J Hand Surg* 1995;20B:146–147.

40. Viegas SF, Yamaguchi S, Boyd NL, et al. The dorsal ligaments of the wrist: anatomy, mechanical properties, and function. *J Hand Surg* 1999;24A:456–468.

41. Viegas SF. The dorsal ligaments of the wrist. *Hand Clin* 2001;17:65–75.

42. Garcia-Elias M, An KN, Cooney WP, et al. Transverse stability of the carpus. An analytical study. *J Orthop Res* 1989;7:738–743.

43. Blevens AD, Light TR, Jablonsky WS, et al. Radiocarpal articular contact characteristics with scaphoid instability. *J Hand Surg* 1989;14A:781–790.

44. Larsen CF, Amadio PC, Gilula LA, et al. Analysis of carpal instability: I. Description of the scheme. *J Hand Surg* 1995;20A:757–764.

45. Watson HK, Ottoni L, Pitts EC, et al. Rotary subluxation of the scaphoid: a spectrum of instability. *J Hand Surg* 1993;18B:62–64.

46. Watson HK, Ryu J. Evolution of arthritis of the wrist. *Clin Orthop* 1986;202:57–67.

47. Short WH, Werner FW, Green JK, et al. Biomechanical evaluation of ligamentous stabilizers of the scaphoid and lunate. *J Hand Surg* 2002;27A:991–1002.

48. Berger RA. The anatomy of the scaphoid. *Hand Clin* 2001;17:525–532.

49. Talaisnik J, Watson HK. Midcarpal instability caused by malunited fractures of the distal radius. *J Hand Surg* 1984;9A:350–357.

50. Freeland AE, McAuliffe JA. Dorsal carpal metacarpal fracture dislocation associated with nondissociative segmental instability. *Orthopedics* 2002;25:753–755.

51. Garcia-Elias M, Dobyns JH, Cooney WP 3rd, et al. Traumatic axial dislocations of the carpus. *J Hand Surg* 1989;14A:446–457.

52. Freeland AE, Rojas SL. Traumatic combined radial and ulnar axial wrist dislocation. *Orthopedics* 2002;245:1161–1163.

53. Mayfield JK, Johnson RP, Kilcoync RK. The ligaments of the human wrist and their functional significance. *Anat Rec* 1976;186:417 428.

54. Mayfield JK, Johnson RP, Kilcoyne RK. Carpal dislocations: pathomechanics and progressive perilunar instability. *J Hand Surg* 1980;5;226–241.

55. Mayfield JK. Patterns of injuries to carpal ligaments: a spectrum. *Clin Orthop* 1984;187:36–42.

56. Mudgal CS, Jones WA. Scapho-lunate diastasis: a component of fractures of the distal radius. *J Hand Surg* 1990;15B:503–505.

57. Geissler WB, Freeland AE, Savoie FH 3rd, et al. Intracarpal soft tissue lesions associated with intra-articular fracture of the distal end of the radius. *J Bone Joint Surg* 1996;78A:357–365.

58. Black DM, Watson HK, Vender MI. Scapholunate gap with scaphoid nonunion. *Clin Orthop* 1987;224:205–209.

59. Vender MI, Watson HK, Black DM, et al. Acute scaphoid fracture with scapholunate gap. *J Hand Surg* 1989;14:1004–1007.

60. Monsivais JJ, Nitz PA, Scully TJ. The role of carpal instability in scaphoid nonunion: casual or causal? *J Hand Surg* 1986;11B:201–206.

61. MacMurtry RY, Youm Y, Flatt AE, et al. Kinematics of the wrist. II. Clinical applications. *J Bone Joint Surg* 1978;60A:955–961.

62. Watson HK, Ballet FL. The SLAC wrist. Scapholunate advanced collapse pattern of degenerative arthritis. *J Hand Surg* 1984;9A:356–365.

63. Ritt MJ, Bishop AT, Berger RA, et al. Lunotriquetral ligament properties: a comparison of three anatomic subregions. *J Hand Surg* 1998;23A:425–431.

64. Ritt MJ, Linschcid RL Cooney WP, et al. Lunotriquetral ligament properties: the lunotriquetral joint: kinematic effects of sequential ligament sectioning, ligament repair, and arthrodesis. *J Hand Surg* 1998;23A:432–445.

65. Shin AY, Murray PM. Biomechanical studies of wrist ligament injuries. In: Trumble TE (ed). *Carpal Fracture-Dislocations.* Rosewood, IL: American Academy of Orthopaedic Surgery, 2002, pp 7–18.

66. Reagan DS, Linscheid RL, Dobyns JH. Lunotriquetral sprains. *J Hand Surg* 1094;9:502–514.

67. Veigas SF, Patterson RM, Peterson PD, et al. Ulnar-sided perilunate instability: an anatomic and biomechanical study. *J Hand Surg* 1990;15A:268–278.

68. Garth WP Jr, Hoffamann DY, Rooks MD. Volar intercalated instability secondary to medial carpal ligament laxity. *Clin Orthop* 1985;201:94–105.

69. Hankin FM, Amadio PC, Wojtys EM, et al. Carpal instability with volar flexion of the proximal row associated with injury to the scapho-trapezial ligament: report of two cases. *J Hand Surg* 1988;13B:298–302.

70. Masquelet AC, Strube F, Nordin JY. The isolated scapho-trapezio-trapezoid ligament injury. Diagnosis and surgical treatment in four cases. *J Hand Surg* 1993;18B:730–735.

71. Johnson RP, Carrera GF. Chronic capitolunate instability. *J Bone Joint Surg* 1986;68A:1164–1176.

72. Louis DS, Hankin FM, Greene TL. Chronic capitolunate instability. *J Bone Joint Surg* 1987;69A:950–951.

73. Siegel DB, Gelberman RH. Radial styloidectomy: an anatomic study with special reference to radiocarpal intracapsular ligamentous morphology. *J Hand Surg* 1991;16A:40–44.

74. Moneim MS, Bolger JT, Omer GE. Radiocarpal dislocation—classification and rationale for management. *Clin Orthop* 1995;192:199–209.

75. Rayhack JM, Linscheid RL, Dobyns JH, Smith JH. Posttraumatic ulnar translocation of the carpus. *J Hand Surg* 1987;12A:180–189.

76. Allieu Y, Garcia-Elias M. Dynamic radial translation instability of the carpus. *J Hand Surg* 2000;25B:33–37.

77. Bauman HW, Messer E, Sennwald G. Measurement of ulnar translation and carpal height. *J Hand Surg* 1994;19B:325–329.

78. Polveche G, Cordonier D, Thery D, et al. An unusual variation of luxation of the wrist: external vertical luxation. Apropos of a case. Review of the literature. *Chir Main Memb Super* 1995;14:159–166.

79. Leung YF, Wai YL, Kam WL, et al. Solitary dislocation of the scaphoid. From case report to literature review. *J Hand Surg* 1998;23B:88–92.

80. Cherif MR, Ben Ghozlen R, Chehimi A, et al. Isolated dislocation of the carpal scaphoid: a case report with review of the literature. *Chir Main* 2002;21:305–308.

12

Management of Scapholunate Instability

William B. Geissler

Arthroscopy has revolutionized the practice of orthopaedics by providing the technical capability to examine and treat intra-articular abnormalities directly with minimal morbidity. The development of wrist arthroscopy was a natural evolutionary progression from the successful application of arthroscopy to other joints. The wrist joint continues to challenge clinicians with an array of potential diagnoses and treatments. Wrist arthroscopy allows direct visualization of the cartilage surfaces, synovial tissue, and particularly the interosseous ligaments under bright light and magnification. This has proven to be a useful adjunct in the management of acute and chronic tears of the scapholunate interosseous ligament.

Though most acute sprains of the wrist with normal radiographic findings resolve after temporary immobilization, the method of choice to evaluate the patient who does not improve is controversial. Tricompartment wrist arthrography has historically been the gold standard for the detection of an interosseous ligament injury.[1] How mechanically significant it is when dye leaks through a perforation in the membranous portion of the interosseous ligament is at issue. However, the capability of wrist arthroscopy to detect and simultaneously treat injuries of the wrist is a major advance. A partial tear of the scapholunate interosseous ligament is difficult to detect with imaging studies, but is readily identifiable arthroscopically.

The indications for wrist arthroscopy continue to expand from Whipple's original description as new techniques and instrumentation develop.[2] Further advance in instrumentation, such as electrothermal shrinkage, will continue to play a role in the management of partial chronic tears of the scapholunate interosseous ligament.

SCAPHOLUNATE DISASSOCIATION

The scapholunate ligament complex involves both intrinsic and extrinsic ligamentous components.[3] The intrinsic portion of the scapholunate interosseous ligament includes the palmar, midsubstance, and dorsal portions. The dorsal portion appears to be the primary biomechanical functioning portion to the interosseous ligament. It is composed of stout transverse fibers to resist rotation. The volar portion of the interosseous ligament is comprised of longer oblique fibers that allow for sagittal rotation. The central fibromembranous portion of the ligament is frequently perforated, particularly in older individuals. Dye from a wrist arthrogram may leak through this perforation, indicating a tear of the ligament, although the thicker volar and dorsal portion of the ligament is still intact and provides stability.[4,5] Thus, a positive arthrogram can cloud the clinical picture. The extrinsic components include the volar radioscaphocapitate, long radiolunate, and short radiolunate ligaments. The extent of injury required to disrupt the normal kinetics of the scapholunate interval is not well understood.

Similar to other ligamentous injuries in the body, the interosseous ligament seems to stretch and then eventually tear. The scapholunate ligament may double in length prior to failure. Mayfield has shown the percent elongation to failure to be up to 225 percent.[6] A spectrum of injury is seen to the interosseous ligament itself. An isolated injury to the scapholunate interosseous ligament itself may not yield scapholunate disassociation and widening on plain radiographs. However, a combined injury to both the intrinsic and extrinsic ligaments will cause scapholunate diastasis.[7] Radiographic abnormalities may not be seen initially until gradual attenuation of the extrinsic ligaments occurs. This may result in delayed detection of scapholunate instability as seen on plain radiographs.

History and Physical Examination

A history of a sudden dorsiflexion injury to the wrist should raise concern of injury to the scapholunate ligamentous complex. Wrist extension and carpal supination are the primary mechanisms of injury to the scapholunate interosseous ligament. Physical examination reveals localized swelling and tenderness directly over the dorsum of the scapholunate interval. The principal provocative maneuver to assess scapholunate instability is the scaphoid shift test. This test evaluates motion of the scaphoid during radial deviation and wrist flexion while pressure is applied to the tubercle of the scaphoid in a volar to dorsal direction. Partial tears to the scapholunate interosseous ligament may produce pain directly over the dorsum of the scapholunate interval with no palpable click. Pain over the scaphoid tubercle as it is palpated is not clinically significant. A complete tear of the scapholunate interosseous ligament results in subluxation of the proximal pole of the scaphoid over the dorsal lip of the distal radius; a palpable shift or click is felt. Both the injured and noninjured wrist should be assessed with the scaphoid shift test to evaluate for inherent laxity, particularly in very ligamentously lax individuals. The radiocarpal joint may be injected with local anesthetic to evaluate for potential shift if pain prohibits the examination.

Radiographs are essential at the initial evaluation to assess the scapholunate articulation. Standard radiographic views include the posteroanterior view in ulnar deviation; an oblique, true lateral; and a clenched-fist views. In the PA view, three smooth radiographic arcs may be drawn to define normal carpal relationships. A step-off in the continuity of any of these arcs indicates an intracarpal instability at the site where the arc is broken. Any overlap between the carpal bones or any joint width exceeding 4 mm strongly suggests a carpal ligamentous injury.

The scapholunate angle is defined by a line tangent to the two proximal and distal convexities of the palmar aspect of the scaphoid. The angle formed by this line and a line through the central axis of the lunate determines the lunate angle. Normal values range between 30 and 60 degrees, with an average of 47 degrees. Angles greater than 80 degrees should be considered a definite indication of scapholunate instability. A so-called Terry-Thomas sign is considered positive when the space between the scaphoid and lunate appears abnormally wide as compared to the opposite wrist. The scapholunate interval should be measured in the middle of the flat medial facet of the scaphoid. Any asymmetric scapholunate gap greater than 5 mm is said to be diagnostic of a scapholunate dissociation. The scaphoid ring sign occurs when the scaphoid has collapsed into flexion and has a foreshortened appearance. The ring sign is present in all cases when the scaphoid is abnormally and palmar flexed, regardless of the etiology. Therefore, the presence of a scaphoid ring sign does not necessarily indicate instability of the scapholunate interval.

On the lateral radiograph, a normal, wide, C-shaped line can be drawn that unites the palmar margin of the scaphoid and radius. When the scaphoid is abnormally flexed, as in a scaphoid dissociation, the palmar outline of the scaphoid intersects the volar margin of the radius and forms an acute angle described as the V-sign.

Management

The management of scapholunate instability is straightforward when, on plain radiographs, signs of scapholunate instability are present in an acute injury. The management of a patient who is clinically suspected of having a scapholunate interosseous ligament injury, yet whose plain radiographs are normal, is controversial. Patients who are clinically suspected of having a scapholunate interosseous ligament injury, but whose radiographs are normal, are immobilized; repeat evaluations are performed at 1 and 3 weeks. Ancillary studies with more radiographs may be considered if the patient continues to be symptomatic by 6 weeks. Ancillary images may include arthrography and magnetic resonance imaging.[8] While MR imaging is surpassing arthrography as the imaging study of choice, satisfactory evaluation requires a sufficiently strong magnet and an experienced radiologist. Several authors have recommended proceeding with direct arthroscopic evaluation rather than further radiographic viewing, due to the sensitivity of the arthroscope to view and to diagnose the severity of injury to the scapholunate interosseous ligament.[9]

The key to arthroscopic treatment of carpal instability is recognition of what is normal and what is pathological anatomy. Both the radiocarpal and midcarpal spaces must be evaluated arthroscopically when carpal instability is suspected. Wrist arthroscopy is usually not considered complete if the midcarpal space has not been evaluated, particularly with a suspected diagnosis of carpal instability.

The scapholunate interosseous ligament is best visualized with the arthroscope in the 3-4 portal. It should have a concave appearance as viewed from the radiocarpal space (Figure 12.1). In the midcarpal space, the scapholunate interval should be tight and congruent without any step-off (Figure 12.2). This is in contrast to the lunotriquetral interval, in which a

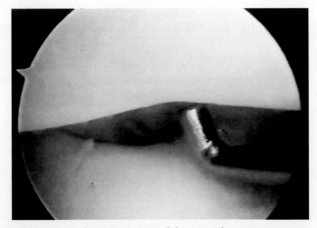

FIGURE 12.1. Arthroscopic view of the normal concave appearance of the scapholunate interosseous ligament as seen from the 3-4 portal in the radiocarpal space.

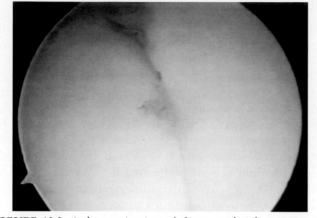

FIGURE 12.2. Arthroscopic view of the normal tight, congruent scapholunate interval as seen from the radial midcarpal portal.

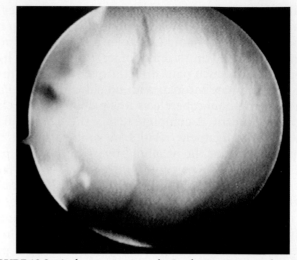

FIGURE 12.3. Arthroscopic view of a Grade I interosseous ligament injury to the scapholunate interosseous ligament as seen from the 3-4 portal in the radiocarpal space. Note that the normal concave appearance at the scapholunate interval has now become convex.

1-mm step-off occasionally is seen, which is considered normal and slight motion is seen between the lunate and triquetrum. When it tears, the interosseous ligament hangs down and blocks visualization with the arthroscope in the radiocarpal space. The normal concave appearance between the carpal bones becomes convex. However, the degree of rotation of the carpal bones and any abnormal motion are best appreciated from the unobstructed view available in the midcarpal space. A limited type of intraoperative arthrogram (poor man's arthrogram) may be performed for the evaluation of carpal instability. After the radiocarpal space has been examined, the inflow cannula, which is usually the 6-U portal, is left in the radiocarpal space. A needle is then placed in either the radioulnar or midcarpal portals. A tear of the interosseous ligament is strongly suspected if a free flow of irrigation fluid is seen through the needle flowing from

the radiocarpal space. An alternative technique is to inject the midcarpal space with air, leaving the arthroscope in the radiocarpal space. If air bubbles are observed between the involved carpal bones, a ligamentous injury is suspected.

A spectrum of injury to either the scapholunate or lunotriquetral interosseous ligament is possible. The interosseous ligament appears to attenuate and then tear from volar to dorsal. Geissler devised an arthroscopic classification of carpal instability and suggested management of acute lesions to the interosseous ligament (Table I).[10] In Grade I injuries, there is loss of the normal concave appearance of the scaphoid and lunate as the interosscous ligament bulges with the convex appearance (Figure 12.3). Evaluation of the

TABLE 12.1. Geissler Arthroscopic Classification of Carpal Instability.

Grade	Description	Management
I	Attenuation/hemorrhage of interosseous ligament as seen from the radiocarpal joint. No incongruency of carpal alignment in the mid carpal space.	Immobilization
II	Attenuation/hemorrhage of interosseous ligament as seen from the radiocarpal joint. Incongruency/step-off as seen from mid carpal space. A slight gap (less than width of a probe) between carpals may be present.	Arthroscopic reduction and pinning
III	Incongruency/step-off of carpal alignment is seen in both the radiocarpal and mid carpal space. The probe may be passed through gap between carpals.	Arthroscopic/open reduction and pinning
IV	Incongruency/step-off of carpal alignment is seen in both the radiocarpal and mid carpal space. Gross instability with manipulation is noted. A 2.7 mm arthroscope may be passed through the gap between carpals.	Open reduction and repair

scapholunate interval from the midcarpal space shows the scapholunate interval still to be tight and congruent. These mild Grade I injuries usually resolve with simple immobilization.

In Grade II injuries, the interosseous ligament bulges similarly to Grade I injuries as seen from the radiocarpal space. In the midcarpal space, the scapholunate interval is no longer congruent. The scaphoid palmar flexes, and its dorsal lip is rotated distal to the lunate (Figure 12.4). This can be better appreciated with the arthroscope placed in the ulnar midcarpal portal looking across the wrist to assess the amount of flexion to the scaphoid.

In Grade III injuries, the interosseous ligament starts to separate, and a gap is seen between the scaphoid and lunate from both the radiocarpal and midcarpal space. A 1-mm probe may be passed through the gap and twisted between the scaphoid and lunate from both the radiocarpal and midcarpal spaces (Figure 12.5). Sometimes the gap between the scaphoid and lunate is not visible until the probe is used to push the scaphoid away from the lunate. A portion of the dorsal scapholunate interosseous ligament is still attached.

In Grade IV injuries, the interosseous ligament is completely torn, and a 2.7-mm arthroscope may be passed freely from the midcarpal space to the radiocarpal space between the scaphoid and lunate (the drive-through sign, Figure 12.6). This corresponds to the widened scapholunate gap seen on plain radiographs with a complete scapholunate dissociation.

When surgical intervention is recommended for scapholunate instability, the wrist is evaluated for a scaphoid shift after satisfactory anesthesia has been obtained. Following this, the wrist is suspended at approximately 10 pounds of traction in a traction tower. It is important to pad the arm and forearm so that the

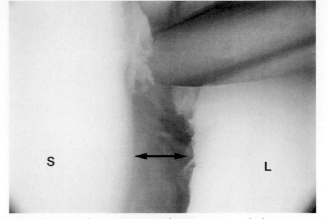

FIGURE 12.5. Arthroscopic view of a Type III scapholunate interosseous ligament tear as seen from the radial midcarpal space. Note the gap between the scaphoid and the lunate. (S = scaphoid, L = lunate).

skin does not touch the metal of the traction tower. This is particularly important when a traction tower has been utilized repeatedly throughout the day and can retain a significant amount of heat. Inflow is provided through the 6-U portal, and the arthroscope with a blunt trocar is introduced through the 3-4 portal. The 3-4 portal is the most ideal viewing portal for visualization of the scapholunate interosseous ligament. A working 4-5 or 6-R portal is then made. The wrist is then systematically evaluated from radial to ulnar. The scapholunate interval is probed. The degree of injury may not be fully appreciated until the tear is palpated with a probe (Figure 12.7). Torn fibers of the scapholunate interosseous ligament, if present, are then debrided with the arthroscope in the 6-R portal, and a shaver inserted into the 3-4 portal. A probe is inserted into the scapholunate interval to note particularly any gap between the scaphoid and lunate. Following arthroscopic debridement of a torn scaphol-

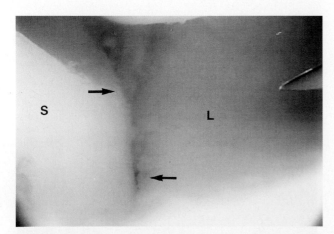

FIGURE 12.4. Arthroscopic view of a Type II scapholunate interosseous ligament injury as seen from the radial midcarpal space. The dorsal lip of the scaphoid is no longer congruent with the lunate as it is palmar flexed. (S = scaphoid, L = lunate).

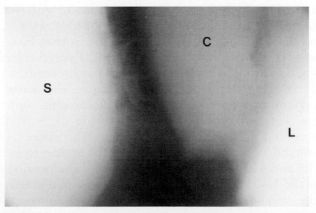

FIGURE 12.6. Arthroscopic view of a Type IV scapholunate ligament-interosseous ligament tear. The scaphoid and lunate are completely separated, and the arthroscope may pass freely between the radiocarpal and midcarpal spaces. The capitate is seen between the scapholunate interval. (S = scaphoid, L = lunate, C = capitate).

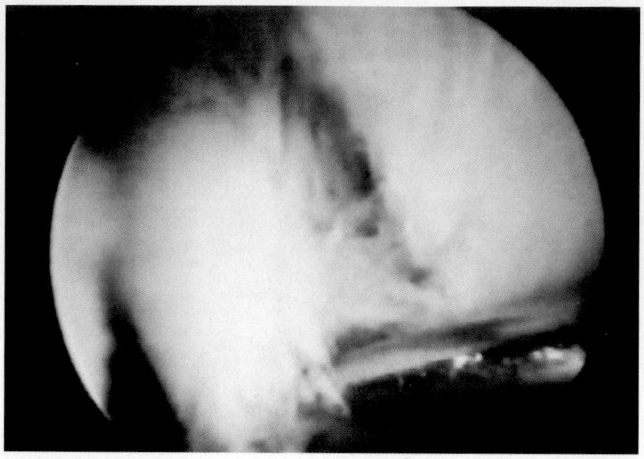

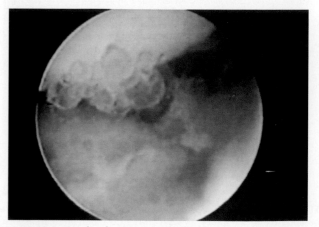

FIGURE 12.7. Arthroscopic view of a Type II scapholunate interosseous ligament tear as seen from the 3-4 portal in the radiocarpal space. A probe is used to palpate the interosseous ligament, and the separation, which was not initially noted, is identified.

unate interosseous ligament from the radiocarpal space, the midcarpal space is then evaluated. The arthroscope is initially placed in the radial midcarpal space. Close attention is paid to any rotational displacement of the scaphoid with the dorsal lip being rotated distal to that of the lunate. This may be best visualized with the arthroscope placed in the ulnar midcarpal portal. Also, any gap where the probe or arthroscope itself can be passed between the carpals is identified.

Patients with a Grade II or Grade III lesion are most ideally suited for arthroscopic assisted reduction and pinning. The arthroscope is placed in the 3-4 portal after the midcarpal space has been evaluated in patients who have a Grade II or III scapholunate interosseous ligament injury. A 0.045 Kirschner wire is inserted through a soft tissue protector or through a 14-gauge needle placed dorsally in the anatomic snuff box to the scaphoid. It is important to use some type of soft tissue protector in order to avoid injury to the sensory branches of the radial nerve. A small incision is made, and blunt dissection is continued down with a hemostat; a soft tissue protector may be placed directly on the scaphoid. The Kirschner wire can then be seen as it enters into the scaphoid with the surgeon looking down the radial gutter with the arthroscope.

In an easier alternative technique, the wrist is taken out of traction and, under fluoroscopic control, the surgeon can begin the Kirschner wire in the scaphoid, aiming towards the lunate. The surgeon can use the previously made portals as landmarks to guide the angulation of the Kirschner wire. The previously made 3-4 and 4-5 portals mark the proximal extent of the scaphoid. The radial midcarpal and ulnar midcarpal portals mark the distal location of the lunate. The surgeon can then aim the Kirschner wire toward the square formed by these four portals, as they mark the location of the lunate. Fluoroscopy then confirms the ideal placement of the wire into the scaphoid so that it will engage the lunate when advanced. The arthroscope is then placed in the ulnar midcarpal portal after the Kirschner wire is confirmed to be in the scaphoid. Placing the arthroscope in the ulnar midcarpal portal allows the surgeon to look across the wrist to better judge the rotation of the scaphoid in relation to the lunate. Additionally, a probe may be inserted through the radial midcarpal space to control the palmar flexion of the scaphoid. The wrist may be extended and ulnarly deviated to help further reduce the palmar flexion of the scaphoid. Occasionally, Kirschner wire joysticks are inserted into the dorsum of the scaphoid and lunate to control rotation of the scapholunate interval. This is particularly useful in Grade III injuries where a gap exists between the scaphoid and lunate. The surgeon then advances the Kirschner wire across the scapholunate interval, aiming for the lunate after the interval has been anatomically reduced as viewed from the midcarpal space. Fat droplets are often seen exiting between the scaphoid and lunate in the midcarpal space as the Kirschner wire is driven across the two carpal bones (Figure 12.8). After the first wire is arthroscopically placed controlling the reduction, two or three additional Kirschner wires are normally placed under fluoroscopic control. All wires are placed between the scapholunate interval, and no wires are placed from the scaphoid into the capitate to violate the pristine articular cartilage of that interval (Figure 12.9).

The wires are left protruding from the skin. The wrist is immobilized in a below-elbow cast, and the pin tracks are evaluated every 2 weeks. The Kirschner wires are then removed in the office at 8 weeks, and the wrist is immobilized for an additional 4 weeks in a removable elbow splint. Physical therapy with range of motion exercises for the fingers is initiated immediately. Range of motion and grip strength of the wrist are initiated at 3 months.

FIGURE 12.8. Fat droplets are seen from the radial midcarpal space as a Kirschner wire is driven across the scapholunate interval.

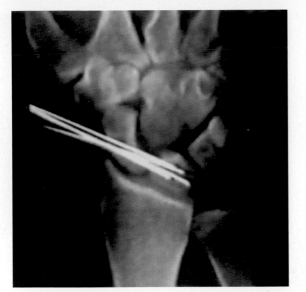

FIGURE 12.9. Anteroposterior radiograph following arthroscopic pinning of the scapholunate interval.

Patients with acute Grade IV injuries to the scapholunate interosseous ligament are best reduced and stabilized through a small dorsal incision to obtain primary repair of the dorsal portion of the scapholunate interosseous ligament. Prior to arthrotomy, the wrist is evaluated arthroscopically for any additional injuries, including potential cartilaginous loose bodies, triangular fibrocartilage complex tears, and possible injury to the lunotriquetral interosseous ligament.

Whipple reviewed the results of arthroscopic management of scapholunate instability, utilizing the previously described techniques in patients who were followed for a duration of 1 to 3 years.[11] In his series, patients were classified into two distinct groups of 40 patients each, according to the duration of symptoms and the radiographic scapholunate gap. Thirty-three patients (83%) who had a history of instability for 3 months or less and had less than 3 mm side-to-side difference in the scapholunate gap had maintenance of the reduction and symptomatic relief. Only 21 patients (53%) had symptomatic relief following arthroscopic reduction and pinning when they had symptoms for greater than 3 months and had more than a 3 mm side-to-side scapholunate gap. Patients with less than 3 months' symptom duration and 3 mm side-to-side scapholunate gap were followed for 2 to 7 years. Whipple found that 85% continued to maintain their stability and comfort in his series. This report emphasized the need for early diagnosis and intervention prior to the onset of fixed carpal alignment and diminished capacity for ligamentous healing.

Management of Chronic Tears

Chronic tears of the scapholunate interosseous ligament lose their intrinsic ability to heal, as shown by the work of Whipple. The management of chronic tears of the scapholunate interosseous ligament is controversial and depends on the severity of the tear. Possible treatment options include simple arthroscopic debridement, ligamentous reconstruction, proximal row carpectomy, intercarpal fusion, or, potentially, wrist fusion as a salvage procedure when secondary degenerative changes are present.

The arthroscopic technique for debridement of partial chronic tears of the scapholunate interosseous ligament is relatively straightforward.[12] The interosseous ligament tear is assessed from both the radiocarpal and midcarpal spaces. Grade I chronic injuries may or may not be symptomatic. Arthroscopic debridement would be indicated primarily for chronic Grade II or Grade III injuries to the scapholunate interosseous ligament. The arthroscope is placed in the 4-5 portal after the degree of tearing to the scapholunate interosseous ligament has been assessed. A shaver is brought into the 3-4 portal to debride the torn fibers of the scapholunate interosseous ligament (Figure 12.10). The goal of management is to debride the unstable tissue flaps back to stable tissue, similar to debridement of a tear to the articular disk of the triangular fibrocartilage complex. Partial access to the volar and dorsal portions of the interosseous ligament is possible with the shaver in the 3-4 portal, but the primary access is the membranous portion to the interosseous ligament.

Weiss examined the role of arthroscopic debridement for the management of partial and complete tears to the interosseous ligaments of the wrist.[13] At an average of 27 months following the procedure, 19 of 29 patients who had a complete tear of the scapholunate interosseous ligament, and 31 of 36 patients who had a partial tear had complete resolution or decrease in wrist symptoms following arthroscopic de-

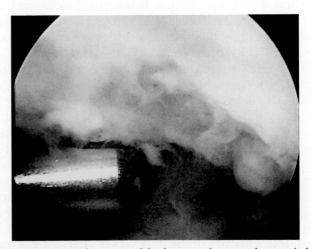

FIGURE 12.10. Arthroscopic debridement of a partial tear of the scapholunate interosseous ligament as seen from the 6-R portal in the radiocarpal space. The shaver is inserted through the 3-4 portal.

bridement. In his series, Weiss also evaluated the results of arthroscopic debridement of the lunotriquetral interosseous ligament. Twenty-six of 33 patients who had a complete tear of the lunotriquetral interosseous ligament and all 43 patients who had a partial tear had complete resolution or decrease in symptoms, at an average of 27 months following the procedure. Patients tolerated debridement of the lunotriquetral interosseous ligament better than debridement of the scapholunate interosseous ligament, due to the lower stress placed on the ulnar side of the wrist. Arthroscopic debridement of complete tears of the scapholunate interosseous ligament had a lower success rate, and other surgical options may need to be considered.

Electrothermal shrinkage may play a role in the management of chronic partial tears of the scapholunate interosseous ligament injuries in the future. Electrothermal shrinkage of tissue has been shown in studies to be beneficial in other joints of the body, particularly the shoulder. However, it is important to note that the use of electrothermal shrinkage is controversial, and studies have a short follow-up. Electrothermal shrinkage is based on the theory that heating the collagen matrix results in shrinkage of the collagen as the structure denatures. Fibroblasts then grow into the shrunken collagen tissue. Several questions still remain unanswered, such as: what is the stability of this disorganized collagen matrix, will the results hold up over time, and will the shrunken tissue act similarly to a normal ligament. The technique is relatively straightforward. The wrist is again initially evaluated from both the carpal and midcarpal spaces, and the grade of injury to the scapholunate interosseous ligament is identified. This technique would be indicated for a chronic partial tear of the scapholunate interosseous ligament. A monopolar or bipolar thermal probe is used. The electrothermal probe is placed in the 3-4 portal, with the arthroscope in the 4-5 or 6-R portal. Following mechanical debridement of the interosseous ligament tear, an electrothermal probe is used to shrink the remaining portion of the interosseous ligament (Figure 12.11). Transverse passes appear to be more effective than longitudinal passes in contracting the interosseous ligament. This involves primarily the membranous portion, as the probe is extended to make contact with the volar capsule and the dorsal portion of the interosseous ligament. The thermal probe is then continued along the dorsal capsule to shrink this structure as well.

It is important that the probe is continuously moving so as not to concentrate all the heat in one particular spot. The entire dorsal capsule should not be painted with the probe, but rather strips of contracture should be made, leaving normal capsule between the areas that make contact with the probe. This

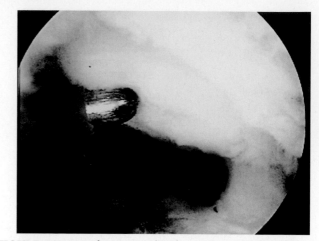

FIGURE 12.11. Arthroscopic shrinkage of a partial tear to the scapholunate interosseous ligament with an electrothermal probe as seen from the 6-R portal in the radiocarpal space. The probe is inserted through the 3-4 portal.

leaves the normal capsule to help vascularize the contracted areas. It is extremely important to increase the flow of the irrigation fluid when using an electrothermal probe. Inflow is provided through a separate portal, and outflow is maintained through the arthroscope. The purpose of increasing the flow is to help disseminate the heat from the probe. The temperature of the irrigation fluid as it leaves the wrist should be monitored. The wattage of the probe may be turned down, and the temperature of the monopolar probe should not exceed 68 degrees centigrade. It is important to remember that the volume of the irrigation fluid in the wrist is quite small, and that the fluid may rapidly heat up. The tissue of the interosseous ligament contracts, but this contraction is not as apparent compared to the glenohumeral capsule.

The arthroscope is then placed back into the radial midcarpal space to evaluate the stability of the scapholunate interval following shrinkage. Generally, less motion is observed in the scaphoid interval following electrothermal shrinkage.

Postoperative management of electrothermal shrinkage for chronic partial tears of the scapholunate interosseous ligament is controversial. There are limited protocols available. Some authors believe immobilization alone is sufficient; others believe in temporary Kirschner wire stabilization while the collagen shrinkage matures. Patients are typically immobilized for approximately 6 to 8 weeks following electrothermal shrinkage. Range of motion and grip strengthening are initiated, similar to the protocol for pinning of acute tears of the scapholunate interosseous ligament at 3 months.

Geissler reviewed the results in 19 patients with isolated chronic interosseous ligament tears to the wrist.[14] A chronic injury was defined as symptoms present greater than 6 months in this study. The follow-up averaged 8 months (range: 6 to 22 months). Grade II tears of the scapholunate interosseous ligament did significantly better when compared to Grade III tears. Of the 6 patients with Grade II tears, there were 4 excellent and 2 good results. In the 4 patients who had a Grade III tear, there was one excellent, one good, one fair, and one poor result. It was noted that this was a preliminary study and that the numbers were small and follow-up was quite short. Further study was recommended.

Wrist arthroscopy plays a limited salvage role in patients with complete chronic tears of the scapholunate interosseous ligament. Wrist arthroscopy can be used to evaluate the degree and extent of articular cartilage degeneration in patients with a scapholunate advanced collapsed wrist.[15] The status of the articular cartilage as determined arthroscopically helps to determine whether a reconstructive procedure, such as ligament reconstruction or capsulodesis versus a salvage procedure (e.g., a 4-corner fusion or proximal row carpectomy), is indicated. Arthroscopic evaluation of the status of the articular cartilage of the head of the capitate is extremely useful in determining the indications for 4-corner fusion versus proximal row carpectomy. In selecting individuals with early slack wrist who desire only minimal arthroscopic intervention, debridement and radial styloidectomy may be an option. This is further described in Chapter 17.

Wrist arthroscopy continues to grow in popularity as a valuable adjunct to the management of wrist disorders. It allows for the evaluation of intracarpal structures in bright light and magnified conditions with minimal morbidity as compared with an arthrotomy. It is extremely sensitive for detecting the spectrum of injury that occurs to the scapholunate interosseous ligament as it stretches and eventually tears.

Improved techniques will continue to emerge as more surgeons are instructed in the use of wrist arthroscopy and better instrumentation is developed.

References

1. Weiss APC, Akelman E, Lambiase R. Comparison of the finding of triple injection cinearthrography of the wrist with those of arthroscopy. *J Hand Surg* 1996;78:348–356.
2. Whipple TL, Marotta JJ, Powell JH. Techniques of wrist arthroscopy. *Arthroscopy* 1986;2:244–253.
3. Berger RA, Landsmeer JMF. The palmar radiocarpal ligaments: a study of adult and fetal wrist joints. *J Hand Surg* 1990; 15:847–854.
4. Cooney WP. Evaluation of chronic wrist pain by arthrography, arthroscopy and arthrotomy. *J Hand Surg* 1993;18:815–822.
5. Chung KC, Zimmerman NB, Travis MT. Wrist arthrography versus arthroscopy: a comparative study of 150 cases. *J Hand Surg* 1996;21:591–594.
6. Mayfield JK, Williams WJ, Erdman AG, et al. Biochemical properties of human carpal ligaments. *Orthop Trans* 1979;3:143.
7. Mead TD, Schneider LH, Cherry K. Radiographic analysis of selective ligament sectioning of the carpal scaphoid: a cadaver study. *J Hand Surg* 1990;15:855–862.
8. Johnstone DJ, Torogood S, Smith WH, et al. A comparison of magnetic resonance imaging and arthroscopy in the investigation of chronic wrist pain. *J Hand Surg* 1997;22:714–718.
9. Adolfsson L. Arthroscopic diagnosis of ligament lesions of the wrist. *J Hand Surg* 1994;19:505–512.
10. Geissler WB, Freeland AE, Savoie FH, et al. Intracarpal soft tissue lesions associated with intraarticular fracture of the distal end of the radius. *J Bone Joint Surg* 1996;78:357–365.
11. Whipple TL. The role of arthroscopy in the treatment of scapholunate instability. *Hand Clin* 1995;11:37–40.
12. Ruch DS, Peopling GG. Arthroscopic management of partial scapholunate and lunotriquetral injuries of the wrist. *J Hand Surg* 1996;21:412–417.
13. Weiss APC, Sachar K, Glowacki KA. Arthroscopic debridement alone for intercarpal ligament tears. *J Hand Surg* 1997;22:344–349.
14. Geissler WB, Haley T. Arthroscopic management of scapholunate instability. *Atlas Hand Clin* 2001;6:253–274.
15. Watson HK, Ballet FL. The SLAC wrist: scapholunate advanced collapse pattern of degenerative arthritis. *J Hand Surg* 1984;9: 358–365.

13

Management of Lunotriquetral Instability

Michael J. Moskal and Felix H. Savoie III

The diagnosis and treatment of ulnar-sided wrist pain can be complex. Wrist arthroscopy is an excellent method to characterize and treat injuries after clinical examination and/or radiographic studies. Arthroscopic evaluation is particularly valuable to examine the anatomy and pathoanatomy of ulnar-sided wrist disorders.[1] Early and accurate diagnosis followed by treatment can significantly improve patient outcome. Wrist arthroscopy facilitates clear characterization of an injury, revealing the quality of the articular surfaces and any associated synovitis, and is the basis for treatment.

Ulnar-sided wrist injuries can result from repetitive trauma or a single traumatic event, such as a twisting injury or a fall on an outstretched hand with a pronated forearm in which a dorsally-directed force causes the wrist to be extended and radially deviated.[2] Intercarpal pronation causes a disruption of the ulnar ligaments by tearing the lunotriquetral interosseous ligament with associated injury to the disk-triquetral and disk-lunate ligaments that leads to greater lunotriquetral instability. It is important to recognize that instability can arise from intrinsic as well as extrinsic ligamentous injury.[3–5] Failure to recognize and treat all the components of a destabilizing injury will lead to a compromised treatment result.

The diagnosis and treatment of ulnar-sided wrist pain and instability can be complex; however, a careful history and physical exam, augmented by ancillary studies when needed, can often elucidate the problem. Physical examination, radiographs, as well as MRI or arthrography, often do not reveal the full extent of an injury. Arthroscopy is an integral part of the injury evaluation and treatment. Arthroscopic evaluation allows precise assessment of the pathoanatomy of an injury and, therefore, specific treatment schemata based upon surgical findings.

For lunotriquetral interosseous ligament tears associated with ulnar-sided wrist pain, pain from a mechanical etiology may be due to impingement of flap-type ligament or fibrocartilage tears and/or dynamic or static joint incongruity of the LT or distal radioulnar joints (DRUJ). The following clinical scenarios are appropriate for arthroscopic treatment.

1. Isolated ligament tears
2. Ligament tears associated with:
   Triangular fibrocartilage complex (TFCC) disorders
   Peripheral traumatic tears
   Degenerative radial or central tears
3. Tears associated with ulnar abutment syndrome

PHYSICAL EXAMINATION

An exam focused toward ulnar-sided pathology is detailed here in brief. The wrist should be routinely inspected and palpated to include the dorsal and volar TFCC. The extensor carpi ulnaris (ECU) is the main anatomic landmark to guide palpation. Just dorsoradial and volar-ulnar to the ECU is the area of capsular attachment of the peripheral TFCC; both areas should be routinely palpated. Additionally, one should palpate the dorsal lunotriquetral joint, extensor carpi ulnaris, extensor digiti quinti, and flexor carpi ulnaris in various positions of forearm rotation.

To further elucidate the nature of a patient's ulnar-sided wrist complaints, the following provocative maneuvers can be performed: lunotriquetral ballottement (compressing the triquetrum against the lunate), shuck test as described by Reagan,[6] shear test as described by Kleinman,[7,8] and distal radioulnar translation (to infer stability).[9,10]

Ulnar deviation should be performed with the wrist in the flexed, extended, and neutral positions. Flexing and extending an ulnar deviated wrist may produce pain associated with crepitus and can be a useful indicator of associated ulnar pathology with LT tears. Finally, pain and/or weakness with resistance to wrist flexion with the forearm in supination increases the suspicion for symptomatic LT tears but also for TFCC tears.

The radiographic evaluation of a painful wrist should include at least a zero-rotation posteroanterior[11,12] and a true lateral of the wrist views. Particular attention should be focused toward ulnar variance,[13,14] lunotriquetral interval and the integrity of the subchondral joint surfaces, and greater and lesser arc continuity;[15] radiolunate and scapholunate angles should be recorded. When the physical examination findings are equivocal, an arthrogram or MRI can be obtained.

ULNAR LIGAMENTOUS ANATOMY

Our approach to LT injuries had evolved from the anatomical concepts of the ulnar ligaments in relationship to the lunotriquetral joint and the TFCC. The lunotriquetral interosseous ligament (LT) is thicker both volarly and dorsally[16] with a membranous central portion. Normal lunotriquetral kinematics is imparted from the integrity of the LT interosseous,[17] ulnolunate (UL), ulnotriquetral (UT),[3–5] dorsal radiotriquetral (RT), and scaphotriquetral (ST) ligaments.[17–19] Severe instability (VISI) requires damage to both the dorsal RT and ST ligaments.[17–19] The TFCC is the primary stabilizer of the distal radioulnar joint via the dorsal and volar radioulnar ligaments;[20,21] it helps to stabilize the ulnar carpus and transmits axial forces to the ulna.[22,23] The TFCC originates from the ulnar aspect of the lunate fossa of the radius and inserts on the base of the ulnar styloid and distally on the lunate, triquetrum, hamate, and fifth metacarpal base. The integrity of the triangular fibrocartilage, volar radiocarpal, as well as dorsal radiocarpal ligaments is visible at arthroscopy. TFCC compromise is often a part of more extensive ulnar-sided injuries.[24] The volar and dorsal aspects of the lunotriquetral ligament merge with the ulnocarpal extrinsic ligaments volarly, and the dorsal radiolunotriquetral ligament dorsally anchors the triquetrum.[25]

The ulnocarpal volar ligaments are composed of the ulnolunate (UL), also known as the disk-lunate; the ulnotriquetral (UT), also known as the disk-triquetral ligaments; and the ulnocapitate. The ulnolunate (UL) and ulnotriquetral (UT) ligaments originate on the volar triangular fibrocartilage complex (TFCC) and insert on the volar lunate and volar triquetrum, respectively, as well as the LT ligament.[26–28] Just palmar lies the ulnocapitate ligament, providing a direct attachment from the ulna to the palmar ulnar ligamentous complex.

The arthroscopic approach to symptomatic LT instability is based upon the contributing factors of the ulnar carpal ligaments to lunotriquetral joint stability. Suture plication of the ulnar ligaments shortens the disk-carpal ligaments and augments the palmar capsular tissue as part of the arthroscopic reduction and internal fixation.

Ligament plication has been implemented to manage capitolunate instability.[29] The central portion of the volar radiocapitate ligament is tethered to the radiotriquetral ligament by a volar approach. UT-UL ligament plication, developed by one of us (FHS), mimics this technique. UT-UL ligament plication has been

used in treating injuries that did not severely destabilize the LT joint and produce a VISI deformity that would require functional compromise of the dorsal extrinsic ligaments (dorsal radiotriquetral and scaphotriquetral). Arthroscopic volar ulnar ligament plication reduces surgical trauma and allows concurrent assessment of its effect while viewing through the radiocarpal and midcarpal joints.

SURGICAL TECHNIQUE

The following is a general approach to arthroscopic stabilization of ulnar-sided instability. It can be used in conjunction with associated pathology, such as ulnar abutment syndrome and TFCC tears when associated with a lunotriquetral interosseous ligament (LTIOL) tear. The 3-4, 6-R, volar 6-U, and the radial and ulnar midcarpal portals are used during arthroscopic capsulodesis and arthroscopic reduction and internal fixation.

An arthroscopic video system should be positioned to allow a clear view of the monitor by the surgeon and assistant. After the limb is exsanguinated, a traction tower is used and 8 to 10 pounds of traction are applied through finger traps with the arm strapped to the hand table. A complete diagnostic radiocarpal and midcarpal diagnostic arthroscopy is performed, typically utilizing the 3-4 and 6-R radiocarpal portals and the radial and ulnar midcarpal portals. Diagnostic radiocarpal arthroscopy should include visualization from the 6-R portal to ensure complete visualization of the LTIOL from dorsal to palmar (Figure 13.1). The LTIOL should be debrided as necessary. In some cases, the addition of a 4-5 portal as either the working or viewing portal can be helpful.

Midcarpal assessment begins with the arthroscope inserted into the radial midcarpal portal and the ulnar

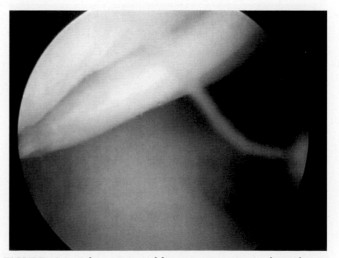

FIGURE 13.1. A lunotriquetral ligament tear as seen from the 6-R portal.

midcarpal portal used as the working portal. The lunotriquetral joint is assessed for congruency and laxity of the triquetrum.

Congruency

1. The lunate and triquetrum should be colinear. If the view of the lunotriquetral joint from the midcarpal radial portal is blocked by a separate lunate facet,[30] place the arthroscope in the midcarpal ulnar portal to gain visualization. Under these conditions, the radial articular edge of the triquetrum should be aligned with the ulnarmost articular edge of the hamate facet of the lunate (Figure 13.2A,B).
2. Although congruent, the LT joint may be unstable due to excessive laxity.

Laxity

1. Assuming it is normal, the scapholunate joint can be used as a reference. Laxity should be assessed both upon triquetral rotation and separation from the lunate.

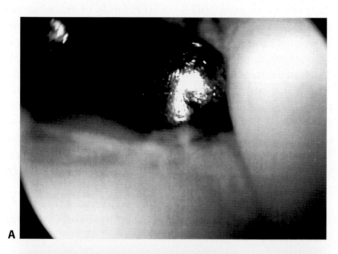

A

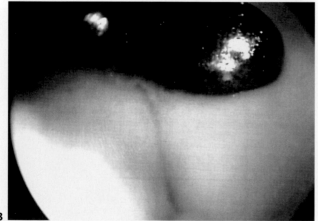

B

FIGURE 13.2. A. An incongruent LT joint as seen from the ulnar midcarpal portal. The probe has been inserted from the radial midcarpal portal. The triquetrum is to the right, and the lunate is to the left. **B.** The same case: The triquetrum has been reduced and stabilized with K-wires and now is congruent with the lunate (left).

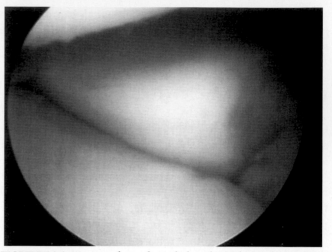

FIGURE 13.3. As seen from the radial midcarpal portal, the dorsal portion of the triquetrum is rotated distally with respect to the dorsal portion of the lunate.

2. Upon midcarpal arthroscopic assessment of an unstable LT joint, the dorsal portion of the triquetrum is often rotated so that its articular surface is distal to the lunate (Figure 13.3). The triquetrum can be translated to a reduced state in which the articular surfaces of the triquetrum and lunate are colinear.
3. An unstable LT joint may have colinear articular surfaces; however, the triquetrum can be ulnarly translated so as to "gap open" the LT joint. The normal SL joint can be used as a reference.

The final midcarpal assessment of the LT joint is the dorsal capsular structures. The dorsal radiocarpal and dorsal intercarpal ligaments attach to the lunate and triquetrum in part. In certain cases, avulsions of the dorsal capsuloligamentous structures have been observed (Figure 13.4).

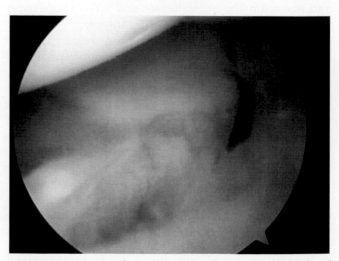

FIGURE 13.4. Viewing from the radial midcarpal portal, the dorsal capsuloligamentous structures have been avulsed from their bony attachment.

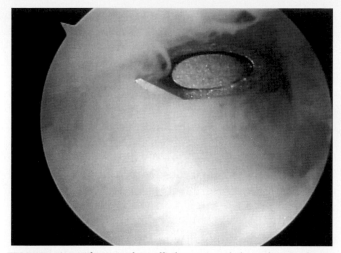

FIGURE 13.5. The spinal needle has entered the radiocarpal joint at the level of the ulnar carpal ligaments. Some fraying of the disk-carpal ligaments is seen that is associated with LT ligament injury.

After the confirmation of LT instability, the arthroscope is placed in the 3-4 portal during disk-lunate to ulnocapitate to disk-triquetral ligament plication. The volar 6-U (V6-U) is established. The V6-U portal is similar to the normal 6-U portal; how-

ever, it is placed just dorsal to the disk-carpal ligaments (Figure 13.5). Care is taken to avoid injury to the dorsal sensory branches of the ulnar nerve during placement.

The interval between the disk-lunate and disk-triquetral ligament identifies the lunotriquetral joint and interosseous ligament. The ligaments are gently debrided. Through the V6-U portal, an 18-gauge spinal needle is passed just volar to the disk-triquetral, ulnocapitate, and disk-lunate entering the radio-carpal joint at the radial edge of the UL ligament just distal to the articular surface of the radius (Figure 13.5). A #2-0 PDS suture is placed through the needle into the joint. The suture is retrieved either sequentially through the 6-R and through the V6-U or directly through the V6-U using a wire loop suture retriever and then tagged as the first plicating suture (Figure 13.6A–C). Similarly, a second plicating suture is placed approximately 5 mm distal to the first so that the suture loops are parallel to the lunate and triquetrum; this is tagged as the second plicating suture (Figure 13.7A–C). Tension on the first stitch often facilitates a second needle passage through the ulnolunate and ulnotriquetral ligaments.

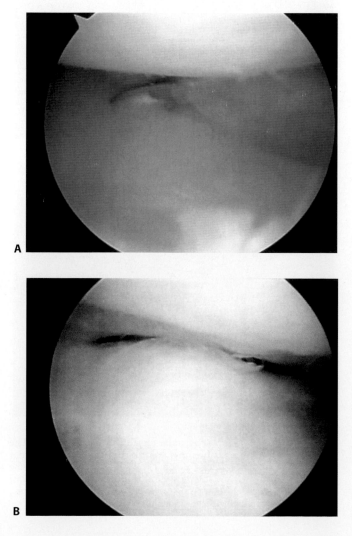

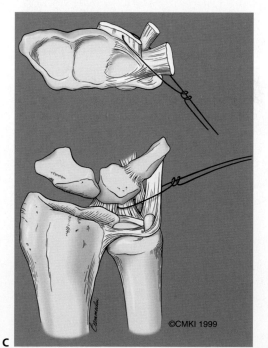

FIGURE 13.6. A. The spinal needle has traversed from ulnar to radial just palmar to the ulnar carpal ligaments. The tip of the needle has reentered the radiocarpal joint radial to the disk-carpal ligament. In the photo, the lunate is above, and the ulnar border of the distal radius (lunate fossa) is seen obliquely at the level of the spinal needle. **B.** A 2-0 PDS suture has been passed through the spinal needle and retrieved out the V6-U portal. The disk-carpal ligaments are visualized with the lunate above. **C.** The suture passage is diagrammatically represented. The disk-triquetral ligament is to the right. The first 2-0 PDS plication suture is passed from ulnar to radial with a spinal needle through the volar 6-U portal. The disk-triquetral, ulnocapitate and disk-lunate ligaments are incorporated in the suture. (**C**, from Christine M. Kleinert Institute for Hand and Microsurgery, Inc., Louisville, Kentucky, with permission.)

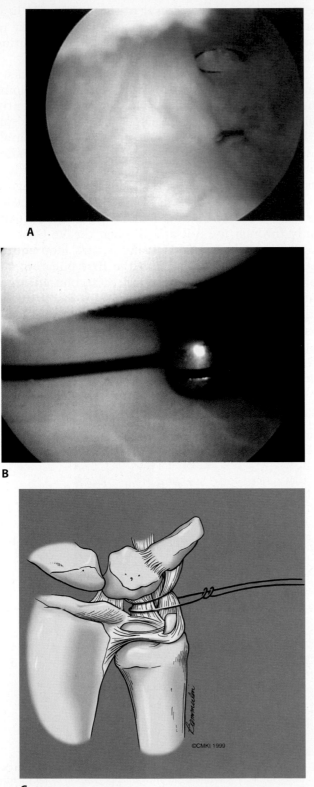

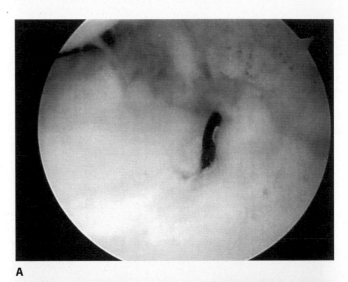

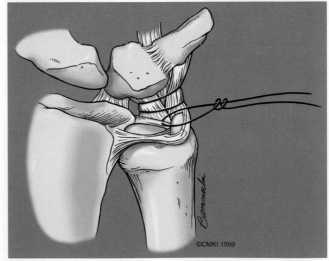

Adequacy of the plication (tension of the stitch) and its effect on LT interval stability should be assessed after each suture passage.

Finally, through the V6-U portal, a spinal needle is passed through the volar aspect of the capsule at the prestyloid recess and then through the peripheral rim of the TFCC. The wire retriever is introduced through the ulnar capsule, and the suture is brought out the V6-U portal to tighten the ulnar capsule (Figure 13.8A,B). The three sets of sutures are tied at the termination of the procedure after the lunotriquetral joint has been congruently reduced and stabilized with K-wires.

Viewing through the midcarpal radial portal, a midcarpal ulnar (MCU) working portal is created. A spinal needle can be placed from ulnar to radial across the distal aspect of the LT joint as a guide for percu-

FIGURE 13.7. A. The disk-triquetral ligament is to the left. The first plicating suture is seen below and to the right (ulnar) exiting ulnarly through the V6-U portal. The spinal needle is seen distal (above), as it is ready to be passed for the second plicating suture. **B.** The second 2-0 PDS plication suture. Tension on the first suture facilitates placement of the second suture, which is placed approximately 5 mm distal to the first suture. **C.** The plication sutures are represented diagrammatically. (**C,** from the Christine M. Kleinert Institute for Hand and Microsurgery, Inc., Louisville, Kentucky, with permission.)

FIGURE 13.8. A. The ulnar capsular tension suture is in place. The suture is passed through the ulnar capsule and through the palmar aspect of the peripheral edge of the TFCC. **B.** Line drawing of the two plication sutures and the prestyloid and TFCC sutures. (**B,** from Christine M. Kleinert Institute for Hand and Microsurgery, Inc., Louisville, Kentucky, with permission.)

taneous pin placement into the triquetrum. The triquetrum is reduced congruent to the lunate articular cartilage with traction on the plication sutures and firm pressure on the triquetrum.

The initial K-wire should be inserted 2 to 3 mm proximal to the spinal needle. Two 0.045 smooth K-wires are placed percutaneously through the lunotriquetral joint (Figure 13.9). The first pin is advanced across the lunotriquetral interval from ulnar to radial under fluoroscopic guidance, and the second pin is placed using the first pin as a guide to placement. After satisfactory reduction of the lunotriquetral joint, traction is released, the forearm is held in neutral rotation, and the plication stitches are tied at the 6-U portal with the knots placed below the skin (Figure 13.10). The peripheral ulnar capsular stitch is retrieved. The K-wires are either cut subcutaneously or bent outside the skin.

LT tears can be seen in combination with TFCC pathology, such as traumatic peripheral tears, in degenerative tears seen in isolation, or as part of ulnar abutment syndrome. In degenerative TFCC tears, the central avascular portion is debrided to a stable rim prior to plication. In traumatic tears, the suture placement through the ulnar capsule and peripheral margin can be extended dorsally after the initial plication sutures are placed.

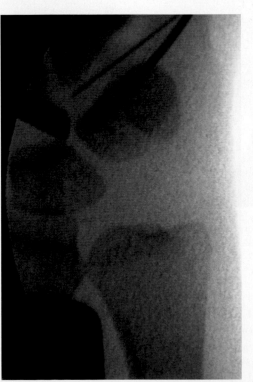

FIGURE 13.9. Pin placement. The viewing portal is in the midcarpal space during arthroscopic reduction and pinning of the lunatotriquetral joint. A needle has been placed into the midcarpal space to act as a guide to K-wire placement. Two to three K-wires are placed.

Patients with lunotriquetral tears often have positive ulnar variance.[6,31,32] In an extension of the initial treatment group, patients with ulnar abutment syndrome with associated lunate chondromalacia, central TFCC perforation, and LT tears have been treated by LT plication stabilization in conjunction with an arthroscopic wafer procedure.

POSTOPERATIVE CARE

Initially, after surgery the patient is placed in a long-arm splint with the elbow flexed at 90 degrees, the forearm in neutral rotation, and the wrist in neutral flexion and extension. At approximately 1 week after surgery, a Muenster cast is applied, with the forearm and wrist in neutral rotation and flexion, respectively. At approximately 6 weeks after surgery, the K-wires are removed. A removable Muenster cast is used for an additional 2 weeks to allow daily gentle flexion, extension, pronation, and supination within a painless arc of motion. Eight weeks after surgery, strengthening exercises are instituted, and work hardening can begin slowly over 8 to 24 weeks postoperatively.

RESULTS

In a case series, we looked at a group of 21 patients, including 7 who were treated as Workman's Compensation claimants and 4 who were competitive athletes who sustained their injuries during sport. All patients complained of ulnar-sided wrist pain, which was invariably increased by use of the wrist. The mean time between the onset of symptoms and treatment was 2.5 years (range, 1 week to 5.5 years). Seventeen patients recalled a specific injury (hyperextension 12, twisting 2, unknown 3), and 4 noted a gradual onset of symptoms. Three patients had additional significant injuries to the affected extremity: elbow dislocation, humeral shaft fracture, and anterior shoulder dislocation.

The patients were uniformly tender over the lunotriquetral joint. Provocative tests for lunotriquetral instability were specifically positive in 9 and for TFCC were positive in 6. Crepitus was produced with pronosupination or ulnar deviation in 10 patients. A VISI instability pattern was not present. The average ingo Mayo wrist score was 50, and increased to an outgo score of 88 at a mean of 3.1 years after surgery with 19 out of 21 patients having excellent and good results and 2 with fair results. The average postoperative scores for the 9 Workman's Compensation claimants or litigants were slightly lower than for the overall group. Three patients had complications that included prolonged tenderness along the extensor carpi ulnaris, and one patient had persistent neuritis of the dorsal branches of the ulnar nerve.

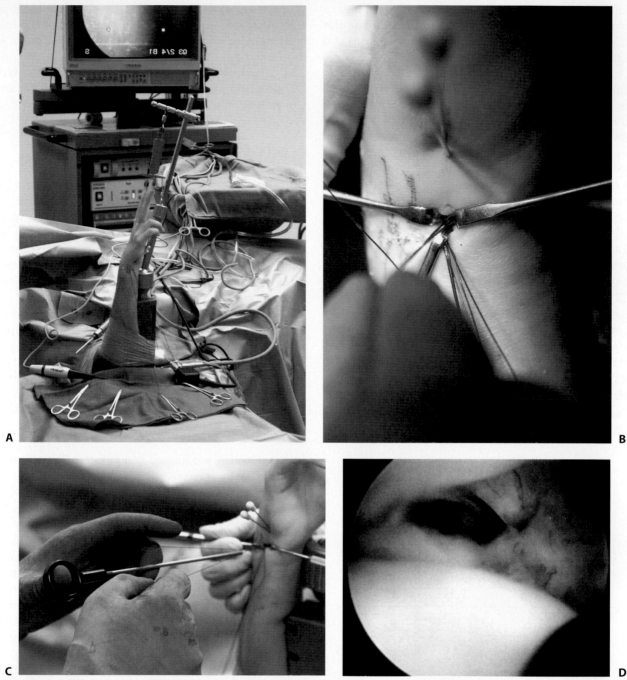

FIGURE 13.10. A. The sutures and K-wires are in place. Traction is taken off the wrist, and the forearm is maintained in neutral rotation. **B.** Retractors can be used to retract soft tissue and protect the ulnar nerve sensory branches. **C.** A knot passer can be used to pass sequential half hitches. **D.** The sutures are seen entering the radiocarpal joint. The knot is seen adjacent to the disk-triquetral ligament.

CONCLUSION

Symptomatic lunotriquetral interosseous ligament tears have been managed by simple arthroscopic debridement, ligamentous repair, and intercarpal arthrodesis. Ligamentous repair or grafting requires an extensile approach, and lunotriquetral joint fusion limits flexion and extension and radioulnar deviation by 14% and 25%, respectively.[33] Arthroscopic ulno-

carpal ligament plication, in addition to LT joint reduction and stabilization, is designed to augment the volar aspect of the LT joint. LT ligament tears are often associated with other pathology, notably ulnar-carpal ligament tears and disruption of the distal radioulnar joint.[34] Furthermore, suture plication of the ulno-carpal ligaments shortens their length to act as a checkrein to excessive lunotriquetral motion perhaps similar to ulnar shortening procedures. Prestyloid recess tightening increases tension in the ulnar DRUJ capsule.

In the presented approach for lunotriquetral instability, postoperative improvement in comfort and function is common. Arthroscopy aided in treatment by comprehensive evaluation of the injured structures and, in many cases, treated multiple concurrent injuries. Arthroscopic stabilization of the lunotriquetral joint is useful for treatment while minimizing motion losses after surgery and surgical exposure.

References

1. Kulick M, Chen C, Swearingen P. Determining the diagnostic accuracy of wrist arthroscopy. Annual meeting of the American Society for Surgery of the Hand, Toronto, 1990.
2. Palmer C, Murray P, SnearlyW. The mechanism of ulnar sided perilunate instability of the wrist. Annual Meeting of the American Society for Surgery of the Hand, Minneapolis, 1998.
3. Horii E, Gacias-Elias M, An K, et al. A kinematic study of lunato-triquetral dislocations. *J Hand Surg* 1991;16A:355.
4. Viegas S, Peterson P, et al. Ulnar-sided perilunate instability: an anatomic and biomechanical study. *J Hand Surg* 1990;15A:268.
5. Trumble T, Bour C, Smith R, et al. Kinematics of the ulnar carpus to the volar intercalated segment instability pattern. *J Hand Surg* 1990;15A:384.
6. Reagan D, Linscheid R, Dobyns J. Lunatotriquetral sprains. *J Hand Surg* 1984;9A:502–514.
7. Kleinman W. Physical examination of lunatotriquetral joint. *Am Soc Surg Hand Corr* 1985;51.
8. Kleinman W. Long-term study of chronic scapho-lunate instability treated by scapho-trapezio-trapezoid arthodesis. *J Hand Surg* 1989;14A:429.
9. Palmer A, Werner F. The triangular fibrocartilage complex of the wrist: anatomy and function. *J Hand Surg* 1981;6:153.
10. Palmer A. Triangular fibrocartilage complex lesions: a classification. *J Hand Surg* 1989;14A:594.
11. Palmer A, Glisson R, Werner F. Ulnar variance determination. *J Hand Surg* 1982;7:376.
12. Gilula L. Posteroanterior wrist radiography: importance of arm positioning. *J Hand Surg* 1987;12A:504–508.
13. Hulten O. Uber anatomische variationen der hand-Gelenk-knochen. *Acta Radiol* 1928;9:155.
14. Steyers C, Blair W. Measuring ulnar variance: a comparison of techniques. *J Hand Surg* 1989;14A:607.
15. Gilula L. Carpal injuries: analytic approach and case exercises. *Am J Radiol* 1979;133:503–517.
16. Bednar J, Osterman A. Carpal instability: evaluation and treatment. *J Am Acad Orthop Surg* 1993;1:10–17.
17. Horii E, Garcias-Elias M, An KN, et al. A kinematic study of luno-triquetral dissociations. *J Hand Surg* 1991;16A:355–362.
18. Reagan DS, Linscheid RL, Dobyns JH. Lunotriquetral sprains. *J Hand Surg* 1984;9A:502–514.
19. Viegas SF, Patterson RM, Peterson PD, et al. Ulnar-sided perilunate instability: an anatomic and biomechanic study. *J Hand Surg* 1990;15A:268–278.
20. Cooney W, Dobyns J, Linscheid R. Arthroscopy of the wrist: anatomy and classification of carpal instability. *Arthroscopy* 1990;6:113–140.
21. Mayfield J. Patterns of injury to carpal ligaments: a spectrum. *Clin Orthop* 1984;187:36.
22. Palmer A, Werner F. Triangular fibrocartilage complex of the wrist: anatomy and function. *J Hand Surg* 1981;6:153.
23. Werner F, Palmer A, Fortino M, et al. Force transmission through the distal ulna: effect of ulnar variance, lunate fossa angulation, and radial and palmar tilt of the distal radius. *J Hand Surg* 1992;17A:423.
24. Melone C Jr, Nathan R. Traumatic disruption of the triangular fibrocartilage complex, pathoanatomy. *Clin Orthop* 1992;275:65–73.
25. Green D. Carpal dislocation and instabilities. In: Green D, ed. *Operative Hand Surgery.* New York: Churchill Livingston, 1988, pp. 878–879.
26. Palmer A, Werner F. Biomechanics of the distal radioulnar joint. *Clin Orthop* 1984;187:26.
27. Garcias-Elias M, Domenech-Mateu J. The articular disc of the wrist: limits and relations. *Acta Anat* 1987;128:51.
28. Melone C, Nathan R. Traumatic disruption of the triangular fibrocartilage complex: pathoanatomy. *Clin Orthop* 1992;275:65–73.
29. Johnson R, Carrera G. Chronic capitolunate instability. *J Bone Joint Surg* 1986;68A:1164–1176.
30. Viegas S, Wagner K, Patterson R, et al. Medial (hamate) facet of the lunate. *J Hand Surg* 1990;15A:564–571.
31. Pin P, Young V, Gilula L, et al. Management of chronic lunatotriquetral ligament tears. *J Hand Surg* 1989;14A:77–83.
32. Osterman A, Sidman G. The role of arthroscopy in the treatment of lunatotriquetral ligament injuries. *Hand Clin* 1995;11:41–50.
33. Seradge H, Sterbank P, Seradge E, et al. Segmental motion of the proximal carpal row: their global effect on the wrist motion. *J Hand Surg* 1990;15A:236–239.
34. Ambrose L, Posner M. Lunate-triquetral and midcarpal joint instability. *Hand Clin* 1992;8:653–668.

14

Management of Distal Radial Fractures

Tommy Lindau

We still have difficulty in predicting the outcome of distal radial fractures 200 years after Colles' historic description, despite several radiographic classifications of the fracture.[1] However, one factor that is known to lead to worse outcomes is intra-articular incongruity of more than 1 mm, which is associated with the development of secondary osteoarthrosis.[2–5] Consequently, anatomical congruency should be restored. Closed reduction solely with fluoroscopic visualization appears inadequate to reestablish the articular congruency.[6,7] Therefore, open reduction through a limited arthrotomy was previously the method of choice, but it was difficult to completely visualize the biconcave articular surface. Consequently, wrist arthroscopy has become an important adjunct in the reduction of these fractures.[8–15] The arthroscopic approach has the benefit of giving an illuminated, magnified view of the fracture system, without the surgical morbidity caused by soft-tissue dissection. Furthermore, we can at the same time detect, and possibly treat, osteochondral loose bodies and associated ligament injuries.[16–18]

INDICATIONS AND CONTRAINDICATIONS

The main indication for an arthroscopy-assisted management of a distal radial fracture is an intra-articular step-off more than 1 mm after attempted closed reduction (Figure 14.1). Signs of complicating associated injuries, e.g. widening of intercarpal joint spaces, a broken carpal arch (the so called Gilula line)[19,20] as well as widening or subluxation of the distal radioulnar (DRU) joint are other indications for arthroscopy.

Open fractures, soft-tissue injuries, incipient carpal tunnel syndrome or compartment syndrome are contraindications for arthroscopy.

SETUP AND PATIENT PREPARATION

The arthroscopy mobile cart (with TV monitor, video camera, video recorder, and light source) is positioned at the foot end of the patient (Figure 14.2A). The fluoroscopy unit or the C-arm radiography is placed on the same side as the hand table.

Axillary block or general anesthesia is recommended for arthroscopy, which preferably is done 2 to 5 days after the trauma. The hand is normally in an upright position, either with an overhead traction boom, as for shoulder arthroscopy, or with a traction tower. The shoulder is in 60 to 90 degrees of abduction and with the elbow flexed to 90 degrees. After exsanguination of the arm, the finger traps are placed on the index and long fingers with a traction of approximately 4 to 5 kg. This traction often facilitates the reduction of the extraarticular fracture component. An elastic dressing is wrapped around the forearm to minimize the risk of extravasation into muscle compartments.

SURGICAL TECHNIQUE

Swelling distorts the normal landmarks for the portals. The 3-4 portal can be approximated by combining a line along the radial side of the long finger together with palpable bony landmarks, such as the tip of the radial styloid and the distal, dorsal rim of the radius and the ulnar head. A needle is introduced at the 3-4 portal, and some of the hemarthrosis is aspirated to confirm proper position after which 5 to 10 mL of saline solution is injected into the joint. The trocar is introduced, and a small joint arthroscope is connected. The procedure starts with an extensive lavage through an outflow portal in the 6-U portal. Blood clots and debris can be removed with a motorized, small joint shaver through the 4-5 or 6-R working portals. Continuous irrigation with saline solution by gravity flow from an elevated bag is used. With this method the intra-articular pressure is kept as low as possible in order to minimize the risk of extravasation of fluid, thus decreasing the risk for postoperative carpal tunnel syndrome and compartment syndrome. After the view has been cleared, the examination starts by evaluating associated injuries to cartilage and ligaments.

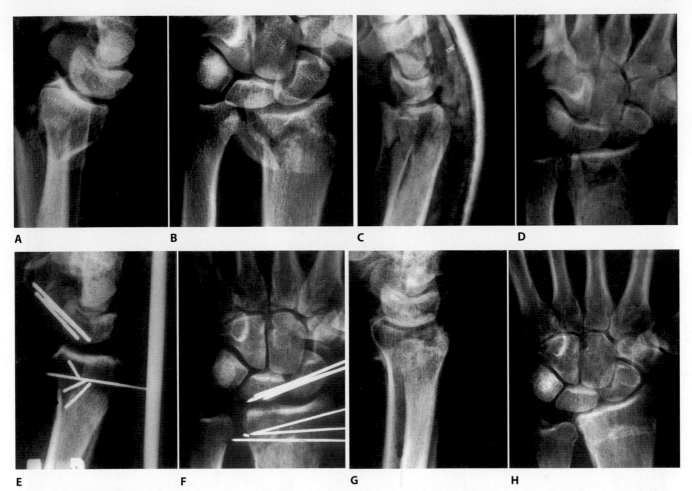

FIGURE 14.1. A 28-year-old male fell from a ladder and sustained a dislocated intra-articular distal radial fracture (**A**, lateral view, (**B**). PA-view). After reduction, there still was a 2-mm incongruency of a die-punch fragment, mainly seen centrally on the lateral view (**C**, lateral view, (**D**). PA view). Arthroscopy-assisted reduction was done, as well as percutaneous pinning of a grade 3 scapholunate (SL) ligament injury (**E**, lateral view, (**F**). PA view). At the one-year follow-up there was no sign of persistent incongruency, secondary osteoarthrosis, or scapholunate dissociation (**G**, lateral view, (**H**). PA view).

Modified Horizontal Wrist Arthroscopy

The standard upright position often leaves a problem after the joint surface is secured. Many fractures have comminution of the metaphysis and need additional treatment (e.g. volar or dorsal buttress plates, external fixator, or bone grafting) as a cancellous support to the cortical treatment. Therefore, I prefer to do the arthroscopy with a modified horizontal technique (Figure 14.2).[21]

The traction is applied on the index and long fingers with the traction force horizontally over a handle on a regular hand table (Figure 14.2B). The wrist is elevated slightly over the hand table and blocked with bars, which hold the forearm in pronation (Figure 14.2C). Arthroscopy with the horizontal technique is sometimes more technically demanding, but is otherwise done as described in the previous and following text (Figure 14.2), with realignment of the joint, as well as assessment and treatment of associated injuries. Hereafter, the horizontal position allows me to

continue with any additional technique that is necessary, without changing the traction or position of the wrist. This secures the reduction of the extra-articular component and facilitates further procedures of the fracture or associated injuries.

ARTHROSCOPY-ASSISTED REDUCTION

General Principles

Most displaced fragments have to be mobilized before they can be repositioned, even if some fragments may be reduced by longitudinal traction alone. This is done either with a probe within the joint (Figure 14.3A) or with an elevator through a 1 to 2 cm separate skin incision over the fracture. K-wires are then placed centrally in each fragment. Depressed fragments are elevated with the combined manipulation with the probe, elevator, and by a "joy-stick" maneuver of the K-wire. Under arthroscopic control, the fracture frag-

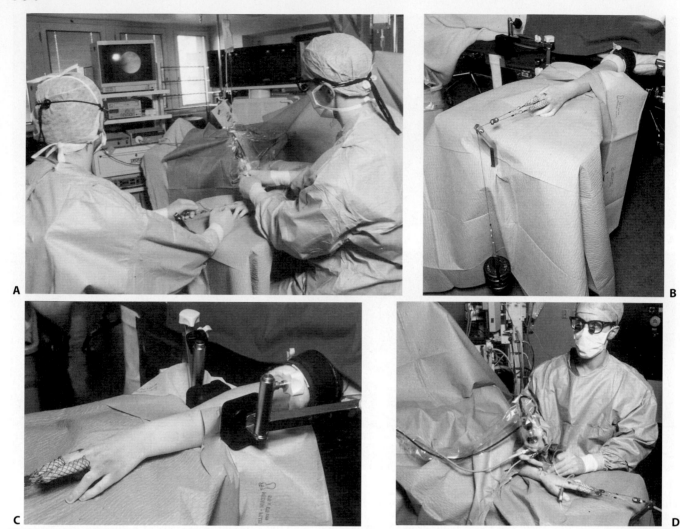

FIGURE 14.2. Modified horizontal arthroscopy technique facilitates complete management of distal radial fractures. **A.** The operating room when horizontal arthroscopy is done, with the mobile cart at the foot end of the patient. **B.** Horizontal traction over a handle on a normal hand table. **C.** The forearm is blocked in pronation with parallel bars. **D.** Arthroscopy with the modified horizontal technique is done with standard instruments.

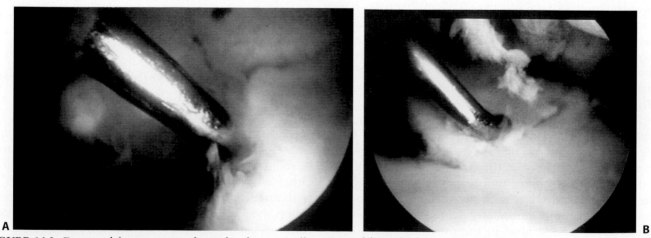

FIGURE 14.3. Depressed fragments are elevated arthroscopically. **A.** This arthroscopic view of the lunate facet shows a depressed "die-punch" fragment (the dorsum of the wrist to the left). The fragment is mobilized with a probe within the joint, while an elevator is used from the fracture outside the joint. **B.** Arthroscopic confirmation of proper congruency after the elevation and fixation of the depressed fragment.

ments are sequentially reduced. I prefer to start with realignment of the ulnar border of the radius, thereby securing the bony congruency of the DRU joint (Figure 14.4A). The next step is to add further fragments to the "ulnar platform" by driving the K-wires from larger to smaller fragments (Figure 14.4B). Afterwards, the realignment of the joint surface is determined arthroscopically (Figure 14.3B), with fluoroscopic confirmation that the pins are in proper position with appropriate length. I prefer to leave the pins outside the skin, as this minimizes the risk of injuries to tendons and the superficial branch of the radial nerve. Finally, the extraarticular fracture component, the cancellous defect, and associated injuries have to be evaluated and additional procedures have to be considered.

Specific Fracture Types

RADIAL STYLOID FRACTURE (CHAUFFEUR'S FRACTURE)

This fracture often has a rotation of the displaced fragment, which often is underestimated (Figure 14.5). Arthroscopically this is seen with "inverted" incongruencies dorsally and volarly (Figure 14.5A). The fragment is best reduced with the wrist in supination. With a K-wire on the tip of the styloid, dorsally in the snuff box, the fragment is reduced, and the wire is driven into the radius. Hereafter, a second K-wire or a cannulated screw is needed for rotational stability (Figure 14.5C).

LUNATE "DIE PUNCH" FRAGMENT

If the fragment is not impacted it is often reduced by traction and some palmar flexion. The reduction can be kept in place with one or two transverse subchondral K-wires placed so as not to penetrate the DRU joint.

If the fragment is impacted, it is disimpacted and mobilized either with a probe within the joint or with an elevator through a 1 to 2 cm separate skin incision over the fracture (Figure 14.3A). When the joint surface is congruent, as determined with arthroscopy (Figure 14.3B), two transverse subchondral K-wires can

secure the position (Figure 14.1). In this situation, additional treatment of the metaphyseal void, by means of bone graft or bone substitution, is needed.

PARTIAL PALMAR FRAGMENTS

As a general guideline, these fragments cannot be reduced by traction due to the strong palmar radiocarpal ligaments, where traction only increases the incongruency. Consequently, they need an open reduction and osteosynthesis with a buttress plate. However, in some cases the fragments might be reduced by loosening the traction and flexing the radiocarpal joint palmarly. In such cases they can be pinned from the dorsal aspect of the distal radius or from the palmar aspect through a limited palmar approach.[13,22]

ADDITIONAL FRACTURE TREATMENT

Cortical Fracture Treatment

DORSAL DISLOCATION

External fixation should be considered in extraarticular, comminuted fractures in order to retain the fracture. In my experience, the fixator is best applied after the intra-articular incongruency has been reduced arthroscopically. Otherwise, the longitudinal bar prevents the possibility of maneuvering the fragments with the "joy-stick" wires. The external fixator is placed while the wrist is still under traction in order to retain the best reduction possible, while keeping the tensile forces under control by the spring scale. Another alternative would be to do an open reduction of the extraarticular component and do the osteosynthesis with, for example, mini-plates and screws.

PALMAR DISLOCATION

In these cases I prefer to start with evaluation of any intra-articular incongruency and assess associated injuries. The modified horizontal technique is especially useful, since the traction is kept after the arthroscopy.

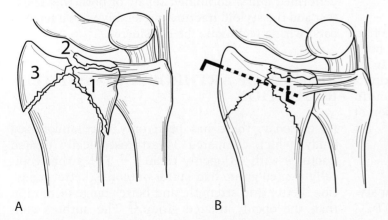

A   B

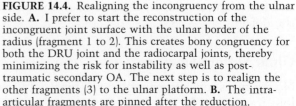

FIGURE 14.4. Realigning the incongruency from the ulnar side. **A.** I prefer to start the reconstruction of the incongruent joint surface with the ulnar border of the radius (fragment 1 to 2). This creates bony congruency for both the DRU joint and the radiocarpal joints, thereby minimizing the risk for instability as well as post-traumatic secondary OA. The next step is to realign the other fragments (3) to the ulnar platform. **B.** The intra-articular fragments are pinned after the reduction.

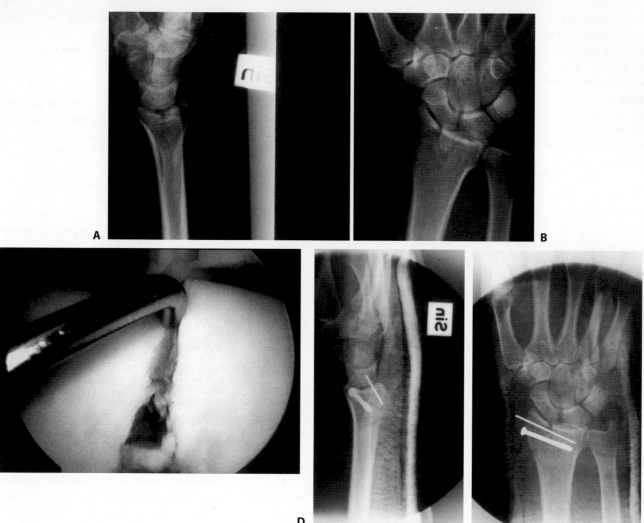

FIGURE 14.5. Radial styloid fractures often have rotational incongruency. **A, B.** Radiographic picture of a radial styloid fracture in a nonosteoporotic patient. **C.** This arthroscopic view shows the frequent finding of rotational incongruency in radial styloid fractures, which is revealed with the "inverted" joint incongruencies palmarly and dorsally (palmar aspect in the bottom with the radial styloid to the right). **D, E.** Radiographic view after realignment of the rotational incongruency and securing the fracture with one cannulated screw and one pin.

By rotating the forearm into supination, it is possible to continue with the standard palmar buttress plating technique without losing the reduction of the fracture.

Cancellous Fracture Treatment

The forces that dislocate and shatter the radius often leave a cancellous defect in the metaphyseal bone when the reduction is completed. The defect can be filled with bone graft or bone substitute by making a small incision between the third and fourth or fourth and fifth compartments, depending on the position of the defect.

Ulnar Styloid Fractures

No studies show any benefits with repair of ulnar styloid fractures. The fracture is associated with TFCC tears[16–18] but not with late clinical instability of the DRU joint,[23,24] at least not in nonosteoporotic patients. However, if a subluxation or even a dislocation is present, I suggest that an arthroscopic evaluation be performed and a combined repair of both the TFCC tear and the styloid fracture, preferably with a tension band wiring technique, be considered.

RESULTS OF ARTHROSCOPY-ASSISTED REDUCTION

As of today, there has been only one randomized study, which compared 34 arthroscopically treated fractures with 48 openly treated.[22] The arthroscopically treated group had better outcome, better reduction, better grip strength, and better range of motion than the openly treated group.[22] The authors concluded that the improved results might result from less soft-tissue scarring, due to less trauma from the arthroscopy-assisted surgery itself as compared with straight dorsal incisions in the openly treated group. Their results support the findings of others, where arthroscopy-assisted reduction has been found to re-align preoperative incongruity with good accuracy and give an excellent or good outcome in about 90% of the patients.[8,11,13,15] Furthermore, with the improved reduction to less than 1 mm intra-articular step-off, we decrease the risk of secondary osteoarthrosis.[2–4,25]

INJURIES ASSOCIATED WITH DISTAL RADIAL FRACTURES

The distal radial fracture in nonosteoporotic patients is most often an intra-articular fracture caused by a severe, high-energy trauma.[26,27] In contrast, the majority of elderly, osteoporotic women have extra-articular fractures,[28] which most often are sustained by falls on level ground.[28–32] Distal radial fractures caused by high-energy wrist trauma have been shown to be very complex injuries with a wide variety of associated tears of the triangular fibrocartilage complex (TFCC) and intercarpal ligaments.[16–18] Most authors have found the TFCC to be the most frequently injured structure, with tears in 49% to 78%.[16–18] However, Mehta et al.[13] found scapholunate (SL) ligament tears to be as frequent as 85%, which is far more than the 32% to 54% SL tears found by others.[16,17] The latter found lunotriquetral (LT) ligament tears to be present in only 15% to 16%.[16,17] Furthermore, subchondral hematomas and other chondral lesions have been found in one-third of nonosteoporotic patients with distal radial fractures.[16]

Chondral Lesions

Acute chondral lesions vary from subchondral hematomas (Figure 14.6A), with or without cracks in the cartilage, to avulsed cartilage flakes (Figure 14.7A), and complete avulsions of the cartilage (Figure 14.6B). They have been found in 19% to 33% of dislocated fractures in nonosteoporotic patients.[13,16] This is important, as subchondral hematoma leads to early onset of mild, radiographic osteoarthrosis (OA).[33] There is no treatment available today for these lesions, but they might explain the development of OA in extra-articular fractures that have been documented in the literature.[24] Most important, together with the associated ligament injuries, they reflect the complexity of distal radial fractures, especially in the nonosteoporotic population.[26]

Triangular Fibrocartilage Complex (TFCC) Injuries

The TFCC is a very complex structure supporting the DRU joint and the ulnocarpal joint. I suggest that we describe tears in this area as central perforation tears, tears of the ulnoradial ligament, or tears of the ulnocarpal ligament. This would facilitate the functional understanding of the different tears, namely as representing possibly destabilizing tears of the DRU joint or not.[26]

CENTRAL PERFORATION TEARS

These tears are located parallel to the sigmoid notch of the radius with a 2 mm rim of membranous substance left between the sigmoid notch and the perforation (Figure 14.8). Central perforation tears are stable and can be debrided with a suction punch. Care should be taken not to be too aggressive, thus jeop-

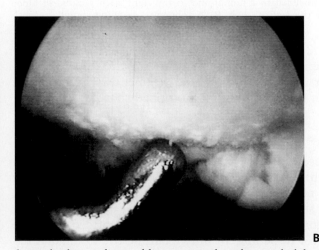

A   **B**

FIGURE 14.6. Subchondral hematoma may cause osteoarthrosis. **A.** A radiocarpal arthroscopic view of a subchondral hematoma (without a macroscopic cartilage destruction) in the scaphoid facet of the radius in a right wrist (dorsal aspect to the right). The scaphoid is seen above, the radial styloid area at the far end and the slightly diagonal palmar radiocarpal ligaments at the palmar end of the joint surface. **B.** This arthroscopic view shows a complete avulsion of the cartilage from the scaphoid. The remaining cartilage is seen to the right.

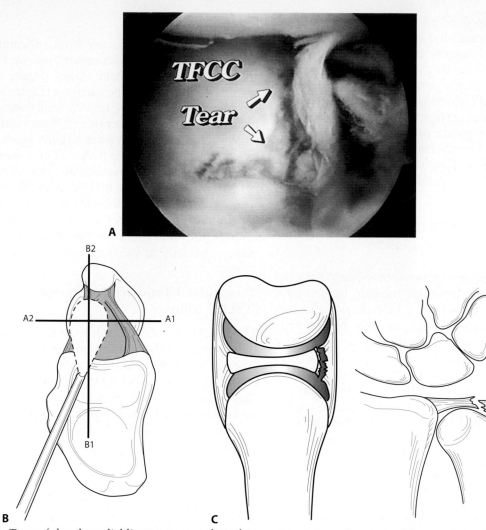

FIGURE 14.7. Tears of the ulnoradial ligament cause clinical instability of the DRU joint. **A.** An arthroscopic view of a dorsal ulnar avulsion tear of the ulnoradial ligament (the transverse, peripheral part of the TFCC; dorsum of the right wrist to the right). The lunate is above with a chondral flake hanging down. The dorsoulnar peripheral tear creates a rough longitudinal line from the lunate facet of the radius below going all the way towards the ulnar styloid, which is not visible arthroscopically. The synovium is imbedded in a hematoma to the right with a cloud of blood over the central disk. **B.** A schematic drawing shows the posi-tion of the arthroscope when examining the dorsoulnar aspect of the radiocarpal joint. The sagittal line A1-A2 and transverse line B1-B2 indicate the cross-sections in **C. C.** These drawings suggest a pathoanatomical continuation of the arthroscopically demonstrated peripheral avulsion tear. The sagittal (left) section has the dorsum to the right, the triquetrum above, and the ulnar head below the dorsally avulsed ligament. The transverse (right) section shows how the peripheral tear penetrates deep into the ligament and probably injures the ligament's insertion in the fovea of the ulnar head.

ardizing the stability by debriding the important palmar and dorsal ulnoradial ligaments. The edges are then smoothed with a motorized shaver.

TEARS OF THE ULNORADIAL LIGAMENT

These can be either avulsion tears from the insertion of the dorsal and palmar edge of the sigmoid notch of the radius or ulnar avulsion tears (Figure 14.7). They can sometimes be hidden behind a capsular blood clot (Figure 14.7). The area should be debrided with the shaver to be able to fully examine the ulnoradial ligament. These tears are associated with late clinical instability of the DRU joint[23] and worse outcome.[23,24] Consequently, they should be repaired.

Radial avulsion tears are often caused by dorsoulnar fracture fragments, but may be true avulsions from the insertion site of the ulnoradial ligament. Fragments should be anatomically restored in order to secure bony congruity of the sigmoid notch and fixate the ligament insertion. A true avulsion at the insertion probably has to be reinserted, either with drill holes through the radius[34,35] or with a suture anchor.

An ulnar avulsion tear is either repaired with 2 or 3 2-0 absorbable (PDS) sutures through the dorsoulnar capsule and extensor carpi ulnaris (ECU) tendon sheath[36-39] or through drill holes of the distal ulna. The repair is protected from supination and pronation for 4 weeks, followed by 2 to 4 weeks in a short-arm cast or VersaWrist splint as suggested by Corso et al.[40]

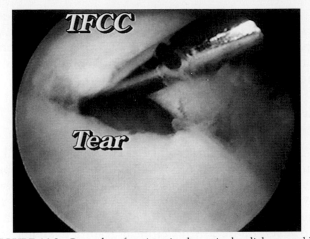

FIGURE 14.8. Central perforations in the articular disk are stable. Radiocarpal arthroscopy here shows a stable central perforation tear in the central articular disk of the TFCC (dorsum of the wrist to the right). The lunate facet of the radius is in the foreground with the probe (1-mm thick) lifting the torn ligament about 2 mm from its insertion in the sigmoid notch of the radius.

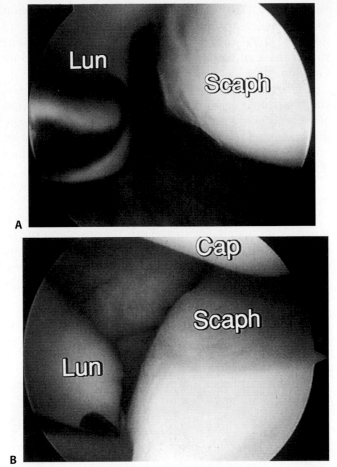

FIGURE 14.9. Scapholunate ligament tears may develop radiographic dissociation. **A.** Arthroscopic radiocarpal view of a complete scapholunate tear showing the ligament avulsed from the proximal scaphoid pole (the dorsum of the wrist is above). A fresh hematoma is seen below, and the probe is lifting the avulsed ligament over the lunate. **B.** The degree of mobility between the scaphoid and lunate can be evaluated with midcarpal arthroscopy. The mobility correlates to the severity of the ligament tear in the radiocarpal joint. Measurements of step-off and diastasis made with a 1 mm probe having a tip length of 2 mm (dorsum of the wrist is above), permit grading of the intercarpal ligament injury (Table 14.1).

TEARS OF THE ULNOCARPAL LIGAMENT

These are rare.[16] Treatment by a palmar open reinsertion technique may be considered.

DEGENERATIVE TEARS

Degenerative tears with different degrees of centrally rounded holes and secondary cartilage afflictions on the ulnar head and the lunate may be found together with the fracture. Sometimes there may be acute tears superimposed on the degenerative tears.[16] The degenerative changes are probably best left alone, as they most often have been asymptomatic prior to the fracture. However, an acute component may need treatment as recommended above.

Intercarpal Ligaments

Under arthroscopic vision, the different structures are thoroughly examined with a probe, and stress tests are done to fully define the ligament tears and the degree of mobility. Registration is done following a standardized protocol. The ligament injuries are classified as partial or complete tears of the radiocarpal joint (Figure 14.9A). The SL ligament is examined in its dorsal, membranous, and palmar portions. In the midcarpal joint, the joint space is examined regarding diastasis and step-off, by means of a probe with a known thickness (e.g., 1 mm) and tip length (e.g., 2 mm) as a reference (Figure 14.9B). The widening and the step-off reflect the degree of mobility, which is not necessarily a pathological laxity, in the afflicted intercarpal joint. Thus, a grading of the intercarpal ligament mobility can be made (Table 14.1).[16]

SL LIGAMENT TEARS

SL ligament injury grade 1-2 (Table 14.1) seems to be a stable injury without the development of radiographic SL dissociation.[33] These tears are probably best treated with just the immobilization needed by

TABLE 14.1. Classification System for Interosseous SL and LT Ligament Injuries and Mobility of the Joints.[16]

	Radiocarpal arthroscopy	Midcarpal arthroscopy	
Grade	Ligament appearance	Diastasis (mm)	Step-off (mm)
1	Hematoma	0	0
2	As above and/or partial tear	0–1	< 2
3	Partial or complete tear	1–2	< 2
4	Complete tear	> 2	> 2

Source: Reprinted from Lindau, Arner, and Hagberg[16], with permission.

the fracture. Debridement in the membranous portion may be necessary in some cases.[41] Currently, we do not have any data that support the proposed treatment to pin these moderate (grade 2) tears, as suggested by Geissler.[10]

SL ligament injury grade 3 (Table 14.1) may be partially unstable, leading to radiographic SL dissociation already after 1 year.[33] I recommend reduction of the diastasis and step-off seen in the midcarpal joint and percutaneous pinning of the SL and SC joints (Figure 14.1).

SL ligament injury grade 4 (Table 14.1) seems to be unstable especially if the scaphoid is flexed.[33,41] Multiple percutaneous pins[42] or, preferably, an open repair is indicated, securing both the insertion of the intercarpal ligament and the dorsal capsule with the extrinsic ligament.[10,41]

LT LIGAMENT TEARS

LT ligament injury grade 1-3 (Table 14.1; Figure 14.10) seems to be a stable injury, but may need debridement.

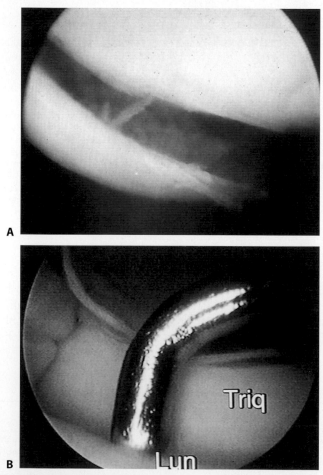

FIGURE 14.10. LT ligament tears develop radiographic dissociation less often. **A.** Radiocarpal arthroscopy reveals an avulsion of the LT ligament from the lunate. The rough undersurface is shown under the avulsed ligament. **B.** Midcarpal arthroscopy permits assessment of the diastasis and step-off between the lunate and the triquetrum, hereby grading the tear (the dorsum of the wrist is up).

LT ligament injury grade 4 (Table 14.1) is an unstable injury, especially if the lunate is flexed.[41] An open dorsal capsulodesis with suture anchors combined with pinning of the LT joint should be considered.[10,41]

Results of Treatment of Injuries Associated with Distal Radial Fractures

We have found SL mobility grade 3 in 14% and LT mobility grade 3 in 6%.[16] No case of grade 4 mobility was found. Preliminary data show that SL mobility grade 3-4 has an increased risk of developing radiographic SL dissociation already after 1 year.[33] However, there are no clinical results available regarding treatment of intercarpal ligament injuries associated with distal radial fractures. Hence, the recommendations given are based upon what is currently known about these conditions. Keep in mind, though, that there are still no randomized studies that support surgical treatment regarding these associated injuries, and that surgery itself adds trauma and possible morbidity. Further randomized studies are needed before advocating treatment algorithms for these injuries.

References

1. Flinkkilä T, Raatikainen T, Hämäläinen M. AO and Frykman's classifications of Colles' fracture. No prognostic value in 652 patients evaluated after 5 years. *Acta Orthop Scand* 1998;69:77–81.
2. Knirk JL, Jupiter JB. Intra-articular fractures of the distal end of the radius in young adults. *J Bone Joint Surg Am* 1986;68:647–659.
3. Axelrod TS, McMurtry RY. Open reduction and internal fixation of comminuted, intraarticular fractures of the distal radius. *J Hand Surg Am* 1990;15:1–11.
4. Trumble TE, Schmitt SR, Vedder NB. Factors affecting functional outcome of displaced intra-articular distal radius fractures. *J Hand Surg Am* 1994;19:325–440.
5. Trumble TE, Culp RW, Hanel DP, et al. Intra-articular fractures of the distal aspect of the radius. *Instr Course Lect* 1999;48:465–480.
6. Auge WK, Velazquez PA. The application of indirect reduction techniques in the distal radius: the role of adjuvant arthroscopy. *Arthroscopy* 2000;830–835.
7. Edwards CC 2nd, Haraszti CJ, McGillivary GR. Intra-articular distal radius fractures: arthroscopic assessment of radiographically assisted reduction. *J Hand Surg Am* 2001;1036–1041.
8. Adolfsson L, Jörgsholm P. Arthroscopically-assisted reduction of intra-articular fractures of the distal radius. *J Hand Surg Br* 1998;23:391–395.
9. Cooney WP, Berger RA. Treatment of complex fractures of the distal radius. Combined use of internal and external fixation and arthroscopic reduction. *Hand Clin* 1993;9:603–612.
10. Geissler WB. Arthroscopically assisted reduction of intra-articular fractures of the distal radius. *Hand Clin* 1995;11:19–29.
11. Geissler WB, Freeland AE. Arthroscopically assisted reduction of intraarticular distal radial fractures. *Clin Orthop* 1996:125–134.
12. Geissler WB, Freeland AE. Arthroscopic management of intra-articular distal radius fractures. *Hand Clin* 1999;15:455–465, viii.

13. Mehta JA, Bain GI, Heptinstall RJ. Anatomical reduction of intra-articular fractures of the distal radius. An arthroscopically-assisted approach. *J Bone Joint Surg Br* 2000;82:79–86.

14. Whipple TL. The role of arthroscopy in the treatment of intra-articular wrist fractures. *Hand Clin* 1995;11:13–18.

15. Wolfe SW, Easterling KJ, Yoo HH. Arthroscopic-assisted reduction of distal radius fractures. *Arthroscopy* 1995;11:706–714.

16. Lindau T, Arner M, Hagberg L. Intraarticular lesions in distal fractures of the radius in young adults. A descriptive arthroscopic study in 50 patients. *J Hand Surg Br* 1997;22:638–643.

17. Geissler WB, Freeland AE, Savoie FH, et al. Intracarpal soft-tissue lesions associated with an intra-articular fracture of the distal end of the radius. *J Bone Joint Surg Am* 1996;78:357–365.

18. Richards RS, Bennett JD, Roth JH, et al. Arthroscopic diagnosis of intra-articular soft tissue injuries associated with distal radial fractures. *J Hand Surg Am* 1997;22:772–776.

19. Bellinghausen HW, Gilula LA, Young LV, et al. Post-traumatic palmar carpal subluxation. Report of two cases. *J Bone Joint Surg Am* 1983;65:998–1006.

20. Biyani A, Sharma JC. An unusual pattern of radiocarpal injury: brief report. *J Bone Joint Surg Br* 1989;71:139.

21. Lindau T. Wrist arthroscopy in distal radial fractures with a modified horizontal technique. *Arthroscopy* 2001;17:E5.

22. Doi K, Hattori Y, Otsuka K, et al. Intra-articular fractures of the distal aspect of the radius: arthroscopically assisted reduction compared with open reduction and internal fixation. *J Bone Joint Surg Am* 1999;81:1093–1110.

23. Lindau T, Adlercreutz C, Aspenberg P. Peripheral tears of the triangular fibrocartilage complex cause distal radioulnar joint instability after distal radial fractures. *J Hand Surg Am* 2000;25:464–468.

24. Lindau T, Hagberg L, Adlercreutz C, et al. Distal radioulnar instability is an independent worsening factor in distal radial fractures. *Clin Orthop* 2000(376):229–235.

25. Kopylov P, Johnell O, Redlund-Johnell I, et al. Fractures of the distal end of the radius in young adults: a 30-year follow-up. *J Hand Surg Br* 1993;18:45–49.

26. Lindau T. Distal radial fractures and effects of associated ligament injuries. Dept of Orthopedics. Lund: University of Lund, 2000:76.

27. Lindau T, Aspenberg P, Arner M, et al. Fractures of the distal forearm in young adults. An epidemiologic description of 341 patients. *Acta Orthop Scand* 1999;70:124–128.

28. Schmalholz A. Epidemiology of distal radius fracture in Stockholm 1981–1982. *Acta Orthop Scand* 1988;59:701–703.

29. Bengner U, Johnell O. Increasing incidence of forearm fractures. A comparison of epidemiologic patterns 25 years apart. *Acta Orthop Scand* 1985;56:158–160.

30. Hove LM, Fjeldsgaard K, Reitan R, et al. Fractures of the distal radius in a Norwegian city. *Scand J Plast Reconstr Surg Hand Surg* 1995;29:263–267.

31. Falch JA. Epidemiology of fractures of the distal forearm in Oslo, Norway. *Acta Orthop Scand* 1983;54:291–295.

32. Robertsson GO, Jonsson GT, Sigurjonsson K. Epidemiology of distal radius fractures in Iceland in 1985. *Acta Orthop Scand* 1990;61:457–459.

33. Lindau T, Adlercreutz C, Jonsson K, et al. Chondral and ligament lesions in distal radial fractures in young adults. One year follow-up in 43 patients with arthroscopic diagnosis. The 7th International Federation of Societies for Surgery of the Hand, Vancouver, Canada, 1998.

34. Sagerman SD, Short W. Arthroscopic repair of radial-sided triangular fibrocartilage complex tears. *Arthroscopy* 1996;12:339–342.

35. Fellinger M, Peicha G, Seibert FJ, et al. Radial avulsion of the triangular fibrocartilage complex in acute wrist trauma: a new technique for arthroscopic repair. *Arthroscopy* 1997;13:370–374.

36. Skie MC, Mekhail AO, Deitrich DR, et al. Operative technique for inside-out repair of the triangular fibrocartilage complex. *J Hand Surg Am* 1997;22:814–817.

37. de Araujo W, Poehling GG, Kuzma GR. New Tuohy needle technique for triangular fibrocartilage complex repair: preliminary studies. *Arthroscopy* 1996;12:699–703.

38. Haugstvedt JR, Husby T. Results of repair of peripheral tears in the triangular fibrocartilage complex using an arthroscopic suture technique. *Scand J Plast Reconstr Surg Hand Surg* 1999;33:439–447.

39. Zachee B, De Smet L, Fabry G. Arthroscopic suturing of TFCC lesions. *Arthroscopy* 1993;9:242–243.

40. Corso SJ, Savoie FH, Geissler WB, et al. Arthroscopic repair of peripheral avulsions of the triangular fibrocartilage complex of the wrist: a multicenter study. *Arthroscopy* 1997;13(1):78–84.

41. Ruch DS, Bowling J. Arthroscopic assessment of carpal instability. *Arthroscopy* 1998;14:675–681.

42. Whipple TL. The role of arthroscopy in the treatment of scapholunate instability. *Hand Clin* 1995;11:37–40.

15

Fixation of Acute and Selected Nonunion Scaphoid Fractures

Joseph F. Slade III, Greg A. Merrell, and William B. Geissler

Techniques in fracture treatment are evolving toward the use of indirect reduction and percutaneous fixation. Several studies have confirmed that scaphoid fractures can also be treated with percutaneous fixation, achieving high rates of union and promising functional outcomes.[1–3] Scaphoid fractures frequently have associated ligamentous injuries that can lead to long-term pain and dysfunction if undiagnosed or untreated. Arthroscopy provides a powerful tool to diagnose and treat these associated injuries. Additionally, it can assist in determining the adequacy of fracture reduction. Lastly, arthroscopy is useful in grading scaphoid fractures and nonunions. This chapter describes our technique treatment of scaphoid fracture and its associated injuries.

INDICATIONS

The indications for arthroscopically assisted repair of scaphoid fractures and nonunions are similar to the indications for open repair, as long as treatment goals can be accomplished. Small joint arthroscopy is used in tandem with mini-fluoroscopic imaging to evaluate and treat scaphoid fractures, ligament injuries, and fracture nonunions. These tools allow for traditionally open techniques to be adapted to minimally invasive procedures, sparing uninjured soft tissue such as stabilizing ligaments (i.e., scapholunate ligament) and the tenuous blood supply necessary for carpal and ligament healing (Figure 15.1A). Indications for treatment of scaphoid injuries have evolved since the successful adaptation of these minimally invasive procedures. These techniques have permitted effective treatment of scaphoid fractures and selected nonunions with a high union rate and minimal complications.[1–3] The indication for arthroscopically assisted treatment of scaphoid injuries can be divided into absolute and relative indications and contraindications (Table 15.1).

CLASSIFICATION AND PREOPERATIVE EVALUATION

The goal of a classification system is to permit accurate communication of an injury and evaluation of

treatment methods. To this end there exist a variety of scaphoid fracture classifications, which do provide a reasonable description of the injury but have been less valuable as tools for evaluation of the efficacy of treatment. Fractures have been classified by anatomic location or direction of the fracture plane.[4] However, the most widely used classification is the Herbert classification, which attempts to classify fractures according to their stability.[5,6] This classification also attempts to classify scaphoid nonunions, but is not detailed enough to be a valuable tool in evaluating treatment results. The causes of treatment failure are multifactorial; among these are included the scaphoid's tenuous blood supply and fracture stability.[7] Unfortunately, standard radiographs are poor tools for effectively evaluating bone stability, displacement, viability, and healing potential.[8] Previous classification systems relied on standard radiographs and did not take into account the arsenal of diagnostic modalities presently available, including computerized tomography (CT); magnetic resonance imaging (MRI); and dynamic imaging with mini-fluoroscopy, arthroscopy, and bone biopsy to direct treatment. Proximal scaphoid fractures are at risk for avascular necrosis. Fracture location can suggest bone viability, but MRI and bone biopsy will provide more accurate assessment. Oblique fractures of the scaphoid have been reported to be unstable, and it is difficult to provide rigid fixation. Correct knowledge of the fracture plane can be important, but standard radiographs are limited. Computerized tomography of the scaphoid fracture will provide better information on fracture plane and displacement.

Utilizing the above tools, fractures are graded using location and a modification of the Herbert scaphoid fracture classification system.[5,6] Ligament injuries are graded using the Geissler classification system.[9] Slade and Geissler developed a classification scheme for management of scaphoid nonunions in Table 15.2. Failed scaphoid healing is defined as failed union by 3 months. Using CT, the gold standard for determining scaphoid union, some authors have determined average scaphoid healing to occur between 3 and 4 months.[8] If union has not occurred by this

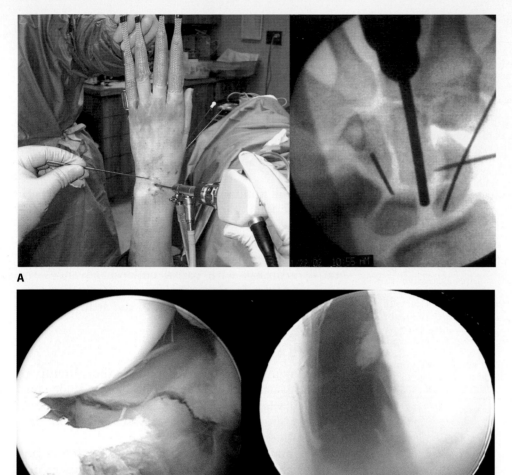

FIGURE 15.1. A. Arthroscope able to be passed through a scapholunate tear. **B.** Evidence of bone bleeding from a proximal pole.

TABLE 15.1. Indications for Treatment.

Absolute indications

Displaced scaphoid fractures
Fractures of the proximal pole
Fractures with delayed presentation
Scaphoid fractures with fibrous unions without displacement
Nondisplaced scaphoid nonunions with minimal sclerosis
Combined injuries including scaphoid fractures
    Distal radius
    Other carpal bones (i.e., capitate fracture)
    Ligament injuries (i.e., transscaphoid dorsal perilunate
      dislocation)
    Polytrauma

Relative indications

Stable scaphoid fractures
Patients desiring early return to work or avocation

Contraindications

Scaphoid nonunions with severe cystic sclerotic changes and
    deformity
Pseudoarthrosis
Avascular necrosis
Nondisplaced pediatric injuries (distal pole)

time with conservative treatment, then surgical repair is recommended. If signs of failed union present earlier, intervention is warranted.

Scaphoid fractures presenting after one month for treatment have a poorer outcome with immobilization alone than those presenting earlier and should be treated with rigid fixation alone (Grade I).[10]

Fibrous unions appear solidly healed, but insufficient remodeling has occurred to resist the stresses of bending and torque (Grade II). Barton explored these fibrous unions, found solid union between the fracture fragments, and determined that healing had occurred. On follow-up, only half proceeded to union.[11] Shah, encountering a similar group of fibrous unions, stabilized them with a compression screw without a bone graft. These all went on to heal.[12] Fibrous scaphoid unions require only rigid fixation to prevent micromotion and to permit bone healing.

Correctly aligned scaphoid nonunions with minimal fracture sclerosis suggest micromotion and early

TABLE 15.2. Treatment Classification System for Scaphoid Nonunion.

I	Scaphoid fractures with delayed presentation for treatment: 4 weeks–12 weeks
II	Fibrous union: minimal fracture line at nonunion interface, no cyst or sclerosis
III	Minimal sclerosis: bone resorption at nonunion interface less than 1mm
IV	Cystic formation and sclerosis: bone resorption at nonunion interface greater than 1 mm but less than 5 mm, cyst, no deformity of lateral radiographs
V	Deformity and/or pseudoarthrosis: bone resorption at nonunion interface greater than 5 mm, cyst, fragment motion, deformity on lateral radiographs
VI	Wrist arthrosis: scaphoid nonunion with radiocarpal and/or midcarpal arthrosis

Special circumstances

PP Proximal pole nonunion. The proximal pole of the scaphoid has a tenuous blood supply and a mechanical disadvantage, which places it at greater risk of delayed or failed union. Because of these difficulties, this injury requires aggressive treatment to ensure successful healing.
AVN Scaphoid nonunion with necrosis is suggested by MRI demonstrating a decrease or absence of vascularity of one or both poles. Bone biopsy can confirm necrosis. Intraoperative inspection of the scaphoid for punctate bleeding is considered definitive.
LI Ligament injury is suggested by static and dynamic imaging of the carpal bones. Arthroscopy is the most sensitive tool for detecting carpal ligament injury.

resorption at the fracture site (Grade III). Small sections of bone may undergo reabsorption, making the fracture gap larger and reducing the overall strain. With gaps less than 1 mm in a stable fracture, healing can proceed across the gap. These nonunions require rigid fixation to achieve union. Wozasek and Ledoux separately reported on nonunions without necrosis or severe sclerosis that healed with rigid fixation without open bone grafting.[13,14] Cosio reported stabilizing nonunions with multiple Kirschner wires and achieved solid union in 80% of patients without open repair and bone graft.[15] A CT scan should confirm that the nonunion front represents only a minimal sclerotic line (less than 1 mm) and is in correct alignment.

Scaphoid nonunions with cystic changes at the fracture represent extensive resorption and nonviable tissue at the fracture site (Grade IV). These nonunions present with sclerotic zones between 1 and 5 mm. Fixation alone of these nonunions offers little success for healing. The large zones of devitalized tissue and the extent of fracture gap are too great a challenge for the local Haversion osteoclast-osteoblast repair system. Minimally, these nonunions require debridement, bone grafting, and rigid fixation. MR imaging should be considered if bone viability of these fracture fragments is of question. CT is required to define the extent of local destruction and confirm correct structural alignment. Both curettage and bone grafting can be accomplished through an arthroscopic portal.

Scaphoid nonunions with pseudoarthrosis and/or deformity require extensive debridement and structural bone grafting for mechanical support (Grade V). These nonunions have extensive bone resorption at the nonunion interface, which is usually greater than 5 mm with large cysts. A flexion deformity is seen on lateral radiographs. These nonunions will require correction of the deformity, interposition of a cortical-cancellous bone graft, and rigid fixation. Arthroscopy will provide valuable information of early signs of arthrosis.

Scaphoid nonunion with wrist arthrosis is a result of dysfunctional carpal motion (Grade VI). Early degenerative changes to the carpus permit the repair of the scaphoid nonunion and treatment of the local arthritis (i.e., radial styloidectomy). Extensive degenerative arthrosis with carpal collapse advances the treatment from fracture repair to wrist salvage procedures, depending on the extent of the arthritis.

Difficult Circumstances

The following circumstances increase the difficulty in achieving successful bone union. These include compromised vascularity and fracture instability due to ligament injuries or inadequate fixation of certain fractures and nonunions.

Proximal pole fractures are the most challenging of all scaphoid injuries, and treatment becomes greatly complicated when treatment results in nonunion. First, the blood supply becomes increasingly compromised the closer the fracture is to the proximal pole. Second, the smaller the fracture fragment the greater the bending forces from the distal scaphoid, which act at the fracture site to produce displacement. Proximal pole fractures should be aggressively fixed to avoid the difficulties of nonunion. Once the native bone of the proximal pole becomes replaced with osteopenic bone or reparative tissue, the challenge to achieve solid union greatly increases.

The presence of avascular necrosis of the scaphoid has been associated with a significant decrease in union rate.[7,12] Fracture necrosis can be difficult to define, but the gold standard remains the MRI.[16] Green evaluated avascular necrosis by direct, open inspection of the nonunion site for punctate bleeding at the time of surgery.[17] Slade has adapted this exam arthroscopically, limiting unnecessary vascular disruption. The proximal pole of the scaphoid is first reamed. The arthroscope is inserted into the base of the scaphoid in the previously drilled bone tract. The tourniquet is deflated, and the cancellous bone is inspected for punctate bleeding (Figure 15.1B). The presence or absence of bleeding bone is recorded, as is the time required for appearance.[18] Revascularization will often proceed with acute fractures if they are rigidly fixed. Nonunions with a large zone of devitalized bone are best treated with a vascular bone bridge. Vascularized bone grafts have increased the union rate and decreased the union time.[19] The introduction of a freshly harvested vascularized pedicle graft serves two purposes. First, the distance required for revascularization is greatly reduced, and second, the stiffness of this new bone as a cortical cancellous graft with the appropriate fixation may provide the stable mechanical construct required for bone healing and revascularization to proceed. This will salvage the wrist from arthrosis, but the trade-off will be limited wrist function.

Ligament injuries associated with scaphoid fractures and nonunion must be identified. Biomechanical studies suggest that torn ligaments result in carpal instability. Cooney reported that scaphoid union was much reduced in the presence of a collapsed scaphoid nonunion with dorsal carpal instability. He documented a 35% failure rate following bone grafting for unstable or displaced scaphoid nonunions.[20,21] Both injuries require evaluation and treatment. Arthroscopic examination of scaphoid fractures and nonunions aids us in staging for defining, identifying, and treating ligament injuries. During arthroscopy, carpal ligament injuries are graded using the Geissler grading system.[9] This system standardizes arthroscopic observation of injuries of the intracarpal ligaments. With a grade I lesion, attenuation of an interosseous ligament is seen with the arthroscope placed in the radiocarpal portal. There is no incongruency between the carpal bones with the arthroscope in the midcarpal portal. With a grade II lesion, there is attenuation of the interosseous ligament at the radiocarpal space and an incongruency between the carpal bones when viewed from the midcarpal portal. In grade III lesions, a separation between the carpal bones is evident from both the radiocarpal and the midcarpal portals. A small joint probe can be passed between the carpal bones, but a 2.7-mm arthroscope cannot be passed. With a grade IV lesion, gapping is sufficient to permit a 2.7-mm arthroscope to be passed between the carpal bones. The arthroscopic findings of increasing carpal gapping correlate with carpal separation as measured on the posteroanterior radiograph. Grade II lesions, which are partial tears, have a measured gapping between 2 and 3 mm. Grade III lesions, complete tears, measure between 3 and 4 mm, and Grade IV lesions are between 5 and 6 mm. Grade IV lesions also demonstrate lateral scapholunate angle greater than 75 degrees. Injuries graded II and III are debrided, reduced and pinned, and loose ligaments are treated with capsular shrinkage. Grade IV injuries are treated similarly, except a small dorsal incision is made and a repair with bone anchors of the dorsal scapholunate interrosseus ligament is performed. The decision to add a dorsal capsulardesis is determined by the degree of instability at the time of repair.

SURGICAL TECHNIQUE

This technique involves the placement of a 0.045-inch guidewire from dorsal to volar along the central axis of a reduced scaphoid fracture or nonunion. The placement of this guidewire and fracture reduction are both fluoroscopically and arthroscopically confirmed. A headless, cannulated compression screw provides rigid fixation and is introduced into the dorsal wrist through a percutaneous incision (Figure 15.2).

Imaging

The injured wrist is imaged with a mini-fluoroscope to identify fracture displacement and ligament injury. At the completion of this survey, the central scaphoid axis is identified. The central axis of the scaphoid is visualized using fluoroscopic imaging. Obtain a posteroanterior view of the wrist. Next, pronate the wrist until the scaphoid becomes a cylinder. This position aligns the proximal and distal poles of the scaphoid. Now flex the wrist 45 degrees, and the scaphoid will be flexed 90 degrees and parallel to the imaging beam. The scaphoid should appear as a circle, and the center of the circle is the central axis of the scaphoid and the exact position for placement of the guidewire. If the scaphoid axis is difficult to image, the central axis can be marked using a Kirschner wire. Using a posteroanterior view of the wrist, locate the distal

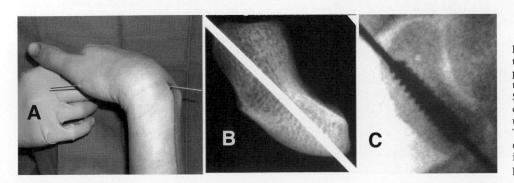

FIGURE 15.2. A, B. The key to the technique is the percutaneous placement of a guidewire along the central axis of a scaphoid. **C.** Scaphoid fracture is repaired via a dorsal percutaneous technique using a standard Acutrak screw. The fixation device is a headless cannulated compression screw implanted through the proximal pole.

scaphoid pole. Place a Kirschner wire into the distal scaphoid pole to the point of central axis. Pronating and flexing the wrist will place the tip of the wire in the center of the circle (Figure 15.3A–C). This will direct the placement of the central axis guidewire. If a mini-fluoroscope is not available, the same image can be obtained using a standard fluoroscope. In this case, the patient should be positioned in the supine position with the arm and elbow extended. The standard fluoroscopy unit is oriented vertically, with the re-

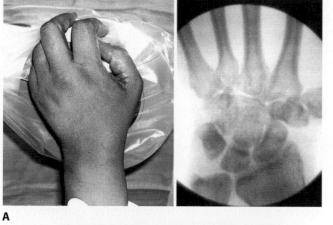

A

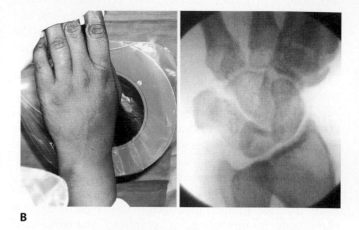

B

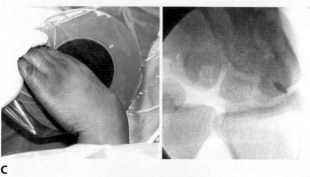

C

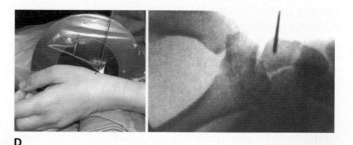

D

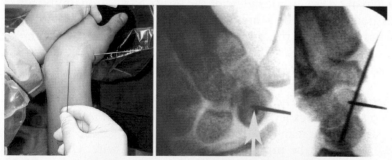

E

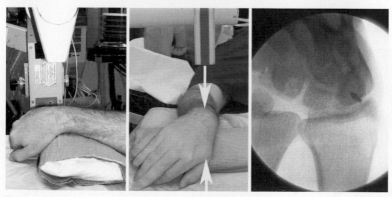

F

FIGURE 15.3. The elbow is flexed, and the imaging beam is perpendicular to the wrist. **A.** A posteroanterior view of the wrist radiograph and picture is demonstrated. **B.** Using fluoroscopy, pronate the wrist until the scaphoid poles are aligned and the scaphoid is viewed as a cylinder. **C.** Now, flex the wrist until the scaphoid cylinder appears as a circle. The central axis of the scaphoid is now in the imaging beam and is the center of the scaphoid circle. **D.** In an alternative technique, a pin is placed in the center of the distal pole of the scaphoid under fluoroscopic control. **E.** The guide pin for the cannulated screw is then placed in the proximal pole of the scaphoid and is aimed toward the distal pin. **F.** The guide pin may be placed in the horizontal position only if a large fluoroscopic unit is available. To obtain the cylinder, the wrist is flexed 45 degrees on a bump and pronated.

ceiving plate horizontal to the floor. A roll is placed under the wrist, flexing the wrist 45 degrees effectively flexes the scaphoid 90 degrees. Simply pronating the flexed wrist in the imaging beam will align the scaphoid pole and reveal the scaphoid central axis (Figure 15.3D–F).

Dorsal Wire Placement

The working distance between a mini-fluoroscopy unit's emission and receiving heads is approximately 14 inches. This limited distance can restrict the targeting of the scaphoid. A double-cut 0.045-inch guidewire is introduced percutaneously at the base of the proximal scaphoid pole using the drill guide improvised from a 14-gauge needle. With the central axis of the scaphoid imaged, the 14-gauge needle is inserted onto the scaphoid proximal pole (Figure 15.4A). The wrist can then be removed from the imaging field and the guidewire introduced through the needle and driven in approximately 1 cm. The position and direction of the wire can be checked and adjusted as needed. If multiple incorrect passes are made, establishing the correct path can be difficult using a 0.045 wire. A stouter 0.062 wire, with its increased stiffness, can be used to establish the correct track. Once the correct path is established, the 0.062 wire can be ex-

changed for the 0.045 guidewire. With the wrist flexed, the wire is driven in a dorsal to volar direction. The wire passes through the trapezium and exits the wrist from the radial thumb border. The central axis of the scaphoid passes through the trapezium. The radial thumb border is a safe zone devoid of neurovascular structures. The wire is then withdrawn until the wrist can be extended without bending the wire (Figure 15.4B). Once the wrist is fully extended, both the position of the wire and the alignment of the scaphoid can be carefully inspected with imaging. Unstable fractures and nonunions require a second parallel wire. Unstable fractures require the stiffness of the additional wire to prevent bending and rotational deformity during reaming and screw placement. Scaphoid nonunions require stabilization so the central axis can be reamed without loss of alignment.

Small Joint Arthroscopy

After positioning the guidewire and confirming fracture alignment by fluoroscopy, an arthroscopic survey is performed. The goal of arthroscopy here is to identify and treat ligament injuries, reduce and stabilize articular joint incongruities, and directly inspect the quality of the reduction in acute fractures. As in acute injuries, arthroscopy is used to identify and treat lig-

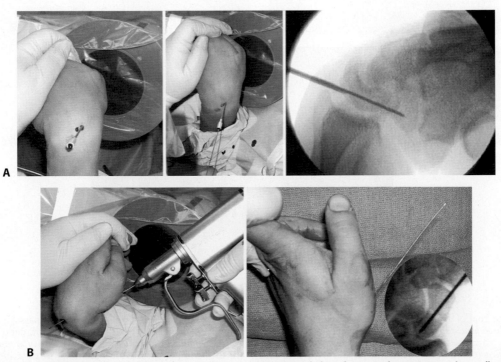

FIGURE 15.4. A. 12- or 14-gauge needle can be used as an improvised drill guide for the 0.045-inch guidewire. After imaging identifies the central axis, the needle is inserted in the scaphoid proximal pole. The wrist can then be removed from the imaging field and the guidewire introduced through the needle and driven approximately 1 cm. Using fluoroscopy, the position and direction of the wire can be checked and adjusted as it is driven in a dorsal to volar direction.

It is critical that the wrist is maintained in a flexed position until the distal end of the wire clears the radiocarpal joint to avoid bending the guidewire. **B.** The wire is withdrawn from the thumb base until the wrist can be extended and mini-fluoroscopy can be used to confirm the guidewire position along the central axis of scaphoid and fracture reduction.

ament and articular injury in scaphoid nonunions. In addition, the fracture site is inspected arthroscopically for evidence of healing, and the articular surface for evidence of degenerative changes.

With the patient in the supine position, the arm is exsanguinated, the elbow is flexed, and the wrist is po-

sitioned upright in a spring-scale-driven traction tower. Twelve pounds of traction is distributed via four finger traps to reduce the possibility of a traction injury. A fluoroscopy unit is placed horizontal to the floor and perpendicular to the wrist as the radiocarpal and mid-carpal joint are identified with imaging (Figure 15.5A,B).

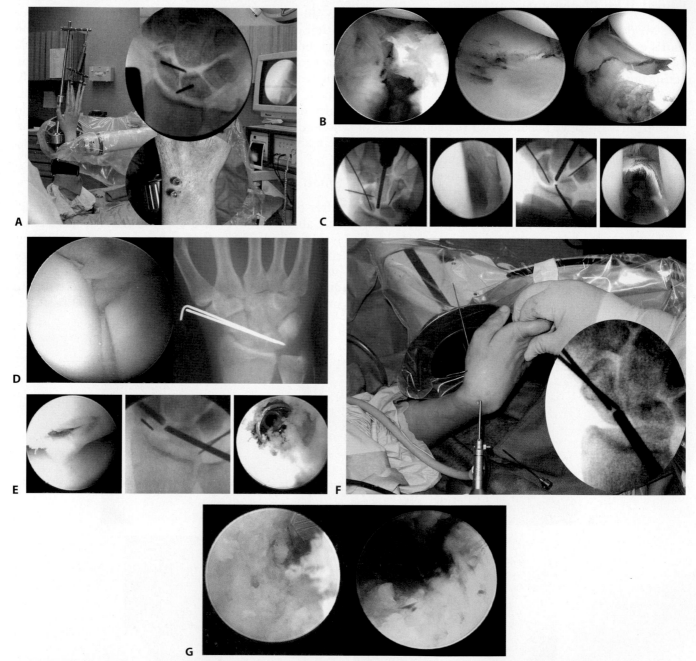

FIGURE 15.5. The goal of arthroscopy is to identify and treat liga-ment injuries, reduce and stabilize articular joint incongruities, and in acute fractures, to inspect the quality of the reduction directly. **A.** The arthroscope is placed in the radial midcarpal row. While large fracture displacements can be detected with fluoroscopy, smaller malalignments could easily be missed. **B.** An arthroscopic radial mid-carpal view, from left to right: displaced scaphoid fracture, minimal displacement of scaphoid, and reduced proximal pole fracture with avulsion of the dorsal lunate. Ligament tears with carpal fractures are not uncommon. **C.** Another radial midcarpal view shows two tears of scapholunate interosseous ligament. On the left is a grade IV tear that will permit passage of a small-joint arthroscope. On the

right is a grade III tear that permits the passage of a 2-mm probe. Small tears and flaps with stable joints are debrided back to a sta-ble rim (I, II). **D.** Partial tears with instability are reduced and pinned (II, III). Complete unstable tears (IV) are open-repaired. **E.** Arthro-scopy is used to confirm complete seating of headless screw. **F.** Small-joint arthroscopy permits the determination of the viability of the proximal scaphoid pole without risking further vascular injury from an open exploration. A small-joint angled arthroscope can be intro-duced into the reaming portal. Using fluoroscopy, its position is guided to the scaphoid base. **G.** With the arthroscope seated in the scaphoid proximal pole and the tourniquet deflated; punctate bleed-ing will soon appear if the bone is viable.

19-gauge needles are introduced into the wrist joint to identify the radiocarpal and midcarpal portals. This maneuver limits iatrogenic injury to the joint, which can result from multiple attempts to introduce a blunt trocar blindly. Once the portals have been successfully located and marked, the imaging unit is removed and the skin alone incised. A small, curved blunt hemostat is used to separate the soft tissue and enter the wrist joint. A blunt trocar is placed at the radial midcarpal portal, and a small-joint angled arthroscope is introduced. Additional 19-gauge needles are inserted to establish outflow. A probe is introduced at the ulnar midcarpal portal, and the competency of the carpal ligaments is evaluated by directly stressing their attachments to detect partial and complete tears. The probe is also placed in the 3-4 portal, immediately proximal to the radial midcarpal portal. With fluoroscopy, the sulcus, which defines the scapholunate ligament, can be identified and probed. With partial tears, the probe will be visualized by the arthroscope in the midcarpal portal as it passes from the radiocarpal joint into the midcarpal joint through a tear in the SLIO (scapholunate interosseous) ligament. Any carpal ligament injuries detected are graded using the Geissler grading system (Figure 15.5C). Grade I and II ligament injuries are treated with debridement and shrinkage alone. Grade III injuries are treated with debridement, and after fracture repair, carpal pinning for 6 weeks (Figure 15.5D,E). Grade IV ligament injuries require open repair of the dorsal SLIO ligament with bone anchors and carpal pinning. The need for the addition of a dorsal capsulardesis tether is determined by the quality of the acute repair after scaphoid fixation. Tears of

the triangular fibrocartilage complex are classified using the Palmer classification, and treated.[22]

Green felt that scaphoid bone viability was best determined at surgery. The scaphoid was directly inspected for punctate bleeding from the proximal scaphoid pole. Avascular necrosis was suspected with the absence of punctate bleeding from the proximal pole.[17] Green's scaphoid bone viability test can be performed arthroscopically, limiting unnecessary vascular and soft tissue injury. Using the central axis guidewire only, the proximal pole of the scaphoid is reamed. The wire is withdrawn to the fracture site, and the small-joint arthroscope is inserted into the base of the scaphoid in the previously reamed bone tract. The tourniquet is deflated, and the cancellous bone is inspected for punctate bleeding (Figure 15.5F,G). Inflow irrigation is momentarily stopped, while the time of the first appearance of bone bleeding is recorded.

Correction of Scaphoid Malalignment

Fractures with displacement are reduced with joy sticks fashioned from percutaneously inserted 0.062-inch Kirschner wires placed dorsally in both fracture fragments. Prior to reduction, the previously placed central axis guidewire is withdrawn volarly across the fracture site, and traction is removed. Often the major deformity observed is a flexion deformity of the fracture fragments. When the dorsal joy sticks are brought together, the flexion deformity of the scaphoid is corrected (Figure 15.6A). These maneuvers can be monitored using either lateral fluoroscopy and/or arthroscopy. With acute injury, it is enough to

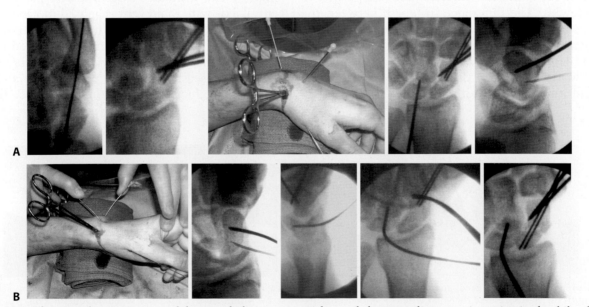

FIGURE 15.6. The central axis wire is withdrawn volarly across the fracture site. **A.** Stout joy sticks, constructed from 0.062 guidewires, are placed percutaneously, dorsally, and perpendicularly into the fracture fragments. **B.** Reduction is achieved using the joy sticks, and fracture alignment is maintained while the volar guidewire is driven from the distal pole into the proximal scaphoid pole, capturing and securing reduction. A difficult fracture can be reduced with a small curved hemostat introduced percutaneously.

reduce the fracture to reestablish normal scaphoid length. This is because there is no loss of volar bone cortex because the volar scaphoid fails in tension with hyperextension injuries. Impacted or severely displaced fractures require the percutaneous insertion of a small, curved hemostat into the fracture site to guide fracture relocation (Figure 15.6B). The hemostat can be introduced through a midcarpal or accessory portal. While the joy sticks maintain reduction, the volar guidewire is driven back proximally and dorsally into the proximal pole to capture the reduction. These fractures are often very unstable and require the placement of a second parallel wire to resist the bending forces and maintain alignment during reaming and screw implantation. Fractures of the scaphoid waist are most likely to result in a humpback deformity from displacement due to forward flexion. Fractures of the proximal pole are more inclined to displace in a translational plane. These fractures are more inclined to displace with disruption of the radioscapho-capitate ligament that crosses and supports the scaphoid waist when uninjured. With fracture reduction secure, the central axis guidewire is adjusted to ensure it is still positioned along the central axis.

Scaphoid Length and Screw Size

At the completion of arthroscopy, with fracture reduction and guidewire position confirmed, the screw size must now be selected. To accomplish this, the scaphoid length must be determined. The wrist is flexed, and the guidewire at the base of the thumb is driven dorsally. The wire is adjusted until the trailing end is in the subchondral bone of the distal scaphoid pole. A second wire of equal length is placed percutaneously at the proximal scaphoid pole and parallel to the guidewire. The difference in length between the trailing end of each wire is the scaphoid length. The screw length selected should be 4 mm less than the scaphoid length. This permits 2 mm of clearance of the screw at each end of the scaphoid, thus ensuring complete implantation without screw exposure (Fig-ure 15.7). The most common complication of percutaneous screw implantation is implantation of a screw that is too long. This complication can be avoided by selecting a screw length that provides for 2 mm of clearance between the screw's end and the proximal and distal scaphoid cortex. The screw length selected is 4 mm shorter than the scaphoid length. This permits the complete implantation of a headless compression screw in bone without exposure.

Now that the length of the screw has been determined, the width must be selected. The forces acting on a scaphoid waist fracture are bending forces. If untreated, this results in a flexed and foreshortened scaphoid. The scaphoid waist fracture can be imaged as two cylinder blocks for the purpose of biomechanical testing. To resist forward bending of these cylinders, the widest possible rod is needed at the fracture site. In selecting a screw type for scaphoid fracture fixation, the most important feature will be the width of the screw at the fracture site. A small increase in the radius leads to a significant increase in strength. In vitro cadaveric biomechanical studies have confirmed that the widest screws provide the strongest fixation. One concern about larger screws introduced dorsally is the consequences of the resulting cartilage defect, but these defects have been shown to heal over with cartilage in time, without degenerative changes.

Percutaneous Bone Grafting

If a scaphoid fracture or nonunion requires bone grafting, introduce a guidewire percutaneously into the scaphoid's proximal pole and drive the wire along the central axis of correctly aligned scaphoid using fluoroscopy. As described earlier, determine the scaphoid's length. Next, introduce a second wire parallel to the central axis wire to prevent scaphoid motion or translation at the fracture site. After introduction of this second wire, maintain the wrist in a flexed position and adjust the central axis wire so that its ends are equally exposed between the dorsal wrist and radial volar thumb. Incise the skin, and introduce the can-

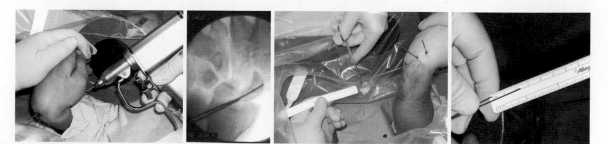

FIGURE 15.7. The wrist is flexed, and the guidewire is advanced dorsally until the trailing end of the volar wire is level with the distal scaphoid cortex. Scaphoid length is determined by placing a second guidewire at the base of the proximal scaphoid, next to the exposed dorsal guidewire. The difference between these wires is the scaphoid length. The screw length is determined by selecting a screw 4 mm shorter than the scaphoid length. This will permit 2 mm of clearance of the screw at each end of the scaphoid and complete implantation without screw exposure to cartilage.

nulated driver percutaneously into the proximal scaphoid along its central axis, using fluoroscopy to monitor the level of reaming. Next, remove the reamer and withdraw the central wire to the level of the fracture site, and curette the nonunion site by introducing the curette via the dorsal drill hole into the nonunion site. Using an 8-gauge bone biopsy needle, harvest bone as cores from either the iliac crest or the distal radius. Next, introduce the 8-gauge bone biopsy cannula over the central axis guidewire into the scaphoid proximal pole and again with the wire to the fracture site. Through this cannula, introduce previously harvested cancellous bone plug until the bone cavity on the radiolucent image has been replaced by a radiopaque image of similar texture to that of the surrounding bone (Figure 15.8).

Alternatively, Geissler devised a cannulated putty pusher system (Acumed, Hillsboro, OR) for injection of demineralized bone matrix or cancellous bone chips for scaphoid nonunions (Figure 15.9). In this system, a guidewire is placed down the center of the axis of the scaphoid, and the bone is drilled. The cannulated trocar is slid over the guidewire into the scaphoid nonunion. The guidewire is removed, the demineralized bone putty (Gens-Sci, Irving, CA) is injected into the cannula, and the trocar pushes the putty into the nonunion site. The guidewire is reinserted as the cannula is removed. The headless cannulated screw is then placed over the guidewire. This system may be used for percutaneous injuries of demineralized bone matrix in other fracture nonunions throughout the body.

After the introduction of bone graft into the scaphoid, advance the central axis guidewire and perform a second drilling prior to screw implantation. Inserting the screw and advancing it into an unprepared graft will force the graft toward the scaphoid cortex and risk exploding out the outer scaphoid cortex. This is avoided by reaming with a sharp drill prior to screw implantation. Implant the headless cannulated screw along the central scaphoid axis. If rigid fixation has not been achieved with screw fixation alone, additional fixation is required. This can be achieved with a 0.062-inch guidewire placed from the scaphoid into the capitate. This will be used to temporarily block midcarpal motion and reduce forces acting on the scaphoid fracture site.

Rigid Fixation with Headless Cannulated Screw

Once the scaphoid is correctly aligned and its length has been determined, the guidewire is adjusted so that its ends are equally exposed between the dorsal wrist and volar radial thumb. This prevents the wire from becoming dislodged during bone reaming and screw

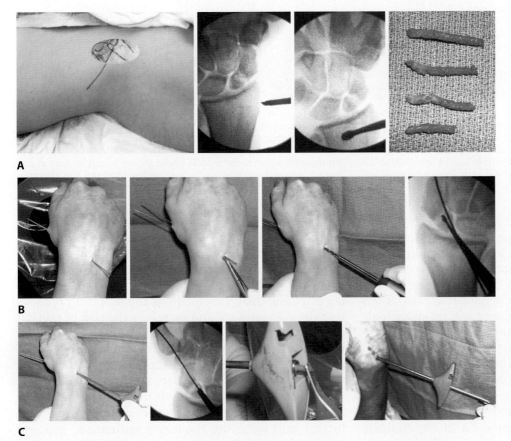

FIGURE 15.8. A. Using a bone biopsy needle, cancellous bone is harvested from the iliac crest or the distal radius. Using fluoroscopy, the nonunion site can be debrided while maintaining the fibrous envelope around the scaphoid nonunion site. **B.** Percutaneously introduce a guidewire along the scaphoid central axis. Hand drill the scaphoid using a cannulated reamer along the scaphoid central axis. Withdraw the reamer and introduce the curette into the scaphoid to the level of the nonunion site. **C.** Introduce an 8-gauge bone biopsy cannula over the central axis guidewire into the scaphoid proximal pole. Through this cannula, introduce a previously harvested cancellous bone plug until the bone cavity has been completely filled.

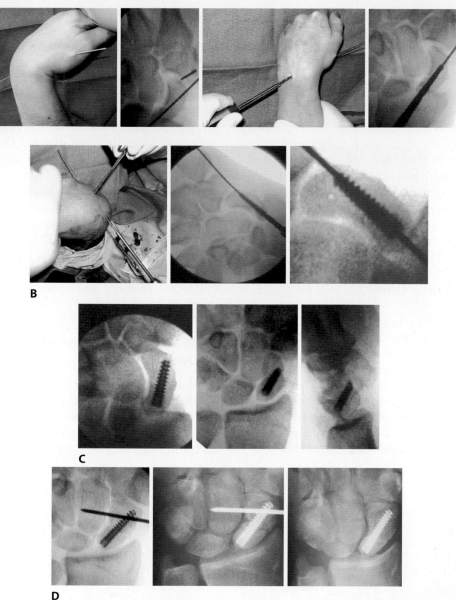

FIGURE 15.9. A. The scaphoid is prepared with a hand reamer. **B.** Fluoroscopy is used to check the position and depth of the drill. It is critical not to ream beyond 2 mm of the opposite cortex. **C.** Fluoroscopy is used to confirm the correct position of the fixation device. If rigid fixation has not been achieved with screw fixation alone, additional fixation is required. **D.** This can be achieved with a 0.062-inch guidewire placed from the scaphoid into the capitate. This will be used to temporaily block midcarpal motion and reduce forces acting on the scaphoid fracture site. In this panel the left picture is an intraoperative photo, the middle photo shows partial healing at one month, and at 2 months future healing has occurred and the midcarpal locking wire is removed to permit wrist rehabilitation.

implantation. It is critical that the wrist maintains a flexed position to prevent the wire from bending. Otherwise, drilling and screw placement will be difficult.

Dorsal implantation of a headless compression screw is recommended for scaphoid fractures of the proximal pole and volar implantation for distal pole fractures, as this permits maximum fracture compression. Fractures of the waist may be fixed from a dorsal or volar approach, as long as the screw is implanted along the central scaphoid axis. Blunt dissection along the guidewire exposes a tract to the dorsal wrist capsule and scaphoid base. The scaphoid is prepared by drilling a path 2 mm short of the opposite

scaphoid cortex with a cannulated hand drill. This will permit the implantation of a headless compression screw completely within the scaphoid. It is critical to use fluoroscopy to check the position and depth of the drill. Overdrilling the scaphoid reduces fracture compression and increases the risk of motion at the fracture site. A standard Acutrak screw is advanced under fluoroscopic guidance along the central axis with the fracture surfaces firmly opposed to within 1 to 2 mm of the opposite cortex. This provides excellent compression. If the screw is advanced to the distal cortex, attempts to advance the screw further will force the fracture fragments to gap and

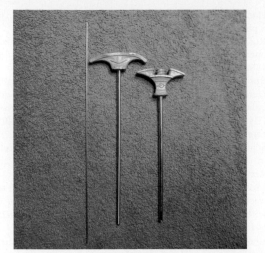

FIGURE 15.10. Cannulated putty pusher system designed by Geissler to inject demineralized bone matrix percutaneously.

separate. With unstable fractures, a joy stick is left in the distal scaphoid fragment for both reaming and screw implantation. As the screw is implanted, a counterforce is exerted through the joy stick, compressing both fracture fragments and ensuring rigid fixation (Figure 15.10).

With small proximal pole fractures or avulsions, there is increasing difficulty in obtaining rigid fixation with headless screw fixation. Having fewer than four screw threads crossing the fracture site leads to a rapid drop-off in pull-out strength.[24] There is also a possible risk of fragmentation with standard screw implantation; under these circumstances a smaller screw should be considered, and the wrist protected. With avulsion injuries, consideration should be given to fixation by temporarily sandwiching the avulsed fracture fragment between the distal scaphoid and lunate with a headless compression screw. This screw will be removed when CT scan confirms healing.

Unstable fractures may not achieve rigid fixation with screw implantation alone, and other temporary constructs may be required. Flexion forces act on the distal scaphoid and extension forces act on the proximal scaphoid through the proximal carpal row.[25] These forces can be balanced by the placement of a 0.062-inch wire from the scaphoid into the capitate. This temporarily blocks midcarpal motion and reduces forces acting on the scaphoid fracture site (Figure 15.9C,D).

Distal scaphoid fractures require the volar implantation of the screw for maximum compression. Guidewire placement and length determination are accomplished in a manner identical to the dorsal technique, except that the central axis carries the guidewire through the trapezium. To prepare the scaphoid for screw placement, both the trapezium and scaphoid are reamed with the cannulated hand drill;

this ensures that the screw is implanted along the central scaphoid axis. This violation of the scaphotrapezial joint is minimal. The remainder of the technique is identical to the dorsal procedure, including screw selection, drilling, and implantation. This volar technique differs from other volar techniques that advocate eccentric screw placement. After screw placement, the guidewire is removed, and wrist fluoroscopy confirms screw position, fracture reduction, and rigid fixation. Arthroscopy at this time can also confirm reduction and complete seating of the screw.

Key Points on Arthroscopic Scaphoid Fixation via a Dorsal Percutaneous Approach

1. Scaphoid fractures and nonunions can be evaluated and graded using imaging (e.g., radiographs, CT, MRI), arthroscopy, and bone biopsy.
2. The central axis of the scaphoid is the key position for the placement of a guidewire in a reduced scaphoid.
3. To identify the central scaphoid axis, the wrist is pronated and flexed until the scaphoid is seen as a circle. The center of the circle is the target point for insertion of the guidewire into the proximal pole of the scaphoid.
4. The guidewire is driven in a dorsal to volar direction, so that the wire exits at the radial base of the thumb.
5. The reduction of the fracture and positioning of the guidewire in the scaphoid are accomplished using mini-fluoroscopy and arthroscopy.
6. Arthroscopy permits the detection, grading, and treatment of carpal bone and ligament injuries.
7. Screw length is determined using two identical parallel wires. The difference in length between these wires is the length of the scaphoid. The screw length is 4 mm shorter than this calculated scaphoid length.
8. Stop reaming 2 mm from the distal cortex of the scaphoid.
9. Implant the screw in the scaphoid at the level to which the scaphoid has been drilled.
10. Rigid fixation may require additional implants.

POSTOPERATIVE CARE

Immediate postoperative care includes a bulky compressive hand dressing and splint. Pain control is managed with narcotics, nonsteroidal antiinflammatory medications, and elevation. The use of thermal cooler pads appears to reduce the need for pain medications. Early finger exercises are encouraged to reduce swelling. The therapist fashions a removable volar splint that holds the wrist and hand in a functional position at the first postoperative visit. All patients are started on a strengthening program. Axially loading the fracture site now secured with an intramedullary screw stimulates healing. Postoperative radiographs are obtained at the first postoperative visit and at 6-week intervals. When fracture healing is suspected, usually at 4 to 6 weeks postoperatively, a CT scan of the scaphoid with 1-mm cuts (PA and lateral) is obtained to evaluate fracture healing. This is repeated every 6 weeks until final union is established. Bridging bone at the fracture site on CT or standard radiographs signifies fracture healing. It is important to understand that patients are often pain free prior to CT evidence of healing. Contact sports and heavy labor are restricted until fracture healing is confirmed by CT. Fractures of the wrist without complete ligament injuries are started on an immediate range of motion protocol, while proximal pole fractures are protected for one month prior to initiation of therapy. We do not routinely cast our scaphoid fractures postoperatively, but candidates for additional protection are evaluated on a case-by-case basis. The postoperative care of scaphoid nonunions is sometimes different from that of acute fractures. For nonunions of the scaphoid wrist, rigid fixation can often be achieved using a stout intramedullary device without additional immobilization. Proximal pole nonunions or wrist nonunions in osteoporetic bone are at a mechanical disadvantage, and rigid fixation can be difficult to achieve. These injuries are protected with a splint or short-arm cast for 4 to 6 weeks until bone union has been established. Only Grade III ligament injuries were protected for 6 weeks. An early strengthening program is also encouraged for early recovery of hand function.

CONCLUSION

At first, percutaneous techniques of scaphoid fracture reduction and fixation may appear daunting. However, with experience, they offer a powerful and versatile capability that is demonstrating promising results in the treatment of notoriously difficult fractures and nonunions. Development of small-joint arthroscopic skill is one of the essential steps in mastering this method of scaphoid fracture treatment.

References

1. Slade JF 3rd, Grauer JN, Mahoney JD. Arthroscopic reduction and percutaneous fixation of scaphoid fractures with a novel dorsal technique. *Orthop Clin North Am.* 2001;32(2):247–261.
2. Bond CD, Shin AY, McBride MT, et al. Percutaneous screw fixation or cast immobilization for nondisplaced scaphoid fractures. *J Bone Joint Surg Am* 2001;83A(4):483–488.
3. Haddad FS, Goddard NJ. Acute percutaneous scaphoid fixation: a pilot study. *J Bone Joint Surg Br* 1998;80(1):95–99.
4. Russe O. Fracture of the carpal navicular. Diagnosis, nonoperative treatment and operative treatment. *J Bone Joint Surg* 1960;42A:759–768.
5. Robbins RR, Ridge O, Carter PR. Iliac crest bone grafting and Herbert screw fixation of nonunions of the scaphoid with avascular proximal poles. *J Hand Surg Am* 1995;20:818–831.
6. Filan SL, Herbert TJ. Herbert screw fixation of scaphoid fractures. *J Bone Joint Surg Br* 1996;78:519–529.
7. Schuind F, Haentjens P, Van Innis F, et al. Prognostic factors in the treatment of carpal scaphoid nonunions. *J Hand Surg Am* 1999;24(4):761–776.
8. Trumble TE, Gilbert M, Murray LW, et al. Displaced scaphoid fractures treated with open reduction and internal fixation with a cannulated screw. *J Bone Joint Surg Am* 2000;82(5):633–641.
9. Geissler WB, Freeland AE, Savoie FH, et al. Intracarpal soft-tissue lesions associated with an intra-articular fracture of the distal end of the radius. *J Bone Joint Surg Am* 1996;78(3):357–365.
10. Langhoff O, Andersen JL. Consequences of late immobilization of scaphoid fractures. *J Hand Surg Br* 1988;13(1):77–79.
11. Barton NJ. Apparent and partial non-union of the scaphoid. *J Hand Surg Br* 1996;21(4):496–500.
12. Shah J, Jones WA. Factors affecting the outcome in 50 cases of scaphoid nonunion treated with Herbert screw fixation. *J Hand Surg Br* 1998;23B:680–685.
13. Ledoux P, Chahidi N, Moermans JP, et al. Percutaneous Herbert screw osteosynthesis of the scaphoid bone. *Acta Orthop Belg* 1995;61(1):43–47.
14. Wozasek GE, Moser KD. Percutaneous screw fixation of fractures of the scaphoid. *J Bone Joint Surg* 1991;73:138–142.
15. Cosio MQ, Camp RA. Percutaneous pinning of symptomatic scaphoid nonunions. *J Hand Surg Am* 1986;11(3):350–355.
16. Trumble TE. Avascular necrosis after scaphoid fracture: a correlation of magnetic resonance imaging and histology. *J Hand Surg Am* 1990;15(4):557–564.
17. Green DP. The effect of avascular necrosis on Russe bone grafting for scaphoid nonunion. *J Hand Surg Am* 1985;10:597–605.
18. Slade JF, Geissler WP, Gutow AP, et al. Percutaneous internal fixation of selected scaphoid non-unions via an arthroscopic assisted dorsal approach. *J Bone Joint Surg Am* in press.
19. Merrell GA, Wolfe SW, Slade JF 3rd. Treatment of scaphoid nonunions: quantitative meta-analysis of the literature. *J Hand Surg Am* 2002;27(4):685–691.
20. Cooney WP, Linscheid RL, Dobyns JH. Scaphoid fractures. Problems associated with nonunion and avascular necrosis. *Orthop Clin North Am* 1984;15:381–391.
21. Cooney WPD, Dobyns JH, Linscheid RL. Nonunion of the scaphoid: analysis of the results from bone grafting. *J Hand Surg Am* 1980;5:343–354.
22. Palmer AK. Triangular fibrocartilage complex lesions: a classification. *J Hand Surg Am* 1989;14(4):594–606.
23. Toby EB, Butler TE, McCormack TJ. A comparison of fixation screws for the scaphoid during application of cyclic bending loads. *J Bone Joint Surg Am* 1997;79A:1190–1197.
24. Gutow A, Noonan J, Westmoreland G, et al. Biomechanical comparison of fixation methods for proximal pole scaphoid fractures. Presenetd at American Society for Surgery of the Hand, Seattle, WA, 2000.
25. Kobayashi M, Garcia-Elias M, Nagy L, et al. Axial loading induces rotation of the proximal carpal row bones around unique screw-displacement axes. *J Biomech* 1997;30(11-12):1165–1167.

16

Management of Articular Cartilage Defects

Christophe Mathoulin and Susan Nasser-Sharif

Cartilaginous defects of the carpus are frequently the source of wrist pain. These defects can increase in size and thickness with wrist movement and function. These lesions are often the result of trauma, but they may occur as part of a degenerative process. We will not discuss the lesions associated with rheumatoid arthritis, as these involve not only cartilage but bone and tendon as well. They are often the result of dislocation or intra-articular synovitis. Wrist arthroscopy allows the diagnosis of these cartilaginous lesions before they may be visible by standard radiographic techniques such as plain radiographs, arthrography, CT scan, or MRI.[1]

It is often difficult to predict the treatment of these articular lesions. Wrist arthroscopy allows the removal of cartilaginous fragments or loose bony particles that may be the source of pain. It also allows debridement of the lesions if they are small. In addition, it allows the localization and the determination of the size of the lesion. This is invaluable when planning treatment.

REMOVAL OF FOREIGN BODIES

Foreign bodies are often the result of cartilaginous or bony lesions. These lesions are usually secondary to repetitive trauma, intra-articular fractures, or metabolic disturbance. Foreign bodies move within the wrist joint. They can cause abnormal contact between the carpal bones and occasionally between the carpal bones and the radius. Finally, their presence may lead to abnormal contact and induce the formation of further cartilaginous lesions. The removal of these foreign bodies is therefore therapeutic, frequently simple, and benefits the patient. The preoperative workup may include plain radiographs, CT scan, and MRI. Often the foreign body is not recognized until the arthroscopy; it is then that removal is possible. Extraction of the body is often made difficult by its size. It is frequently necessary to break the body into pieces using a forceps or bur. In order to accomplish this, it is sometimes helpful to fix the fragment temporarily by placing a needle transcutaneously. Foreign bodies

in the radiocarpal joint are often secondary to fractures, pseudoarthrosis, necrosis of the proximal pole of the scaphoid, or necrosis of the lunate as seen in Kienbock's disease. Foreign bodies can also be seen after a scapholunate or lunotriquetral dissociation (Figure 16.1). Finally, ulnar abutment resulting from a distal radius fracture with subsequent shortening may also lead to cartilaginous debris, especially on the dorsomedial surface of the lunate.

At the level of the midcarpal joint, cartilaginous fragments are often seen secondary to scaphotrapezotrapezoid arthritis (Figure 16.2). In addition, the sequellae of scaphoid pseudoarthrosis or scapholunate dissociation leading to the classic scaphoid nonunion advanced collapse (SNAC) or scapholunate advanced collapse (SLAC) wrist will often lead to cartilaginous fragments within the joint.

Rarely, there may be cartilaginous fragments in the distal radioulnar joint. This may occur if there has been a dislocation of the distal radioulnar joint with bone or cartilage fragments that detach and become lodged between the radius and the ulnar head.

Removal of the foreign bodies is only one of the therapeutic solutions possible using wrist arthroscopy.[1] If there is an associated mechanical synovitis, a synovectomy should be undertaken as well as an arthroscopic washout. The treatment of the associated cartilaginous lesions is the final touch during the arthroscopy. The intra-articular washout often helps to diminish the pain, particularly when the lesion is small and posttraumatic. It is also more effective if the lesion is recent.

DIAGNOSIS AND TREATMENT OF INTRA-ARTICULAR LESIONS

Preoperative Planning for Conventional Open Surgery

It is not unusual to have normal plain radiographs and yet to find a cartilaginous lesion in a contact zone between two bones that is responsible for the pain. It is not uncommon that the surgical plan needs intraop-

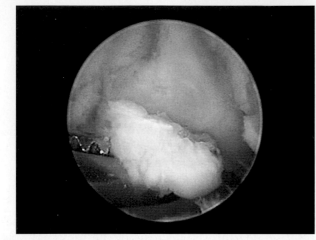

FIGURE 16.1. Removal of foreign body in radiocarpal joint after scapholunate dissociation with small fragment of dorsal lunate.

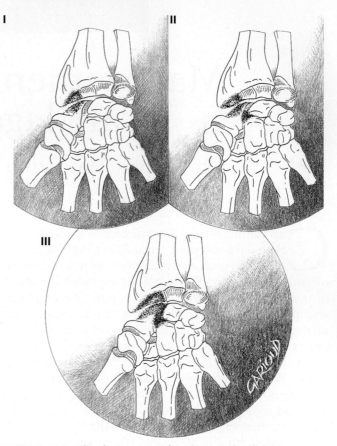

FIGURE 16.3. The three stages of evolution of arthritis in SNAC or SLAC wrist.

erative modification because of a cartilaginous lesion that was not noticed preoperatively on plain radiographs. This may change a simple curative surgery into a palliative effort. Wrist arthroscopy, simple to perform and with few postoperative complications, allows one to avoid this situation. It is very useful in treating certain disease processes. For example, the evolution of arthritis in the classic SNAC or SLAC wrist is always the same (Figure 16.3). The first lesions are seen on the radial styloid and the lateral surface of the scaphoid. The next step involves the head of the capitate along with the deep surface of the scaphoid proximal pole and the space between the scaphoid and the lunate. In the end, the entire scaphoid fossa of the radius becomes involved in the arthritic process, along with the lateral surface of the scaphoid. At a later stage, one that is rarely attained, the whole radiocarpal joint may be involved.

KIENBOCK'S DISEASE

Kienbock's disease of the lunate often necessitates a complex surgical approach aimed at reducing pain and revascularizing the lunate. A CT scan or MRI is often needed. Nevertheless, these may be alarming and may convince the surgeon to proceed with a palliative procedure when it is possible to attempt a bony reconstruction. Wrist arthroscopy allows one to evaluate the cartilage of the carpal bones, including the proximal row, especially the lunate. We use the 3-4 portal to place the arthroscope and the 4-5 portal to place the instruments. By flexing and extending the wrist, one can study the proximal row as well as the scapholunate and lunotriquetral ligaments. It is often useful to switch the positions of the arthroscope and the probe. Sometimes the classic tests suggest that there is no bony support, yet during arthroscopy one can see that the cartilage of the lunate is healthy (Figure 16.4A–C). The act of placing the wrist in traction in order to perform the arthroscopy may diminish the load on the lunate and allow it to assume a more normal shape. This will give the proximal row a normal configuration. With the help of a probe, one can feel that there is no bony support for the lunate cartilage. By using the radial midcarpal portal, one can examine the cartilage of the midcarpal joint, especially that of

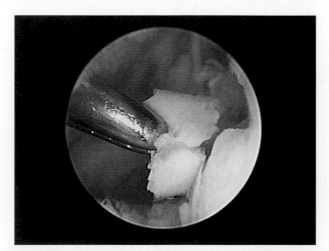

FIGURE 16.2. Removal of small piece of bone in scaphotrapezio-trapezoid joint secondary to STT arthritis.

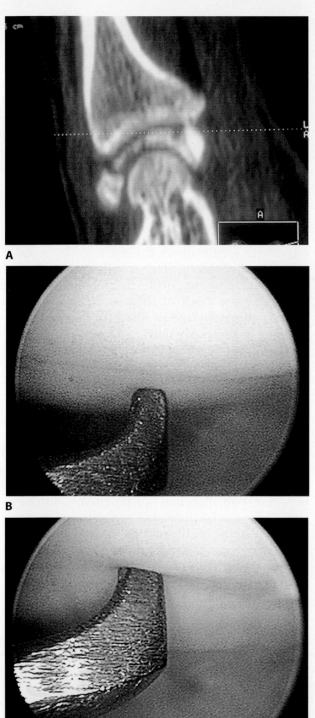

PSEUDARTHROSIS OF THE SCAPHOID

The treatment of pseudoarthrosis of the scaphoid is difficult and controversial. The treatment options are varied and range from simple screw fixation to reconstruction with a vascularized bone graft. Nevertheless, before undertaking the task of reconstruction, one must ensure that the articular surfaces are intact. Placing the arthroscope in the 3-4 portal will allow the exploration of the articular surface of the radial styloid and the dorsolateral surface of the scaphoid. By using the radial midcarpal portal, the arthroscope allows the examination of the distal cartilage of the scaphoid, as well as the cartilage of the capitate and the lunate. If there is isolated involvement of the radial styloid, a styloidectomy may be performed during the same operative sitting. It is also possible to discover a capitate devoid of cartilage with mirror lesions on the lunate. This type of lesion is a contraindication to reconstruction of the scaphoid.

DISSOCIATION OF THE SCAPHOLUNATE OR LUNOTRIQUETRAL LIGAMENTS

Rupture of the scapholunate or lunotriquetral ligaments leads to an alteration of the biomechanics of the wrist with changes in the zones of contact. This often leads to arthritis. Reconstructive options are difficult and controversial. Before considering the reconstructive options, one must evaluate the state of the cartilage of the carpal bones and the radius. With the help of the classic 3-4 and 4-5 radiocarpal portals, or the 6-R radiocarpal and the radial midcarpal portals, one can explore without difficulty the entire cartilaginous surface of the carpus. One can search for lesions of the radial styloid, as well as lesions between the scaphoid and the lunate and between the lunate and triquetrum (Figure 16.5). If there is a significant disruption of the scapholunate ligament, one is able to "drive through" the

FIGURE 16.4. A. Tomodensitometry showing complete bony destruction of lunate in Kienbock's disease. **B.** Arthroscopic view showing the normal aspect of cartilage in radiocarpal joint, with a normal scapholunate joint. **C.** Arthroscopic view showing a depression in lunate cartilage because there is no bony support.

the lunate. In cases where the cartilage is normal between the scaphoid and the lunate, and between the scaphoid and the triquetrum, a bony reconstruction with revascularization can be considered.

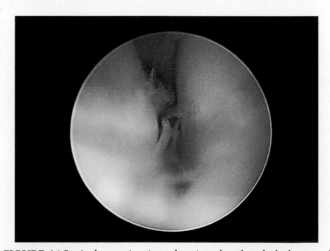

FIGURE 16.5. Arthoscopic view showing the chondral change of the scapholunate in the midcarpal joint. In this beginning stage, there are only fringes without cartilaginous defect.

scapholunate interval from the radiocarpal to the mid-carpal joint. The presence of arthritis is a contraindication to ligament reconstruction.

THE SPECIAL CASE OF DISTAL RADIOULNAR JOINT INVOLVEMENT

After a fracture of the distal radius, the radius may shorten, and this can lead to an abutment between the ulnar head and the lunate. Depending upon the degree of abutment and the amount of radial shortening, an ulnar shortening osteotomy may be indicated. It is important to ensure that the cartilage between the distal radius and the ulnar head is intact before repositioning the ulna. In order to do this, one may perform a classic arthroscopy of the radiocarpal joint, as well as of the distal radioulnar joint. To accomplish arthroscopy of the distal radioulnar joint, one must use a portal that enters the distal radioulnar joint directly. This portal is 1.5 cm proximal with respect to the 4-5 portal.

PROXIMAL ROW CARPECTOMY

It is possible to consider performing a proximal row carpectomy (PRC) using an arthroscope, even if this is a long and difficult procedure. Prior to proceeding with a PRC, regardless of the method, it is important to examine the cartilage of the head of the capitate. It is impossible to consider a PRC if the distal row shows articular involvement. Arthroscopy of the radiocarpal joint allows inspection of the lunate fossa in order to ensure that the cartilage is intact. Resection of the involved arthritic bones can be accomplished through the arthroscope, with the understanding that this is only a temporary solution. A bur is used to resect the bone until the subchondral bone is reached. One morcelizes the bone in order to resect it completely without damaging the surrounding cartilage. The advantage of this technique is that it prevents damage to the extrinsic ligaments and allows early mobilization. These indications are rare.

Shaving of Cartilaginous Lesions

Direct visualization permitted by arthroscopy has led to classification of cartilaginous lesions (Table 16.1). This differs from the classic radiographic classification,[2] which is based on lesions visible on plain ra-diographs. This implies complete loss of cartilage and focuses on subchondral lesions and associated bony changes. Arthroscopy allows the diagnosis of chondropathy long before these bony changes occur. The treatment options are therefore different, and this classification allows for the prevention of progression of these lesions. This classification, modified from Outerbridge's classification, takes into consideration cartilaginous lesions that are evaluated by direct vision, often before they can be detected radiographically (Figure 16.6).[3,4]

GRADE 1

This is composed of simple depression of the cartilage often with continuity of the surface. The probe demonstrates that the cartilage is soft; at this stage, there is no specific treatment for the chondropathy (Figure 16.7). In some cases, if there is a zone of increased stress, a preventive procedure may be performed. For example, a radial styloidectomy may be indicated if there is grade 1 chondropathy involving the proximal lateral cartilage of the scaphoid.

GRADE 2

This is the stage where the cartilage develops fringes. The cartilage begins to break down due to friction. These fringes float inside the joint (Figure 16.8). This is the stage where shaving may be helpful. The goal of shaving is to reduce the friction during movement between two irregular cartilaginous surfaces. By smoothing the cartilaginous surfaces, one also has the chance to diminish the normal inflammatory response that follows cartilage breakdown. As with grade 1 chondropathy, it is important to eliminate the cause of the chondropathy whenever possible.

GRADE 3

In this stage the cartilage detaches in a flap that can contain some subchondral bone (Figure 16.9). The cartilaginous flap is often posttraumatic. Treatment of this flap depends on the underlying bone and the remaining cartilage. If removal is attempted, it should be done with a suction punch or fine scissors (Figure 16.10). The fragment is then removed like a foreign body. A shaver is used only to smooth the cartilage depression.

GRADE 4

This consists of a cartilaginous defect with exposed underlying subchondral bone (Figure 16.11). At this stage, a shaver is useless. Certain authors suggest drilling the subchondral bone in order to promote bleeding. The goal is to have the clot transform to a patch of fibrocartilage. We reserve this technique for lesions less than or equal to 5 mm. With the help of

TABLE 16.1. Classification of Cartilaginous Lesions.

Grade	Description
I	Localized cartilage softening
II	Fibrillated articular surfaces
III	Thicker flap of cartilage
IV	Full-thickness defect of cartilage

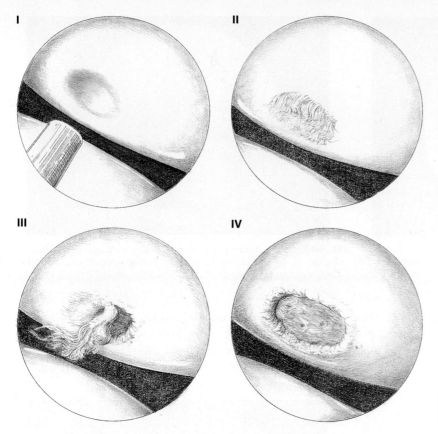

FIGURE 16.6. Diagram showing the four grades of arthroscopic classification of cartilaginous lesions.

a shaver and a curette, the edges of the defect are debrided. A small bur is used to produce bleeding in the subchondral bone. The wrist is completely immobilized for one week and is then placed in a splint for 3 weeks in order to limit movements that put pressure on the treated area.

Shaving is not a treatment by itself. It allows the debridement of fringes or flaps of cartilage (grade 2 or 3) (Figure 16.12A,B). If the cause of the lesion was a direct blow, then the improvement after shaving is definitive. If, however, the cause has abnormal pressure between two bony surfaces, then shaving is only temporarily effective.[5–7] In this case, shaving is not a cure. Shaving should be combined with another classic treatment such as stabilization of the bony pieces or another secondary palliative procedure. A denervation associated with a lavage-shaving can be an elegant solution for certain cases of advanced chondropathy. Oc-

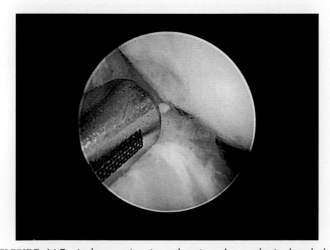

FIGURE 16.7. Arthroscopic view showing the grade 1 chondral change of the scaphoid in the radiocarpal joint. In this stage, there is a simple depression with continuity of cartilage.

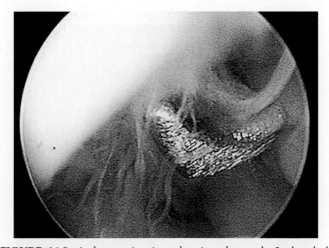

FIGURE 16.8. Arthroscopic view showing the grade 2 chondral change of the scaphoid in the radiocarpal joint. In this stage, fringes of cartilage float into the joint.

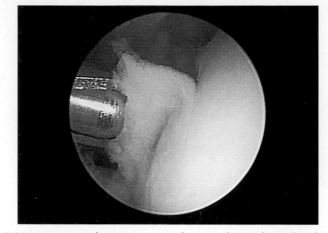

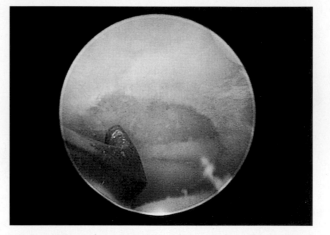

FIGURE 16.9. Arthroscopic view showing the grade 3 chondral change of the distal scaphoid in the midcarpal joint with a flap of cartilage.

FIGURE 16.11. Arthroscopic view showing the grade 4 chondral change of proximal trapezium in scapotrapeziotrapezoid joint. There is a cartilaginous defect, and the subchondral bone is exposed.

casionally, arthroscopy permits the treatment of the cause of the chondropathy. In such cases, arthroscopy is the only intervention.

Specific Cases

RADIAL STYLOIDECTOMY

Cartilaginous lesions may involve the radial styloid and the adjacent scaphoid. These lesions can appear following a direct blow or a fracture of the scaphoid. The most frequent cause, however, is a dissociation of the scapholunate ligament (disruption or distension). The scaphoid, therefore, regularly abuts the radial styloid. This leads to changes in the cartilage and subsequent pain. Weight-lifting frequently leads to this type of injury. At the end of a throwing arc, the arm is under tension, with the wrist in radial deviation supporting a significant weight, often greater than 100 kg. This position leads to multiple repetitive mi-

crotraumas to the radial styloid. Arthroscopy allows for the diagnosis of these lesions. The arthroscope is placed in the 3-4 radiocarpal portal. One can find a grade 2 lesion of the radial styloid and grade 1 of the

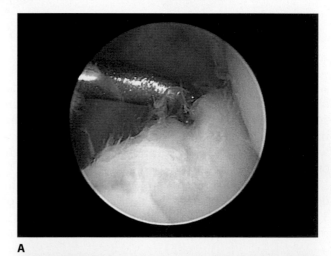

A

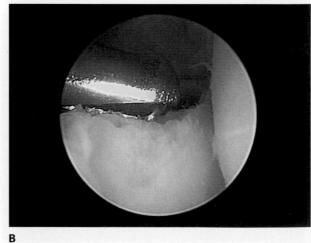

B

FIGURE 16.12. A. Arthroscopic view showing the grade 2 chondral change of the distal scaphoid in the STT joint. **B.** Arthroscopic view showing the distal scaphoid cartilage after debridement by shaving.

FIGURE 16.10. Arthroscopic view showing the removal of cartilaginous flap with a shaver.

scaphoid. Using a 1-2 radiocarpal portal, a bur is placed to perform the styloidectomy under direct vision. The arthroscopic approach allows for immediate mobilization and relief of pain.

RESECTION OF THE DISTAL ULNA

Shortening of the radius often follows a fracture of the distal radius, which can lead to abnormal contact between the distal ulna and the lunate. This abutment is worsened with radial deviation and leads to deterioration of the cartilage, with subsequent pain. The arthroscope is placed in the 3-4 portal to make the initial evaluation. It is not rare to see grade 4 changes on the lunate. If the wrist is ulnar positive by less than 5 mm, then one can propose a distal ulnar resection using the arthroscope. A bur is placed in the 6-R radiocarpal portal. This allows the resection to take place under direct vision (Figure 16.13A,B). It is frequently necessary to switch the positions of the arthroscope and the bur during the procedure. There are two important rules during this procedure. First, in order to achieve a complete resection, pronation and supina-

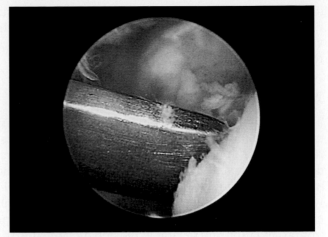

FIGURE 16.14. Arthroscopic view showing the resection of scapho-trapezoidal exostoses with a small chisel.

tion of the wrist are mandatory. By pronating and supinating, one avoids leaving irregular bony prominences. Second, the distal radioulnar joint must be preserved. Placing the arthroscope in the 6-R position allows evaluation of the adequacy of ulnar resection by comparing it to the height of the distal radius.

RESECTION OF EXOSTOSES OF THE STT JOINT

Arthritis involving the scaphotrapeziotrapezoid joint is often very painful. The usual treatment is an arthrodesis of the STT joint. This modifies the carpal dynamics and may lead to the appearance of arthritic changes proximally. Another treatment consists of resection of the trapezium. Wrist arthroscopy can permit the debridement of this joint; in particular, it allows for the resection of painful exostoses that often bridge the scaphotrapezial and the scaphotrapezoidal joints. The arthroscope is placed in the radial midcarpal portal. Using a needle, the STT joint is localized. Instruments are then placed in the STT portal (1-2 midcarpal portal) created at the site of the needle. This is situated ulnar to the extensor pollicis longus (EPL), along the axis of the radial border of the index metacarpal. With the help of a bur or small chisel, the exostosis is resected (Figure 16.14). It is often located at the dorsal aspect of the STT joint. The resection of the exostosis does not cure the arthritis, but it may lead to significant improvement in the pain. In addition, no postoperative immobilization is necessary.

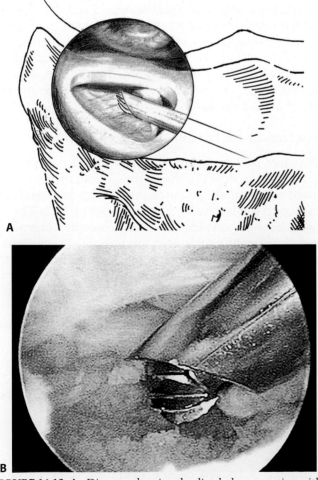

FIGURE 16.13. A. Diagram showing the distal ulnar resection with a bur under arthroscopic control. **B.** Arthroscopic view showing distal ulnar resection with a bur.

ARTHROSCOPIC ARTHROPLASTY FOR PROXIMAL POLE NONUNION

Pseudoarthrosis and necrosis of the proximal part of the scaphoid lead to radioscaphoid arthritis, which progressively spreads to the whole wrist and causes carpal collapse: scaphoid nonunion advanced collapse

(SNAC) wrist. A novel implant that adapts to the kinematics of the carpus has recently been proposed.[8] In view of the quality of the reported results, we decided to try placing the implant by arthroscopy.[9]

Adaptative Proximal Scaphoid Implant

This implant (pyrolitic carbon) is distinctive in that its ovoid shape allows it "adaptive" mobility when the first row of carpal bones move.[9,10] Frontally, the small radius corresponds to the scaphoid area of the radius, and from the side view the large radius forms an ovoid, of which the large curve is anteroposterior, and the small curve is frontal. By rotating on these two axes during frontal deviation and flexion-extension movements, the APSI copies the movements of the proximal scaphoid exactly and becomes integrated in a corroborating and synchronous way with the kinematics of the carpal bones (Figure 16.15). Because of this 3-dimensional reorientation during the movements of the wrist, the implant remains stable in the physiological amplitudes and does not require any form of fixation to the distal scaphoid or periprosthetic encapsulation.

Surgical Technique

All patients in our series were operated on as outpatients under local regional anesthesia using a pneumatic tourniquet.

The arm is laid flat on an arm table, and axial traction is applied to the forearm and wrist using a wrist tower. The strength of the traction is usually 7 kgf. After drawing the different bone parts on the carpus, the wrist is filled with about 10 cc of saline solution. At first, the arthroscopic guide and the arthroscope are positioned in the radiocarpal joint using the 6-R radiocarpal portal. Exploration of the joint is performed, locating any possible associated lesions. After locating the proximal pole, a 3-4 radiocarpal portal is performed. This surgical approach is slightly larger than usual, about 1.5 cm, so that the proximal pole can be withdrawn and the implant put in place. The maximum width of the implant is 1 cm. The arthroscope can easily be positioned in this surgical approach, allowing direct access to the area of nonunion. A radial midcarpal surgical approach is used to analyze carti-

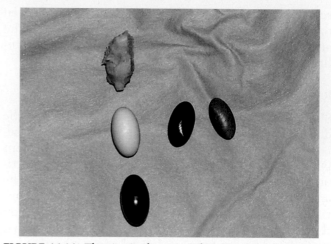

FIGURE 16.16. The size is chosen on the operating table by positioning the test implant next to the resected proximal pole. It is interesting to check the similar shape of resected proximal pole, the large test implant, and the definitive prosthesis.

lage and to monitor the positioning of the implant. After examining the proximal pole, the remaining cartilage is analyzed. First, the luno radial area is analyzed in order to check that the cartilage between the lunate and the radius is sound. Then the quality of the cartilage between the distal scaphoid and the capitate is evaluated. It is always surprising to see good articular cartilage at this interval. When considering the age of the lesion, one would expect to see much more extensive cartilage degeneration. Finally, the state of the cartilage between the head of the capitate and the distal face of the lunate is analyzed.

RESECTION OF THE PROXIMAL PART OF THE SCAPHOID

Proximal pole resection is a relatively easy procedure, depending on how old the lesion is. Sometimes we are faced with a small, necrosed proximal pole, weakly attached to the lunate by a few ligament fibers. The attachments are divided under arthroscopic control using instruments such as a surgical blade and small scissors. The detached proximal pole is easily withdrawn with forceps. In certain cases, it is necessary to use a bur to resect the proximal pole. A radial styloid osteotomy is recommended to remove a painful contact between the styloid and the remaining distal part of the scaphoid.

PLACING THE IMPLANT

First, the test implant is tried. There are three sizes:

- Small: length 16 mm, width 8 mm
- Medium: length 17 mm, width 9.1 mm
- Large: length 18 mm, width 10 mm

The size is chosen on the operating table by positioning the test implants next to the resected proximal pole (Figure 16.16). The test implant is then put

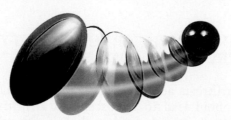

FIGURE 16.15. Diagram showing the adaptative mobility of the proximal pole implant according to the wrist motion.

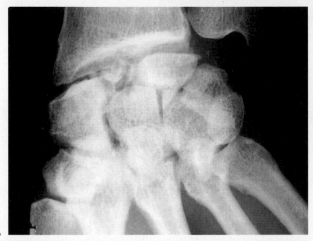

FIGURE 16.17. A. Clinical case: Adult 42 years old with proximal pole necrosis, without wrist arthritis. The pain was permanent, disabling, and the range of motion decreased (30 degrees of extension, 15 degrees of flexion). **B.** Clinical case: At one year after arthro-scopy, pain had completely disappeared. The APSI was stable. The carpal height seemed better, and the range of motion increased to 60 degrees in flexion-extension.

into the radiocarpal joint in place of the proximal pole, and it is very satisfying to see how well this implant puts itself into the correct position. After checking the correct congruence of the test implant by arthroscopy, it must be taken out. It is replaced very easily by the definitive prosthesis, still under arthroscopic control. After removing the arthroscope, forced wrist movements are carried out to confirm that there is no dislocation.

Postoperative Care

Only the 3-4 radiocarpal portal is closed. A protective dressing is put in place for 8 days. Mobility is started immediately, letting the patient choose the movements he or she wishes to make depending on postoperative pain. If necessary, rehabilitation can start after the third week.

Results

Our series is short. We have operated on only nine patients. All were operated on as outpatients under local regional anesthesia using a pneumatic tourniquet. The average age was 49 (range 40 to 81 years old). None of our three elderly patients had postoperative immobilization. In younger people, we needed to place a volar splint in half of the cases. We had one case of palmar implant dislocation in the youngest patient 6 days postsurgery. After intra-articular replacement and cast immobilization for 6 weeks, the patient finally had a very good result. Our average follow-up was 17 months

(range 6 to 32 months). The range of motion improved in all cases (Figure 16.17). Pain disappeared completely after 3 months. We haven't collected follow-up data long enough yet to check these encouraging results. Arthroscopic arthroplasty for proximal pole scaphoid nonunion is a safe and reliable procedure.

References

1. Whipple TL. *Arthroscopic Surgery. The Wrist.* Philadelphia: J.B. Lippincott, 1992, pp. 82–84.
2. Goldberg D, Menkes CJ. L'arthrose de la main In: Jubiana R, (ed.) *Traite de Chirurgie de la Main.* Paris: Masson, 1995, pp. 586–596.
3. Outerbridge RE. The etiology of chondromalacia patellae. *J Bone Joint Surg* 1961;43B:752–757.
4. Dougados M, Ayral X, Listrat V. The SFA system for assessing articular cartilage lesions at arthroscopy of the knee. *Arthroscopy* 1994;10:69–77.
5. Slater RB, Simmonds DF, Malcolm BW, et al. The biological effect of continuous passive motion on the healing of full-thickness defects in articular cartilage. *J Bone Joint Surg Am* 1980;62(8):1232.
6. Bleton R, Alnot JY, Levame JH. Possibilités thérapeutiques de l'arthroscopie dans les poignets douloureux chroniques. *Ann Chir Main* 1993;12(5):313–325.
7. Bain G, Roth J. The role of arthroscopy in arthritis: ectomy procedure. *Hand Clin* 1995;11:51–59.
8. Pequignot JP, Lussiez B, Allieu Y. Implant adaptatif du scaphoïde proximal. *Chir Main* 2000;2:276–285.
9. Mathoulin CL. Arthroscopic arthroplasty for proximal pole scaphoid nonunion In: Geissler WB, (ed.) *Atlas of Hand Clinics.* Philadelphia: WB Saunders Co., 2001, pp. 341–358.
10. Chen LT, Vincent J, Hetherington B, Reed S. A review of pyrolitic carbon: application in bone and joint surgery. *J Foot Ankle Surg* 1993;32(5):490–498.

17

Radial Styloidectomy

David M. Kalainov, Mark S. Cohen, and Stephanie Sweet

Excision of the radial styloid gained recognition in 1948 when Barnard and Stubbins[1] reported on ten scaphoid fracture nonunions treated with bone grafting and radial styloidectomy. The procedure has since been advocated to address radioscaphoid arthritis developing from a variety of injuries, including previous fractures of the radial styloid and scaphoid, and arthritis related to posttraumatic scapholunate instability.[2–8]

Resection of the radial styloid has also been a useful adjunct to other procedures where there is potential for impingement between the styloid process and distal scaphoid or trapezium.[9–15] Authors have included discussion of successful radial styloidectomy in descriptions of proximal row carpectomy, midcarpal arthrodesis, and triscaphe fusion procedures. On occasion, an individual may be too physically unfit or unwilling to undergo an extensive operation to address a symptomatic scaphoid nonunion or scapholunate dissociation. A limited radial styloidectomy may be a reasonable alternative in these cases.

ANATOMY

The radial styloid is positioned slightly volar to the midcoronal plane of the radius. The bony excrescence is the origin for the palmar extrinsic ligaments integral to carpal stability.[16–18] The radioscaphocapitate ligament averages 7 mm in width and originates only 4 mm from the tip of the styloid process. The long radiolunate ligament is approximately 10 mm wide and starts 10 mm proximal to the tip of the styloid (Figure 17.1).

Three basic types of styloid osteotomies have been described: short oblique, vertical oblique, and transverse (Figure 17.2). The potential for symptomatic carpal instability has been associated with the size and shape of the excised bone fragment. Siegel and Gelberman[18] performed a cadaveric study to assess the effect of these three styloidectomy configurations on extrinsic carpal ligament integrity. The short oblique osteotomy was the least damaging, with removal of only 9% of the radioscaphocapitate origin; this styloidectomy was found to leave the long radiolunate ligament attachment site intact. The vertical oblique osteotomy removed 92% of the radioscaphocapitate and 21% of the long radiolunate ligament origins. The transverse osteotomy was the most invasive, detaching 95% of the radioscaphocapitate and 46% of the long radiolunate ligament origins.

In another cadaveric model, Nakamura et al[19] examined the effects of increasingly larger oblique styloidectomies on carpal stability. They concluded that the procedure should be limited to a 3- to 4-mm bony resection. With axial loading, significantly increased radial, ulnar, and palmar displacements of the carpus were detected after removing 6-mm and 10-mm styloid segments. The 6-mm cut violated the radioscaphocapitate ligament origin, whereas the 10-mm cut removed the radioscaphocapitate and a portion of the long radiolunate ligament origins. Only an insignificant change in carpal translation was detected after a 3-mm osteotomy.

Other ligament attachments to the radial styloid include the radial collateral ligament, the dorsal radiocarpal ligament, and the radioscapholunate ligament.[16] The radial collateral ligament originates radially from to the tip of the styloid process and inserts into the waist and distal pole of the scaphoid. This structure represents the lateralmost margin of the radioscaphocapitate ligament and is removed in all styloidectomy procedures. No adverse effects have been reported in the literature. The dorsal radiocarpal ligament has a broad origin from the distal radius, beginning radial to the level of Lister's tubercle and coursing distally to its insertion into the triquetrum. Violation of a portion of the dorsal radiocarpal ligament following styloidectomy may potentially affect carpal stability, but this has not been described. The radioscapholunate ligament is a vascular structure with limited mechanical function. The ligament originates from the palmar aspect of the distal radius, in between the long and short radiolunate ligaments, and merges with the scapholunate interosseous ligament distally.

OPEN TECHNIQUE

The radial styloid may be excised as an adjunct to another carpal procedure; the styloid is approached

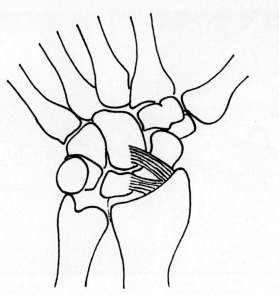

FIGURE 17.1. The radioscaphocapitate and long radiolunate ligament origins.

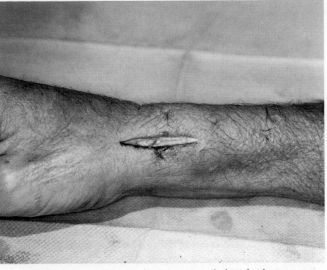

FIGURE 17.3. Exposure for an open radial styloidectomy.

through the same incision or a separate incision in these cases. With an isolated styloidectomy, a straight incision is made between the first and second extensor tendon compartments (Figure 17.3). The incision is centered over the tip of the styloid process, with care taken to protect the dorsal branch of the radial artery and small branches of the radial sensory and lateral antebrachial cutaneous nerves.[13]

The extensor retinaculum and periosteum are incised longitudinally over the palpable styloid. The tip is exposed by subperiosteal dissection, preserving the palmar attachments of the radioscaphocapitate and long radiolunate ligaments. A small, straight os-

teotome is used to remove 3 mm to 4 mm of the tip at an oblique angle (Figure 17.4). The cut should be parallel to the projected course of the radioscaphocapitate ligament and perpendicular to the distal radius articular surface (Figure 17.5).

Periosteum is reapproximated over the debrided styloid using absorbable sutures. The skin edges are repaired with subcuticular sutures in an effort to minimize scar formation. A bulky gauze dressing is applied, and the wrist is supported in neutral alignment with a volar plaster splint.

ARTHROSCOPIC TECHNIQUE

Finger traps are placed over the index and long fingers, and the hand is suspended in an overhead traction

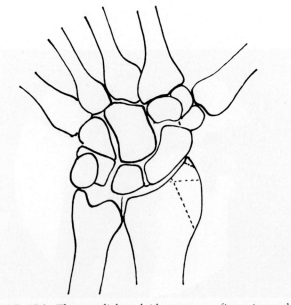

FIGURE 17.2. Three radial styloidectomy configurations: short oblique, vertical oblique, and transverse.

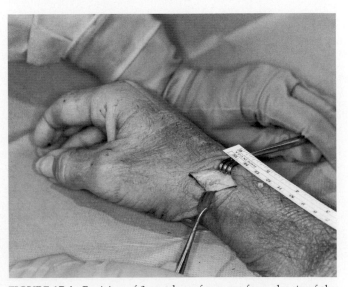

FIGURE 17.4. Excision of 3-mm bone fragment from the tip of the radial styloid.

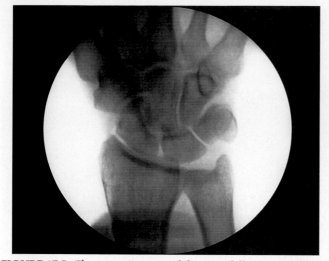

FIGURE 17.5. Fluoroscopic image of the wrist following an oblique radial styloidectomy.

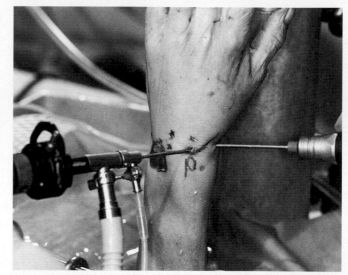

FIGURE 17.7. Resection tool in the 1-2 portal and arthroscopic camera in the 3-4 portal.

device. The arm is secured to the extremity table with a well-padded strap for countertraction. The major external landmarks and the positions of the portals that may be used in examining the wrist and performing the styloidectomy are shown in Figure 17.6.[14,15]

Eight to 10 pounds of traction are applied to the fingers to distract the wrist joint. The 3-4 portal is established to accommodate the arthroscopic camera. Outflow is achieved by placing an 18-gauge needle or small plastic cannula through the 6-U portal. A complete examination of the wrist is performed.

The 1-2 portal is then established for access to the radial styloid (Figure 17.7). A limited resection of 3 mm to 4 mm of the styloid tip is performed using a covered bur (2.9 mm to 3.5 mm) and/or full-radius shaver (2 mm to 2.9 mm). A small osteotome or pituitary rongeur may be helpful in removing hard

subchondral bone. Use of a laser device may also be considered.[20] The radioscaphocapitate and long radiolunate ligaments are visualized directly with the camera and adequate bone resection is confirmed with a mini-fluoroscopy unit (Figure 17.8). The procedure may be converted to an open technique if visualization is compromised.

The portal sites are either left open or closed with sutures. A bulky gauze dressing and volar plaster splint are applied with the wrist in neutral alignment.

REHABILITATION

Following an isolated radial styloidectomy, the dressing, splint, and sutures are removed after 1 week. A

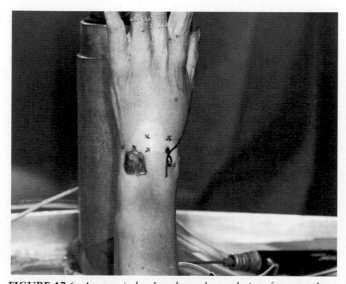

FIGURE 17.6. Anatomic landmarks and portal sites for an arthroscopic wrist examination and radial styloidectomy.

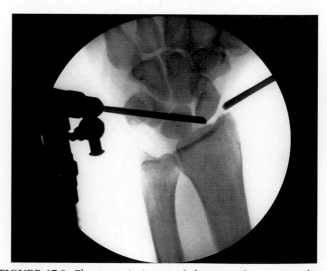

FIGURE 17.8. Fluoroscopic image of the wrist during an arthroscopic radial styloidectomy.

gradual return to work and sport activities is permitted. Assistance from a hand therapist may be helpful for instruction on wrist motion and grip strengthening exercises. The period of wrist immobilization will be necessarily extended if a concurrent procedure precludes early joint motion.

COMPLICATIONS

Complications inherent to any orthopedic procedure apply to both open and arthroscopic radial styloidectomies (e.g., infection, joint stiffness, keloid formation). Specific problems that may result from a radial styloidectomy include injury to the dorsal branch of the radial artery and neuropraxia or neurotmesis of local sensory nerves (i.e., dorsal branches of the radial sensory and lateral antebrachial cutaneous nerves). A complex regional pain syndrome may develop following any nerve injury, necessitating intensive therapy and pain management intervention. An incomplete radial styloidectomy may also be problematic, with persistent complaints of radial-sided wrist pain. Excessive bony resection is potentially disastrous, resulting in ulnar translation of the carpus and symptoms of wrist joint instability.

A radial styloidectomy is contraindicated when there is preexisting ulnar translation of the carpus or incompetence of the radioscaphocapitate and long radiolunate ligaments. This procedure alone will not adequately address arthritic changes that extend beyond the distal radioscaphoid articulation (i.e., degenerative arthritis involving the lunatocapitate joint secondary to chronic scapholunate instability or an untreated scaphoid nonunion). A concurrent operation to address the midcarpal arthritic changes should be considered in these cases.

RESULTS

We reviewed 7 patients who underwent an arthroscopic or arthroscopically assisted radial styloidectomy between 1992 and 1997. Three patients had scaphoid nonunions with posttraumatic arthritis involving the radioscaphoid articulation, 2 patients had radioscaphoid arthritis developing after a healed scaphoid fracture, one patient had arthritic changes involving the radioscaphoid articulation secondary to a scapholunate ligament injury, and one patient had isolated arthritis of the radioscaphoid joint of unknown cause. All these patients elected surgery after failing to experience pain relief with conservative treatment measures.

In addition to a radial styloidectomy, one individual underwent arthroscopic removal of nearly the entire scaphoid bone, and another individual underwent arthroscopic excision of the scaphoid proximal pole; both patients presented with scaphoid nonunions. Temporary wrist immobilization was implemented postoperatively in all cases.

The mean follow-up period for these 7 patients was 29 months (range 3 to 57 months). The Mayo modified wrist scores[21] increased from an average of 62 points preoperatively to 75 points postoperatively. Two patients reported no residual pain, and 5 patients described only mild, occasional pain. Six patients returned to regular employment activities, whereas one patient was able to work but was unemployed. None of the patients described difficulty performing activities of daily living.

CONCLUSION

Arthroscopic radial styloidectomy is a useful treatment for symptomatic arthritis localized to the distal radioscaphoid articulation, either as an isolated technique or as an adjunct to another carpal procedure. The procedure is minimally invasive with the potential for temporary pain relief and improved hand function. The details of the technique are important to review in order to avoid injury to cutaneous nerves, the dorsal branch of the radial artery, and the palmar radiocarpal ligaments. The bony resection should be limited to 3 mm to 4 mm, preserving the origins of the radioscaphocapitate and long radiolunate ligaments.

References

1. Barnard L, Stubbins SG. Styloidectomy of the radius in the surgical treatment of non-union of the carpal navicular: a preliminary report. *J Bone Joint Surg* 1948;30A:98–102.
2. Smith L, Friedman B. Treatment of ununited fracture of the carpal navicular by styloidectomy of the radius. *J Bone Joint Surg* 1956;38A:368–376.
3. Sprague B, Justis EJ. Nonunion of the carpal navicular: modes of treatment. *Arch Surg* 1974;108:692–697.
4. Herness D, Posner MA. Some aspects of bone grafting for nonunion of the carpal navicular: analysis of 41 cases. *Acta Orthop Scand* 1977;48:373–378.
5. Stark HH, Rickard TA, Zemel NP, et al. Treatment of ununited fractures of the scaphoid by iliac bone grafts and Kirschner-wire fixation. *J Bone Joint Surg* 1988;70A:982–991.
6. Osterman AL, Mikulics M. Scaphoid nonunion. *Hand Clin* 1988;14:437–455.
7. Ruch DS, Chang DS, Poehling GG. The arthroscopic treatment of avascular necrosis of the proximal pole following scaphoid nonunion: case report. *Arthroscopy* 1998;14:747–752.
8. Watson HK, Ballet FL. The SLAC wrist: scapholunate advanced collapse pattern of degenerative arthritis. *J Hand Surg* 1984;9A:358–365.
9. Watson HK, Ryu J, DiBella A. An approach to Kienbock's disease: triscaphe arthrodesis. *J Hand Surg* 1985;10A:179–187.
10. Rogers WD, Watson HK. Radial styloid impingement after triscaphe arthrodesis. *J Hand Surg* 1989;14A:297–301.
11. Minamikawa Y, Peimer CA, Yamaguchi T, et al. Ideal scaphoid angle for intercarpal arthrodesis. *J Hand Surg* 1992;17A:370–375.
12. Atik TL, Baratz M. The role of arthroscopy in wrist arthritis. *Hand Clin* 1999;15:489–494.

13. Cooney WP, DeBartolo T, Wood MB. Post-traumatic arthritis of the wrist. In: Cooney WP, Linscheid RL, Dobyns JH. (eds). *The Wrist: Diagnosis and Operative Treatment.* St. Louis: Mosby, 1998, pp. 588–629.

14. Osterman AL. Wrist arthroscopy. In: Green DP, Hotchkiss RN, Pederson WC, (eds.) *Green's Operative Hand Surgery.* 4th ed. New York: Churchill Livingstone, 1999, pp. 207–222.

15. Savoie FH 111, Field LD. Diagnostic and operative arthroscopy. In: Gelberman RH, (ed). *The Wrist,* 2nd ed. Philadelphia: Lippincott Williams & Wilkins, 2002, pp. 21–35.

16. Berger RA. The ligaments of the wrist: a current overview of anatomy with considerations of their potential functions. *Hand Clin* 1997;13:63–82.

17. Blevens AD, Light TR, Jablonsky WS, et al. Radiocarpal articular contact characteristics with scaphoid instability. *J Hand Surg* 1989;14A:781–790.

18. Siegel DB, Gelberman, RH. Radial styloidectomy: an anatomical study with special reference to radiocarpal intracapsular ligamentous morphology. *J Hand Surg* 1991;16A:40–44.

19. Nakamura T, Cooney WP III, Lui WH, et al. Radial styloidectomy: a biomechanical study on stability of the wrist joint. *J Hand Surg* 2001;26A:85–93.

20. Nagle DJ. Laser-assisted wrist arthroscopy. *Hand Clin* 1999;15: 495–499.

21. Cooney WP, Linscheid RL, Dobyns, JH. Triangular fibrocartilage tears. *J Hand Surg* 1994;19A:143–154.

Excision of Dorsal Wrist Ganglia

William B. Geissler

Ganglia are the most common tumors of the hand, representing approximately 50% to 70% of all soft tissue hand tumors.[2] The dorsal wrist ganglion is by far the most common cyst, accounting for 60% to 70% of all hand and wrist ganglia.[2] Ganglia are more common in females.[2] They usually appear between the second and fifth decades of life, but also have been reported in children. A specific traumatic event is described in 10% to 50% of cases, and repetitive microtrauma also appears to be an etiologic factor.[3]

The origin of dorsal ganglia is usually over the dorsum of the scapholunate interosseous ligament. The dorsal ganglion usually appears as a cystic mass, distal and ulnar to the extensor pollicis longus tendon, between the third and fourth dorsal compartments. However, the cyst may present anywhere along the dorsum of the wrist, connected by a long pedicle. It can even track radially and present on the volar aspect of the wrist, although its source is the dorsum of the scapholunate interosseous ligament. Careful palpation of the cyst is important to show the extent of the cyst and the direction and origin of the pedicle.

Occult dorsal ganglia can be palpated only with the wrist in volar flexion.[4] Comparison with the opposite wrist is often necessary. An occult dorsal ganglion may be the cause of dorsal wrist pain with normal radiographs. Its proximity to the posterior interosseous nerve explains the exquisite tenderness that may be present with occult ganglia. The differential diagnosis may include extensor tendon tenosynovitis, Kienböck's disease, and scapholunate interosseous ligament injury.

The etiology and pathogenesis of ganglia continue to be controversial. Mucoid degenerative changes in collagen tissue were initially proposed by Letterhaus in 1893 and popularized by Carp and Stout in 1938.[2] Collections of mucin secondary to collagen breakdown product collect and expand into the soft tissues. Fibrous tissue around the mucin becomes compacted, forming a pseudocapsule. Electromicroscopic studies have shown that the wall is made of compressed collagen fibers, without evidence of a true epithelial or synovial lining.[5] Angelides and Wallace believe that microtrauma or rotation becomes a stimulating factor for production of hyuronic acid.[6] This process is initiated at the synovial capsule interface. Mucin collects and dissects throughout the attached joint capsule to collate and form the subcutaneous cyst itself.

Angelides and Wallace defined the origin of the dorsal ganglia to be at the dorsum of the scapholunate interosseous ligament.[6] This area of transition between the dorsal capsule and the interosseous ligament may serve as a tortuous duct that acts as a one-way valvelike mechanism. McEvedy injected ganglia with contrast dye and found no communication with the joint itself.[3] Andren and Eiken injected the wrist joint in their series of ganglia and found a significant percentage of ganglia filled with dye from the joint, which would suggest a one-way valvelike effect from the wrist.[7] Watson et al reported on 17 patients who developed rotary subluxation of the scaphoid following scaphoid excision.[8] They concluded that dorsal ganglia are a secondary manifestation of scapholunate instability.

Patients with dorsal ganglia usually present with a mass on the back of the hand and complain of a constant, dull ache that may be due to the location of the ganglion and its proximity to the posterior interosseous nerve.[9] Patients complain of increased pain with wrist extension, particularly in large ganglia. Some patients also complain of weakness of grip. The mass may have appeared suddenly or gradually and may change size with time.

The natural history with spontaneous resolution of ganglia has been reported to be between 28% and 58%.[2,10] The success of nonoperative management of dorsal ganglia is approximately 50%.[5,11,12] Previous treatment recommendations included rupturing the cyst with a Bible, a ganglion mallet, or with the physician's thumb.[3] Aspiration, with or without the use of cortisone, has reported a success rate of 35% to 50%.[11–13]

Surgical excision of the cyst with its ganglion stalk and surrounding capsule has reduced the recurrence rate to approximately 15% or lower.[14] A vertical or transverse incision may be made directly over the ganglion, although most surgeons recommend a transverse incision. The dorsal sensory branches of the radial nerve are identified and protected. The extensor pollicis longus and extensor carpi radialis brevis tendons are retracted radially, and the extensor communis tendons are retracted ulnarly, exposing the dorsal ganglion. Draining the ganglion, particularly if it is quite large, makes dissection around the ganglion easier. The ganglion and its stalk with capsular attachments are then sharply excised. It is very important to visualize the scapholunate interosseous ligament and excise the mucin-filled duct in the superficial portion of the ligament without cutting the ligament and causing scapholunate instability. If the origin of the duct is not excised, a high recurrence rate can be expected. The joint capsule is not closed, and early range of motion is encouraged. The key to open excision is identification of the stalk and its excision at the base of the scapholunate interosseous ligament.

Open excision of dorsal ganglia is not a benign procedure, although it has lowered the recurrence rate. There can be significant surgical morbidity from what the patient may perceive as a relatively benign surgery. Patients are trading a bump for a scar. They may experience numbness distally and around the incision due to involvement with the dorsal sensory branches. Particularly, patients may complain of wrist stiffness, usually with wrist flexion. This may be due to prolonged immobilization, or closure of the capsular defect rather than the dorsal capsule remaining open. Osterman and Raphael initially reported on arthroscopic excision of a dorsal ganglion.[15] The initial study was based on the clinical experience of a 36-year-old patient with a combined 1 cm, asymptomatic dorsal ganglion and a symptomatic tear of the triangular fibrocartilage complex (TFCC). The patient asked if the dorsal ganglion could be excised at the same time as the arthroscopic management of the TFCC tear. It was found that the ganglion ruptured when the 3-4 portal was established. Follow-up of the patient showed the ganglion had not returned after 2 years.

Arthroscopic excision of dorsal ganglia does have several advantages. Most important, it allows for a more rapid return of range of motion. This can be a significant advantage to the mother of young children, who requires both hands as soon as possible to care for her children. Similarly, the self-employed professional or manual laborer who cannot afford any down time may frequently inquire about arthroscopic excision and early range of motion. Other patients frequently would prefer to trade a portal for the bump, rather than a surgical scar. Theoretically, the patient may be less likely to experience numbness around a portal as compared to around a scar.

INDICATIONS

Surgical indications for a symptomatic dorsal ganglion include at least one failed attempt at aspiration. The key surgical indication is that the ganglion is symptomatic. Ganglia that are asymptomatic are followed

nonoperatively. The ideal ganglion for arthroscopic surgery is a single-lobe ganglion located between the third and fourth dorsal compartments. This is the most typical location for a dorsal ganglion and presents the lowest risk of injury to the extensor tendons during arthroscopic excision of the dorsal capsule and stalk.

Occult dorsal ganglia are particularly amenable to arthroscopic excision. Open excision of occult dorsal ganglia frequently requires a significant amount of blunt dissection to localize and identify the ganglion. This blunt dissection may lead to increased scarring and decreased range of motion, particularly in flexion. Arthroscopic excision and excising the ganglion from inside out eliminates this considerable amount of dissection and potential scarring. It also allows for identification and management of any additional intra-articular pathology of the wrist.

Patients whose ganglia appear in atypical locations are more controversial. Ganglia with long stalks that appear between the dorsal extensor tendons may still be arthroscopically excised, but close attention to protection of the tendons is essential. A typical ganglion that presents between the first and second dorsal compartments is usually excised to prevent injury to the radial artery and the dorsal sensory branch of the radial nerve. If the tendon is multilobulated, open excision is preferred. Arthroscopic excision of volar ganglia is further described in Chapter 6.

SURGICAL TECHNIQUE

Small-joint arthroscopy instrumentation is used. The wrist is suspended to place 10 pounds of traction in a traction tower. A traction tower is useful because it both provides traction and helps stabilize the wrist. The bony and soft tissue landmarks are identified and marked after the wrist is suspended. It is important to note the location of the extensor carpi radialis brevis, extensor pollicis longus, and extensor digitorum communis tendons. It is important to mark the location of these tendons prior to injecting inflow into the wrist, because the tendons are less palpable as the wrist swells during the procedure.

An inflow cannula is introduced through the 6-U portal. It is important that the skin only is excised by pulling the skin against the tip of a number 11 scalpel blade to limit potential injury to the dorsal sensory branch of the ulnar nerve. This nerve is at risk for laceration and neuroma formation with introduction of the 6-U portal. Blunt dissection is continued down with a small hemostat, and an inflow cannula is introduced through the 6-U portal into the prestyloid recess. A tourniquet is rarely required when separate inflow is provided through the 6-U portal. Alternatively, inflow may be provided through the arthroscopic cannula at the surgeon's preference. A 2.7-mm arthroscope is initially placed in the 6-R portal, not the standard 3-4 viewing portal. The 6-R portal lies just radial to the extensor carpi ulnaris tendon. This provides excellent visualization of the dorsal distal portion of the scapholunate interosseous ligament and capsule (Figure 18.1). Usually, a small amount of dorsal synovitis obscures adequate visualization of the dorsal capsule as it intersects the dorsal portion of the scapholunate interosseous ligament. An 18-gauge needle is then introduced through the ganglion into the radiocarpal joint. The ganglion itself is usually located distal to the traditional location of the 3-4 portal. The needle, therefore, is introduced at a much more oblique angle than is usual for a 3-4 portal (Figure 18.2). The needle should be seen at the junction of the dorsal capsule at the level of the scapholunate interosseous ligament.

A pearl-like ganglion stalk may be arthroscopically identified at the very distal aspect of the scapholunate interosseous ligament, as can be seen from the radiocarpal space (Figure 18.3). Osterman and Raphael reported that the stalk of the ganglion was identified arthroscopically in their series 61% of the time.[15] Others have described the identification of the stalk with far less frequency.[16] It is not vital to identify the stalk of the ganglion. The key is to place the portal through the ganglion itself and enter at the junction of the dorsal aspect of the capsule with the scapholunate interosseous ligament. Once an ideal location has been identified with a needle, a portal is made, again by incising the skin with the tip of a number 11 blade and bluntly dissecting with a hemostat. A 2.9-mm, full-radius or end-cutting resector is then placed through this working portal, through the ganglion, and into the radiocarpal space (Figure 18.4). Just as in open excision, the goal of arthroscopic excision is to excise the base of the stalk from its origin at the scapholunate

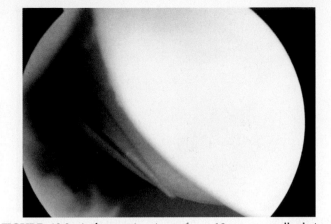

FIGURE 18.2. Arthroscopic view of an 18-gauge needle being passed through a ganglion cyst into the radiocarpal space, as seen from the 6-R portal. Note the oblique angle of the needle as the ganglion arises distal to the normal location of the 3-4 portal.

interosseous ligament. Approximately a 1 × 1 cm section of dorsal capsule and its attachment to the interosseous ligament is resected. Care must be taken not to injure the overlying extensor tendons. However, small-joint shavers are not very aggressive compared with their larger counterparts, and it is fairly difficult to excise through an extensor tendon with a small-joint shaver or joint punch. Once a shaver is introduced, the dorsal capsule at its insertion to the scapholunate interosseous ligament is excised, leaving an approximately 1 × 1 cm defect (Figure 18.5). A small-joint punch is particularly useful to excise the dorsal capsule; it saves time once the capsular defect has been created by the shaver (Figure 18.6).

The tendon of the extensor carpi radialis brevis should be identified to ensure that full-thickness debridement of the dorsal capsule has been achieved (Figure 18.7). It is easily recognizable by its longitudinally

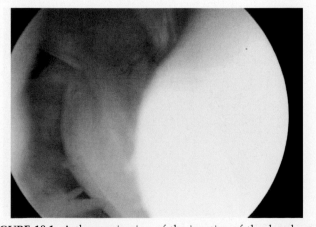

FIGURE 18.1. Arthroscopic view of the junction of the dorsal capsule and the scapholunate interosseous ligament, where a dorsal ganglion usually arises, as seen with the arthroscope in the 6-R portal.

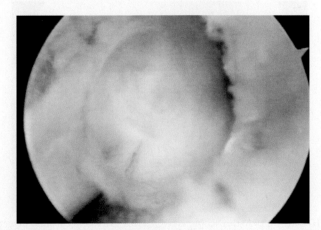

FIGURE 18.3. Arthroscopic view of the "pearl" at the ganglion stalk, as seen in a left wrist from the 6-R portal.

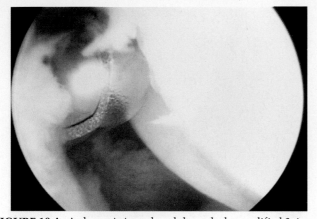

FIGURE 18.4. A shaver is introduced through the modified 3-4 portal through the ganglion cyst to enter the joint at the junction of the scapholunate interosseous ligament and the dorsal capsule, as seen from the 6-R portal.

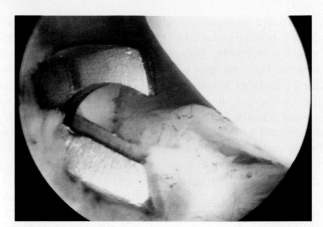

FIGURE 18.6. A small arthroscopic wrist punch is useful to enlarge the capsular defect.

running fibers and slightly different color as compared to the dorsal capsule. It is very important to recognize this structure to ensure that full-thickness debridement of the dorsal capsule has been achieved. The gelatinous fluid of the ganglion may occasionally be seen intra-articularly as the cyst is decompressed.

Following resection of the dorsal capsule, the ganglion should be palpated and felt to be decompressed. A key to improved visualization of the dorsal capsule at its junction with the scapholunate interosseous ligament is to place the wrist in extension in the traction tower. For the majority of time during a wrist arthroscopy, the wrist is in slight flexion to help gain access to the wrist for introduction of the instrumentation. However, to improve visualization at the junction of the dorsal capsule with the scapholunate interosseous ligament, the wrist is placed in slight extension. This will significantly improve visualization in this area, particularly after debridement of any synovitis in this area. Following resection of the dor-

sal capsule, it is important to palpate the ganglion to ensure that the ganglion itself has ruptured. This is particularly useful in a multilobular ganglion. If the ganglion is still palpable, further resection may be required, or the ganglion may be aspirated.

Following arthroscopic excision of the dorsal ganglion, the remaining structures of the wrist should be evaluated, particularly the scapholunate and lunotriquetral interosseous ligaments. The 3-4 portal is usually closed with a Steri-Strip, and the other portals are left open. The wrist is placed in a volar splint, which is then removed at the next clinic visit. Rarely is physical therapy required. The patient is encouraged in a range of motion program after the first week, and strengthening exercises are initiated 4 weeks postoperatively.

RESULTS

Arthroscopic ganglion excision allows simultaneous evaluation of the wrist for other intra-articular ab-

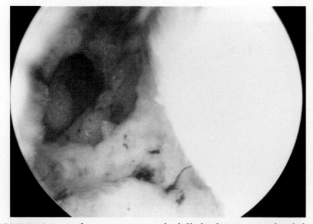

FIGURE 18.5. Arthroscopic view of a full-thickness capsular defect after shaving at the origin of the dorsal ganglion stalk, as seen from the 6-R portal.

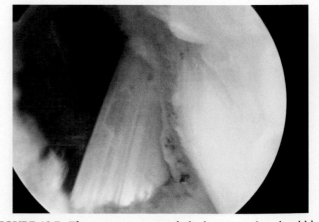

FIGURE 18.7. The extensor carpi radialis brevis tendon should be visualized through the capsular defect to ensure a full-thickness debridement of the capsule has been performed.

normalities. Osterman and Raphael reported that 50% of their initial 18 patients had other intra-articular abnormalities.[15] These included 2 patients with perforations of the scapholunate interosseous ligament and 3 patients with laxity of the scapholunate interosseous ligament. Two patients had tears of the triangular fibrocartilage complex, one had radial chondromalacia, and one patient had triquetral hamate chondromalacia. In their series, which averaged a 16-month follow-up, no patients had any recurrence, and the average return to work was 3.5 weeks.

We have reviewed our results in arthroscopic excision of dorsal ganglia in 25 patients with more than a 1-year follow-up (range: 12 to 26 months).[16] There were 19 female and five male patients. There was one recurrence in this group. This recurrence occurred early in our study and was felt to be secondary to inadequate identification of the stalk of the ganglion. The ganglion itself needs to be palpated after excision of the stalk to make sure that the sac has fully ruptured. Subjectively, the patient required minimal pain medication and started early range of motion 1 week following excision.

COMPLICATIONS

The primary complication to arthroscopic gangliectomy is potential recurrence. This would be secondary to inadequate resection of the origin of the stalk and capsule, which may occur early in the surgeon's learning curve. Resection of this key structure is vital, just as it is in open excision. It is important to shave any synovitis away from the dorsal capsule to help with visualization of the potential stalk in the intersection of the dorsal capsule of the scapholunate ligament. Again, extension of the wrist, when the wrist is in the traction tower, particularly improves visualization at this key area. Although visualization of the stalk is not necessary and will not be possible every time, this does make excision easier. Visualization of the extensor carpi radialis brevis tendon is an excellent landmark to ensure that a full-thickness debridement of the dorsal capsule has been achieved to lower the risk of recurrence. The rate of recurrence in the preliminary studies of excision of dorsal ganglia is extremely low compared with open excision and may prove a substantial benefit of undertaking this procedure arthroscopically.

It is vital to palpate the extraarticular sac to make sure it is ruptured. This is particularly true when the sac is multilobulated. Following excision, it is helpful to take the wrist out of traction and to palmar flex the wrist to ensure that the sac cannot be palpated and has ruptured.

The dorsal extensor tendons are at risk during arthroscopic excision of the dorsal ganglion. However, this risk is quite minimal with close attention to detail. The standard small-joint arthroscopy punches are not wide enough to capture the entire extensor tendon in one cut. It would take multiple passes to achieve a full-thickness cut to the extensor tendon. Also, the consistency of the extensor tendon is much firmer than the dorsal capsule, and it should have a different feel if the tendon is about to be cut with a shaver or punch.

One disadvantage of arthroscopic excision of dorsal ganglia is the required operating room time. The actual surgical time in our institution has been similar to that of open excision. However, the additional time needed to set up the arthroscopic traction equipment is longer compared to open excision. If only an occasional wrist arthroscopic procedure is performed, the operating room personnel may not be as familiar with the equipment, and this can prolong operating room time to set up for the case. Open excision of dorsal ganglia is traditionally performed under intravenous regional anesthesia, whereas arthroscopic excision may need to be performed under axillary or general anesthesia until the operating room personnel are proficient in setting up the equipment.

CONCLUSION

Arthroscopic excision of dorsal ganglia is a reasonable alternative to open excision, with decreased postoperative morbidity. Arthroscopic excision has been shown to equal, if not lower the risk of recurrence, as compared with open excision. This lower risk of recurrence in preliminary studies, combined with more rapid improvement in postoperative range of motion is a significant advantage over open excision. Arthroscopic excision allows precise identification and excision of the stalk of the ganglion from the scapholunate interosseous ligament under magnified conditions. It allows protection of the scapholunate interosseous ligament as it is directly visualized under bright light and in well-magnified conditions. This may potentially lower the risk of injury to the interosseous ligament as compared to open excision.[17] Simultaneous arthroscopic evaluation of the radiocarpal and midcarpal spaces allows detection and management of any additional intra-articular pathology that may be extant. This also allows the patient to trade a bump for a portal rather than a scar, which is pleasing to those patients who feel cosmesis is important.

References

1. Angelides AC. Ganglions of the hand and wrist. In: Green D (ed) *Operative Hand Surgery*, 2nd ed. New York: Churchill Livingstone, 1988, pp. 2281.
2. Carp L, Stout AP. A study of ganglion with special reference to treatment. *Surg Gynecol Obstet* 1938;47:460–468.

3. Nelson CL, Sawmiller S, Phalen GS. Ganglions of the wrist and hand. *J Bone Joint Surg* 1972;5A:1459–1464.

4. Sanders WE. The occult dorsal carpal ganglion. *J Hand Surg* 1987;10B:257–260.

5. Psaila JV, Mansel RE. The surface ultrastructure of ganglia. *J Bone Joint Surg* 1978;60B:228–233.

6. Angelides AC, Wallace PF. The dorsal ganglion of the wrist: its pathogenesis, gross anatomy and surgical treatment. *J Hand Surg* 1976;1:228–235.

7. Andren L, Eiken O. Arthrographic studies of wrist ganglions. *J Bone Joint Surg* 1971;53A:299–302.

8. Watson HK, Rogers WD, Ashmead DF. Re-evaluating the cause of the wrist ganglion. *J Hand Surg* 1989;14A:812–817.

9. Dellon AL, Seif SS. Anatomic dissection relating the posterior interosseous nerve to the carpus and etiology of dorsal wrist ganglion pain. *J Hand Surg* 1978;3:326–332.

10. McEvedy BV. Simple ganglia: a review of modes of treatment and an explanation for the frequent failures of surgery. *Lancet* 1965;266:135.

11. Richman JA, Gelberman RH, Engher WD, et al. Ganglions of the wrist and digits: results of treatment by aspiration and cyst wall puncture. *J Hand Surg* 1987;12A:1041–1043.

12. Zubowicz VN, Ischii CH. Management of ganglion cysts of the hand by simple aspiration. *J Hand Surg* 1987;12A:618–620.

13. Holm DC, Pandey SD. Treatment of ganglia of the hand and wrist with aspiration and injection of hydrocortisone. *Hand Clin* 1973;5:63–68.

14. Clay NR, Clement DA. The treatment of dorsal wrist ganglia by radial excision. *J Hand Surg* 1988;13B:187–191.

15. Osterman AL, Raphael J. Arthroscopic resection of dorsal ganglions of the wrist. *Hand Clin* 1995;11:7–12.

16. Geissler WB. Arthroscopic excision of dorsal wrist ganglia. *Tech Hand Upper Extr Surg* 1998;2:196–201.

17. Crawford GP, Taleisnik J. Rotary subluxation of the scaphoid after excision of dorsal carpal ganglion and wrist manipulation: a case report. *J Hand Surg* 1983;8A:921–925.

19

Wrist Arthrolysis

Riccardo Luchetti, Andrea Atzei, and Tracy Fairplay

Wrist stiffness is a complication either from trauma (with or without extra- and/or intra-articular fractures) or surgery.[1] Rehabilitation of the wrist is the treatment of choice when a patient presents with wrist stiffness of over 3 to 6 months' duration. Wrist manipulation under anesthesia may be used in cases in which a rehabilitation regime has failed to produce increased wrist range of motion. However, this procedure can also be dangerous, provoking further damage such as ligament or bone lesions (ulnar head fracture). Surgical arthrolysis is an alternative option that can be performed via open surgery or arthroscopy. Surgical arthrolysis is rarely performed in cases of flexion-extension rigidity, but it is frequently used for distal radioulnar joint (DRUJ) wrist rigidity in which pronosupination range of motion (ROM) is affected.[2] This joint is easier to reach than the radiocarpal joint, and rehabilitation is initiated immediately after surgery.

Arthroscopic arthrolysis is a new procedure that allows the surgeon to treat all the wrist joints without running the risk of causing secondary damage to the articulations involved and, at the same time, permitting immediate postoperative mobilization.[3–8] The use of this technique to treat posttraumatic wrist stiffness began in the early 1990s.[9,10] An improvement of wrist ROM was seen after arthrography. This stimulated enthusiasm among surgical specialists to further research its surgical efficiency,[10] which they hypothesized was due to the effect of the fluid that was injected into the joint, and thus causing joint distension. In addition, other authors[11–14] had already demonstrated that knee, elbow, and shoulder rigidity due to adhesive capsulitis or arthrofibrosis could be successfully treated by arthroscopic arthrolysis.

INDICATIONS

Improvement of arthroscopic instruments, technique, and knowledge of arthroscopic wrist anatomy have led to the application of this technique in a much wider range of wrist pathologies. Indications for arthroscopic wrist arthrolysis include all cases in which rigidity has occurred following prolonged immobilization after trauma (fractures or dislocations) or surgery. Pain is almost always present with articular rigidity. The causes of the rigidity could be intra- and/or extra-articular (Table 19.1). Localization of joint stiffness depends on the damaged site. Radiocarpal (RC), midcarpal (MC), and DRUJ rigidity can be present individually or in association with each other.

The most frequent clinical pathological conditions are adhesive capsulitis and arthrofibrosis of the wrist. Capsulitis is due to ligament and/or capsule contractures, and wrist arthrofibrosis is usually due to osseous band fibrosis of the radius and/or first row carpal bone(s) from a radius articular fracture. These two conditions can be associated in the same case. Wrist rigidity can also be a consequence of injury to the wrist bones and/or ligaments, for example, a 4-corner intercarpal arthrodesis, a proximal row carpectomy, or reconstruction of the scapholunate interosseus ligament. Wrist rigidity can also be associated with other pathologies of the wrist, such as median nerve compression, stenosing tenovaginitis of the flexor tendons, or even an injury to the dorsal terminal root of the posterior interosseous nerve.

We must not forget that all hand articulations are susceptible to articular rigidity, as we frequently see in the first carpometacarpal (CMC) joint; even in this case, arthroscopic arthrolysis is a possible treatment of choice.

SURGICAL TECHNIQUE

RC, MC, and DRUJ portals are the arthroscopic surgical approaches of choice. Most recently two volar RC portals (radial and ulnar) have also been added.[15] Wrist arthrolysis must be performed by using both traditional and more elaborate instruments (Table 19.2).

Although arthroscopy starts at the level of the RC joint, the MC joint should always be thoroughly evaluated. When there is a loss of pronosupination articular range of motion, arthrolysis of the distal radioulnar joint must also be performed.

In the most difficult cases, it is impossible to recognize the normal arthroscopic anatomy of the wrist (Figures 19.1 and 19.2). Difficulties could be encountered in performing triangulation with the instruments. Synovitis, fibrosis, and adhesions can obstruct

TABLE 19.1. Possible Causes of Secondary Wrist Rigidity (extra- and/or intra-articular).

Post-trauma	Post-surgery	After immobilization
Fracture	Dorsal wrist ganglia recurrences	Prolonged immobilization
Fracture-dislocation	Treatment of scaphoid fracture or nonunion	Incorrect wrist immobilization
Dislocation	Intercarpal arthrodesis (4 bones fusion, etc)	
Ligament lesions	Ligament reconstruction (SL ligament, etc)	
	Proximal row carpectomy	

the visual field; therefore, they must be removed with caution, ensuring that no damage occurs to the surrounding structures. Obviously, the surgeon's ability is of utmost importance.

Radiocarpal Joint

All the portals (1-2, 3-4, 4-5, 6-R, and 6-U) are used, including the volar, when needed. Fibrotic adhesions are initially removed with the appropriate instruments: motor engine, laser, and radiofrequency instruments. This procedure is frequently sufficient to improve wrist ROM. When needed, the volar and/or dorsal radiocarpal ligaments must be resected from the border of the radius to improve wrist ROM (Figure 19.3). Miniblade, laser, or radiofrequency instruments are used to resect the ligament. Dorsal capsulotomy sometimes may require a volar approach. It is very important to remember that the volar and dorsal ulnar ligaments must not be resected. Ulnar translation of the carpal bones has not been demonstrated after resection of the radial ligaments.[4]

Limited articular steps of the radius (less than 1 mm) must be leveled, when possible (Figure 19.4). Triangular fibrocartilage complex (TFCC) central tears are also treated: the flap is removed and the borders are cleaned. When the patient presents with an ulnar plus wrist, it must be treated with wafer arthroscopic resection. The loose bodies must be removed if they are found inside the articulation. At the end of the surgery, wrist manipulation is performed to evaluate its range of motion and to determine if there has been an improvement in articular excursion.

Midcarpal Joint

The approach for this articulation is via the four portals (RMC, UMC, STT, and TH), thus making it possible to verify if there is involvement of the MC joint that could be contributing to wrist stiffness. Arthro-

scopy of this joint is much easier to perform, and synovitis is the most frequently found pathology in this zone. It is usually localized to the level of the STT and TH joints. Commonly, one sees an associated capitate and hamate chondritis. This also can cause the patient to have wrist pain. Debridement of the MC joint is performed in order to improve painless joint movement. MC joint arthroscopy does not require that ligament resection be performed.

Distal Radioulnar Joint

It is very unusual to have good visibility of this joint even in normal conditions. Stiffness of this joint is due to synovitis and fibrosis, which in turn increase the difficulty of performing the arthroscopy. In cases when this particular joint arthroscopy begins to take a prolonged amount of time and becomes quite tedious, it is convenient to introduce a dissector into the proximal portal and to detach the adhesions between the ulnar head and the sigmoid fossa, or resect the volar capsule from the bone. The dissector can also be introduced through the distal portal; then one should perform resection of the adhesions between the ulnar head and the ulnar surface of the TFCC. These maneuvers usually result in a good pronosupination wrist ROM improvement.

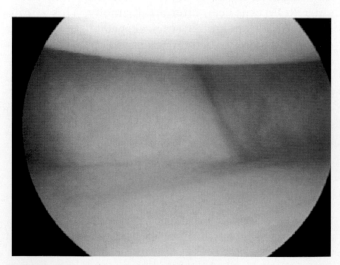

FIGURE 19.1. Arthroscopic normal appearance of volar ligaments (RSC and LRL ligaments). (Reprinted from *Atlas Hand Clinics*, 6(2):371–387, R. Luchetti, A. Atzei, and B. Mustapha, Arthroscopic wrist arthrolysis, pp. 371–387, © 2001 with permission from Elsevier Science.)

TABLE 19.2. Instruments for Arthroscopic Arthrolysis.

Motor powered	Suction punch
Full radius blade	Mini-scalpel (banana blade)
Cutter blade	Laser
Razor cut blade	Radiofrequency
Barrel abrader	Dissector and scalpel

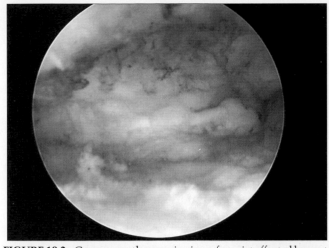

FIGURE 19.2. Common arthroscopic view of a wrist affected by post-traumatic stiffness (fibrotic bands between the radius and the carpal bones). (Reprinted from *Atlas Hand Clinics*, 6(2):371–387, R. Luchetti, A. Atzei, and B. Mustapha, Arthroscopic wrist arthrolysis, pp. 371–387, © 2001 with permission from Elsevier Science.)

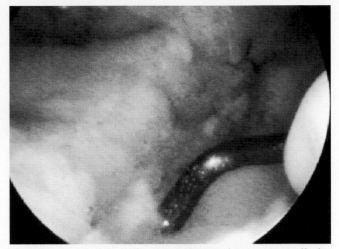

FIGURE 19.4. Evidence of an articular postfracture step-off after the joint debridment. (Reprinted from *Atlas Hand Clinics*, 6(2):371–387, R. Luchetti, A. Atzei, and B. Mustapha, Arthroscopic wrist arthrolysis, pp. 371–387, © 2001 with permission from Elsevier Science.)

Technical Notes

Portals for introducing inflow and/or outflow, instruments, and the arthroscope must frequently be shifted. It is advisable to set the water inflow pressure at 35/45 mmHg or more. Outflow is not necessary for all the joints.

Pre-, intra-, and postoperative fluoroscopic evaluation must be performed to verify the position and the anatomy of the wrist. Pre- and immediate postoperative wrist motion must be evaluated to determine if there has been an improvement.

POSTOPERATIVE REHABILITATION

Rehabilitation is started immediately after surgery. Sometimes pain control may require an analgesic. The

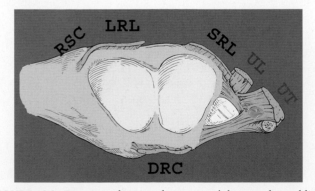

FIGURE 19.3. Drawings showing the extent of the capsular and ligament release of the wrist. RSC (radioscaphocapitate), LRL (long radiolunate), SRL (short radiolunate), DRC (dorsal radiocarpal). The ulnar ligaments, UL (ulnar lunate) and UT (ulnar triquetral) must not be sectioned. (Reprinted from *Atlas Hand Clinics*, 6(2):371–387, R. Luchetti, A. Atzei, and B. Mustapha, Arthroscopic wrist arthrolysis, pp. 371–387, © 2001 with permission from Elsevier Science.)

physical therapist plays a vital role in evaluating the patient's capacity to perform all the wrist range of motion exercises and in instructing the patient in antiedema techniques that should be followed diligently at home for the first 7 days after surgery. In cases of severe edema, the therapist should begin a tenacious antiedema program consisting of the use of contrast baths to aid in stimulating the vasodilatation-vasoconstriction mechanism of the patient's hand and forearm. The temperatures of the baths are 35 to 38 degrees C and 10 to 15 degrees C. The patient submerges the hand and forearm initially in the cool bath for 1 minute and then in the warm bath for 5 minutes. This exercise is repeated continuously for 30 minutes. The patient should begin and end by submerging the hand in the cool bath. Once the contrast bath technique has finished, the therapist should immediately apply distal-proximal functional compressive bandaging to each finger, hand, wrist, and midforearm (Figure 19.5), to aid in lymph drainage and venous return. Lymph drainage massage should be done, following the bandaging, to the entire upper extremity with the patient in a supine posture.

If the patient shows very limited wrist range of motion and the initial onset of edema, it is appropriate to begin a home range of motion program using a continual passive movement device (CPM) to help in maintaining the wrist ROM that was obtained during surgery and to increase blood circulation to the area, thus decreasing edema and the eventual onset of wrist stiffness (Figure 19.6). Pronation-supination and flexion-extension exercises are performed for almost 3 months, gradually increasing the number of repetitions and amount of resistance applied. Aquatic rehabilitation is the initial treatment of choice. The patient is instructed to perform nonresisted hand-

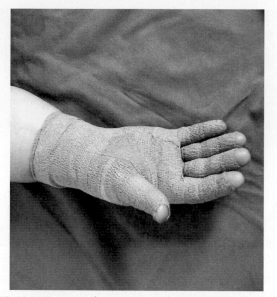

FIGURE 19.5. Functional compressive bandaging preventing the onset of stagnant distal edema of the hand.

more than half a kilo of resistance and slowly increase this resistance and the number of repetitions being performed, always respecting the pain threshold and avoiding the onset of excessive muscular fatigue.

Return to work is limited up until 3 months or in relationship to the job requirements. A palmar wrist splint is used to protect the articulation when the subject must perform heavy labor activities. Work-hardening and endurance-strengthening exercises using isokinetic and isotonic rehabilitation equipment can be initiated 1 month after surgery under the strict supervision of a physical therapist (Figure 19.7A,B). Patient protocols are individualized depending on the strength requirements they need to obtain in order to perform their jobs. It is advisable that the physical therapist do an on-site ergonomic evaluation of the patient being rehabilitated, and quantify the forces required of the patient's entire upper extremity in order to perform work duties.[16]

grasping activities in tepid water, such as squeezing a sponge for 10 minutes four times a day. It is also important that the hand and forearm are not submerged for a long period of time in water that is either too hot or too cold, since excessive vasodilation or constriction is counterproductive during the healing process. The patient eventually progresses to performing all wrist exercises in all planes of motion, in the water, with associated hand exercises in which the fingers are in both the closed-fist or open-palm positions. The patient can gradually progress to exercising in antigravity postures out of water. The patient is instructed on how to perform passive, active, and active assisted exercises. It is advisable to begin the patient with no

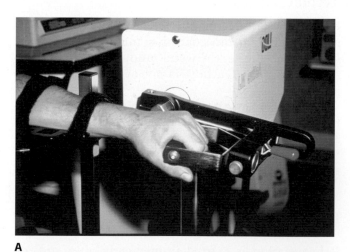

A

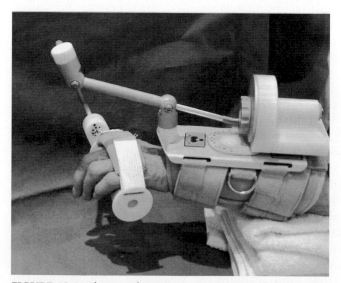

FIGURE 19.6. The use of a continuous passive mobilizer helps to maintain the wrist range of motion that has been obtained during arthroscopic surgery.

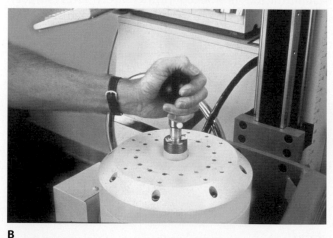

B

FIGURE 19.7. A, B. Isokinetic rehabilitation can be started 1 month after surgery. **A.** Isokinetic exercise for improving both strength and endurance of wrist flexors and extensors. **B.** Isokinetic work simulation is done to re-integrate the entire upper extremity to assume the correct kinematic postures during specific work postures.

TABLE 19.3. Preoperative and Postoperative Evaluation Parameters.

Mayo Wrist Score (Preop)
  Pain (VAS)
  Wrist ROM (degrees)
  Grip strength (Kg or %)
  Work status
DASH questionnaire (Postop)

PERSONAL CLINICAL EXPERIENCE

The authors' clinical experience was initiated in 1988, and up until now we have operated on 43 cases. The first case operated on was to reduce first CMC joint rigidity due to prolonged immobilization after conservative treatment of a Bennett fracture. Arthroscopic arthrolysis of the patient's first CMC joint allowed recovery of complete wrist range of motion without pain. All the other cases involved wrist rigidity secondary to immobilization after wrist fracture or surgery.

In our control series study, 18 patients (13 males and 5 females, with a mean age of 38 years) were included: one of our cases was operated on bilaterally and successively required an additional right wrist arthroscopic arthrolysis in order to reach the same level of improvement as that of the contralateral side. Seventeen cases followed wrist fractures, and one followed open surgery for triangular fibrocartilage complex (TFCC) tear (type 1B).

Criteria for Inclusion

Criteria for inclusion in this study were:

- Wrist stiffness with or without pain.
- Decreased grip strength.
- Unsuccessful results from rehabilitation after 3 to 6 months.

Method of Evaluation and Results

Preoperative and postoperative evaluation of all the patients were done using the Mayo Wrist Score criteria.[17,18] The DASH questionnaire was included in the postoperative checkup (Table 19.3). All the cases were clinically reevaluated at a mean follow-up of 32

TABLE 19.4. Results of Arthroscopic Wrist Arthrolysis for 18 Patients/19 Cases.

	Preop (mean)	Postop (mean)
Pain (VAS)	7	1
Flexion/extension (degrees)	84	107
Rad/ulnar deviation (degrees)	48	49
Prono/supination (degrees)	132	156
Grip strength (Kgs)	27	36

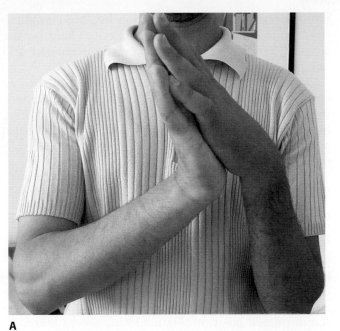

A

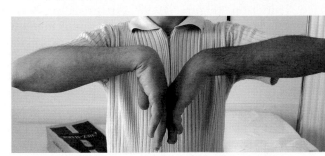

B

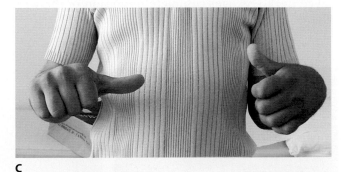

C

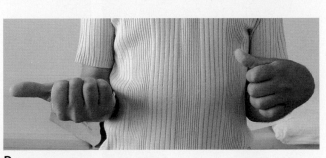

D

FIGURE 19.8. A–D. Distal radius fracture treated with reduction and cast immobilization. Left wrist remained stiff in flexion and in semipronated position after 4 months of rehabilitation.

months (range from 2 to 140 months). No complications were documented. One case failed because the surgical indications were not correctly evaluated, and one patient was deceased.

In all cases, pain was significantly diminished or completely absent, and wrist ROM and grip strength were improved (Table 19.4). The average modified Mayo Clinic Wrist Score improved from 39 (preoperative) to 87 (postop), and the DASH questionnaire obtained an average of 21 points.

Clinical Cases

CASE 19.1

A 26-year-old man with a distal radius fracture of the left wrist was treated with reduction and prolonged plaster cast immobilization in a Cotton-Loder position for 40 days. After 4 months of rehabilitation, the wrist remained completely stiff in flexion and in a semipronated position (Figure 19.8). X-rays taken after 3 months showed osteoporosis and articular wrist space reduction (Figure 19.9). Arthroscopic wrist arthrolysis was performed after 4 months of rehabilitation, obtaining improvement of flexion-extension and pronosupination wrist ROM (Figure 19.10).

CASE 19.2

A 29-year-old woman had limitation in right wrist pronation ROM after a surgical repair of TFCC tear (Figure 19.11). Wrist ROM before surgery was 0 degrees pronation (Figure 19.12). Flexion-extension and supination were normal. Arthroscopic arthrolysis allowed her to recover complete pronation of the wrist (Figure 19.13).

DISCUSSION

Verhellen and Bain[5] demonstrated that arthroscopic arthrolysis cannot harm the median nerve and the radial artery because these important anatomical structures are at a safe distance from the site of ligament resection (from 5 to 6 mm).

Comparison between previous experiences regarding the improvement of wrist ROM after arthroscopic wrist arthrolysis is reported in Table 19.5.

In respect to Verhellen and Bain[5] and Osterman and Culp[6] our cases had a greater preoperative wrist ROM, but the final results of wrist motion were almost the same. Our indication for selecting surgical candidates is based on the subject's level of wrist rigidity that is associated with pain. Wrist rigidity alone is not considered to be important enough to require arthroscopic arthrolysis, but when rigidity is associated with pain, this surgical technique is strongly indicated.

An additional arthroscopic arthrolysis of the same wrist can also be performed again, if required (one case of this nature occurred in our study), based on the clinical results and degree of range of motion improvement. Reoperation is well accepted by patients since the surgery does not take a long time and it is not painful, but most of all because the patient is able to see immediate improvements in wrist motion.

Arthroscopy can reveal associated soft tissue tears that are considered to be the cause of the wrist pain. In our cases, we frequently found loose bodies, arthrofibrosis, chondritis and osteochondritis, partial tears of the intercarpal ligaments (SL, LT, and TFCC) and/or a minimal articular step, which were not evident in the X-ray and/or MRI (Figure 19.4). This con-

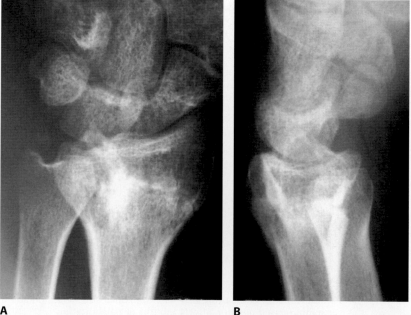

A   **B**

FIGURE 19.9. A, B. X-rays taken after 3 months of rehabilitation; osteoporosis and articular wrist space reduction are visible.

Arthroscopic arthrolysis of other joints, such as the first CMC joint, can also be contemporaneously performed.

Based on our experience, we suggest that ulnar avulsion of the TFCC (type 1B) or a complete lesion of the SL ligament must not be treated simultaneously to this technique since they require prolonged immobilization that is contrary to the immediate rehabilitation that is initiated after arthroscopic arthrolysis. Therefore, it is important to discuss with the patient the surgical procedure indicated. It is mandatory that the wrist be mobilized and that the patient initiate rehabilitation immediately after an arthroscopic arthrolysis procedure.

One must remember that if there is an underlying SL ligament tear in addition to the wrist rigidity, the surgeon will not be able to obtain good results from performing an arthroscopic arthrolysis. The injury to this ligament is predominantly hidden by wrist rigidity; only after the wrist has undergone an arthrolysis can the clinical manifestations of wrist instability due to ligament tear become apparent. The improvement

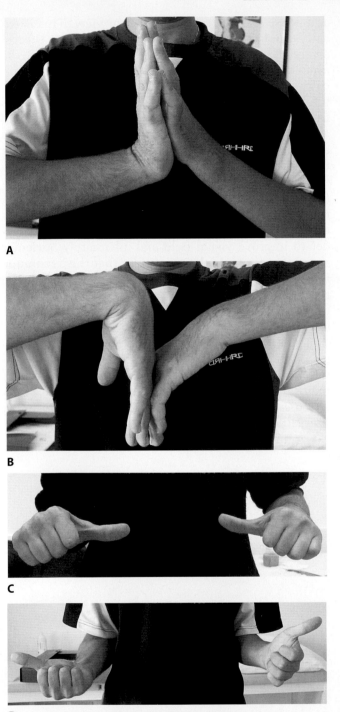

FIGURE 19.10. Both (**A, B**) flexion-extension and (**C, D**) pronation-supination are improved after arthroscopic arthrolysis.

firms the validity of arthroscopy in comparison to other methods.[19,20] Moreover, during the operation, it is possible to treat all these conditions, thus improving both wrist pain and rigidity at the same time.

Conversion to open surgery is suggested only when it is necessary to surgically treat the DRUJ, when difficulty is encountered during the arthroscopy. Other surgical approaches are adopted to treat associated soft tissue tears or pathologies, such as carpal tunnel syndrome (CTS) and partial or total wrist denervation.

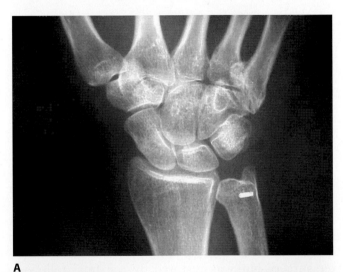

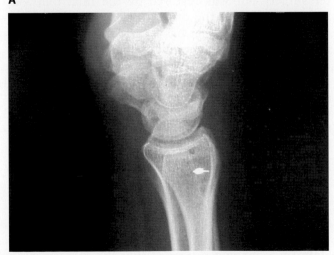

FIGURE 19.11. A, B. TFCC tear of right wrist was surgically repaired.

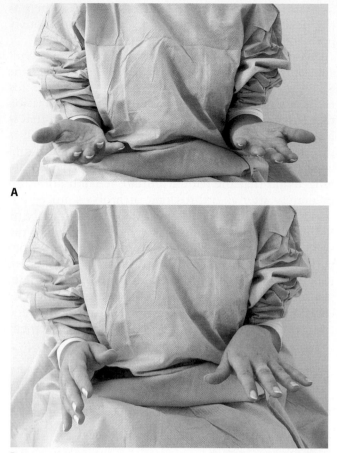

A

B

FIGURE 19.12. A, B. Wrist range of motion was 0 degrees pronation before arthroscopy; flexion-extension and supination were normal.

and dense and obstructs the field of view. This is exactly what occurred in one of our cases that successively ended in a radiocarpal ankylosis. These are the types of cases that should not be treated arthroscopically since they easily end up with residual wrist rigidity. In addition, a radiologic wrist exam, 3 to 6 months from the time of fracture, does not always demonstrate all the various underlying problems; when surgeons see a preserved articular space, they tend to be eager to perform a surgical arthroscopic arthrolysis. Unfortunately, the underlying difficulties become quite evident during the surgery, and if one is able to perform the wrist arthrolysis, the tenaciously adherent bands and the osteofibrotic bridges must be detached in order to improve visual field and, ultimately, articular range of motion. At the same time that this technique is being performed, it becomes quite evident that the radial surface is no longer completely covered by cartilage and there is the presence of osteochondral lesions of various severity.

Even if a proper physical therapy program is followed, it is quite common for fibrotic bridges to reform in a few months and provoke partial or complete radiocarpal ankylosis. It is also possible to find extra-articular wrist rigidity that has been caused by reflex sympathetic dystrophy. In these cases, wrist arthrolysis must be associated with the release of extra-

of wrist range of motion that is obtained during wrist arthrolysis can be inconsistent.

In a previous study (Figure 19.14), we found that intraoperative increase of wrist flexion-extension ROM was followed by a temporary decrease soon after surgery but was restored by the final follow-up reevaluation.[3] On the other hand, pronation-supination improvement that has been obtained during surgery is almost always maintained postoperatively.

Rigidity of the wrist does not always involve the radiocarpal joint (flexion-extension) by itself. DRUJ (pronosupination) rigidity is more frequently encountered, and it can be isolated (Case 19.2) or associated with the radiocarpal joint (Case 19.1). When the rigidity of the DRUJ is isolated, ROM recovery after surgery is easier to obtain than flexion-extension ROM, and this improvement has been maintained.

COMPLICATIONS

Unfortunately, it can happen that the surgeon is unable to perform a wrist arthroscopic arthrolysis due to the presence of an osteofibrotic band that is too thick

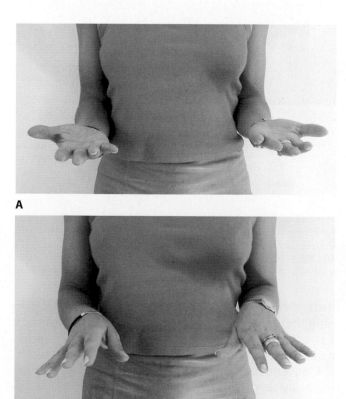

A

B

FIGURE 19.13. A, B. Arthroscopic arthrolysis restored complete pronation of the wrist.

TABLE 19.5. Comparison of Previous Studies in Literature.

Publications	No. cases	Follow-up months	Preop Flex/Ext (mean degrees)	Postop Flex/Ext (mean degrees)
Pederzini et al., 1991	5	10	44/40	54/60
Verhellen and Bain, 2000	5	6	17/10	47/50
Osterman and Culp, 2000	20	32	9/15	42/58
Luchetti, Atzei, Mustapha, 2001	19	32	46/38	54/53

articular soft tissue adhesions. Surgery in these cases must be approached with extreme caution since the root of the wrist rigidity is much more complex than just a localized articular dysfunction.

The surgeon can also run into unpleasant technical situations during surgery such as the breakdown of instruments, including tweezers, scissors, miniscalpel or motorized instruments.[21]

When the patient reports that wrist pain has reappeared or has never completely disappeared after surgery, the surgeon should take note that there can still be an underlying articular pathology that has not been uncovered. Often, the pain can be due to intrinsic ligament tears (SL or LT) that had not been taken into consideration preoperatively. The use of articular instruments and motorized instruments can cause unwanted osteoarticular lesions (chondral scuffing, ligament injuries etc.) that can manifest themselves postoperatively in the form of pain or wrist instability.

CONCLUSION

Arthroscopic arthrolysis is a promising surgical option for the treatment of wrist rigidity after trauma or surgery. Reasons for performing arthroscopic wrist arthrolysis include the following:

- It is safe and requires a minimal amount of invasive surgery.

- It allows the surgeon to precisely identify the real causes of intra-articular rigidity and pain.
- It does not preclude the possibility of performing another surgical procedure in the future that requires prolonged immobilization.
- It does not preclude the possibility of converting an arthroscopic arthrolysis into an open surgery.

It must be remembered that arthroscopic arthrolysis is a difficult procedure to perform and must be done by a skilled and well-trained arthroscopic surgeon.

References

1. Altissimi M, Rinonapoli E. Le rigidità del polso e della mano. Inquadramento clinico, valutazione diagnostica e indicazioni terapeutiche. *Ital J Orthop Traumatol* 1995;21(3):187–192.
2. af Ekenstam FW. Capsulotomy of the distal radio-ulnar joint. *Scand J Plast Surg* 1988;22:169–171.
3. Pederzini L, Luchetti R, Montagna G, et al. Trattamento artroscopico delle rigidità di polso. *Il Ginocchio* 1991;XI–XII:1–13.
4. Bain GI, Verhellen R, Pederzini L. Procedure artroscopiche capsulari del polso. In: Pederzini L, (ed) *Artroscopia di Polso*. Milano: Springer-Verlag Italia, 1999, pp. 123–128.
5. Verhellen R, Bain GI. Arthroscopic capsular release for contracture of the wrist. *Arthroscopy* 2000;16:106–110.
6. Osterman AL, Culp RW, Bednar JM. The arthroscopic release of wrist contractures. Scientific Paper Session A1, American Society for Surgery of the Hand Annual Meeting, Boston, 1999.
7. Luchetti R, Atzei A. Artrolisi artroscopica nelle rigidità posttraumatiche. In: Luchetti R, Atzei A (eds.) *Artroscopia di Polso*. Fidenza: Mattioli 1885 Editore, 2001, pp. 67–71.
8. Luchetti R, Atzei A, Mustapha B. Arthroscopic wrist arthrolysis. *Atlas Hand Clin* 2001;6(2):371–387.
9. Maloney MD, Sauser DD, Hanson EC, et al. Adhesive capsulitis of the wrist: arthrographic diagnosis. *Radiology* 1988;167:187–190.
10. Hanson EC, Wood VE, Thiel AE, et al. Adhesive capsulitis of the wrist. Diagnosis and treatment. *Clin Orthop Rel Res* 1988;234:51–55.
11. Sprauge N, O'Connor RL, Fox JM. Arthroscopic treatment of post operative knee fibroarthrosis. *Clin Orthop Rel Res* 1982;166:125–128.
12. Jones GS, Savoie FH. Arthroscopic capsular release of flexion contractures of the elbow. *Arthroscopy* 1993;9:277–283.
13. Warner JJ, Allen AA, Marks PH, et al. Arthroscopic release of post-operative capsular contracture of the shoulder. *J Bone Joint Surg* 1996;79A:1151–1158.
14. Warner JJ, Answorth A, Marsh PH, et al. Arthroscopic release for chronic, refractory adhesive capsulitis of the shoulder. *J Bone Joint Surg* 1995;78A:1808–1816.
15. Doi K, Hattori Y, Otsuka K, et al. Intra-articular fractures of the distal aspect of the radius: arthroscopically assisted reduc-

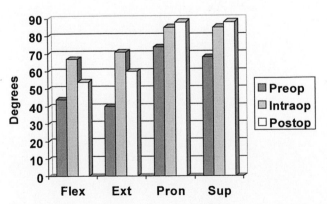

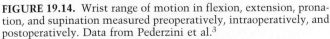

FIGURE 19.14. Wrist range of motion in flexion, extension, pronation, and supination measured preoperatively, intraoperatively, and postoperatively. Data from Pederzini et al.[3]

tion compared with open reduction and internal fixation. *J Bone Joint Surg* 1999;81A:1093–1110.

16. Travaglia-Fairplay T. Valutazione ergonomica dell'ambiente industriale e sua applicazione per screening di pre-assunzione e riabilitazione work-hardening. In: Bazzini G (ed.) *Nuovi Approcci alla Riabilitazione Industriale*. Pavia: Fondazione Clinica del Lavoro Edizioni, 1993, pp. 33–48.

17. Cooney WP, Bussey R, Dobyns JH, et al. Difficult wrist fractures. Perilunate fracture-dislocations of the wrist. *Clin Orthop* 1987;(214):136–147.

18. Krimmer H. Gegenuberstellung der mediokarpalen Teilarthrodese und der Totalarthrodese des Handgelenkes durch Scorebewertung. In: Krimmer H (ed.) *Der posttraumatische karpale kollaps*. Berlin: Springer 2000, pp. 48–57.

19. Cerofolini E, Luchetti R, Pederzini L, et al. MR. Evaluation of triangular fibrocartilage complex tears in the wrist: comparison with arthrography and arthroscopy. *J Comput Assist Tomogr* 1990;14:963–967.

20. Zlatkin MB, Chao PC, Osterman AL, et al. Chronic wrist pain: evaluation with high resolution MR imaging. *Radiology* 1989; 173:723–729.

21. Luchetti R, Atzei A. Insuccessi nelle tecniche artroscopiche. *Riv Chir Mano* 2001;38(2):180–187.

20

Small-Joint Arthroscopy in the Hand and Wrist

Richard A. Berger

Ten years ago, small-joint arthroscopy in the hand and wrist was tantamount to a technique searching for a purpose. Today, small-joint arthroscopy has found its way into virtually every arthroscopist's armamentarium. Reductions in the dimensions of arthroscopic equipment and improvements in our understanding of the internal anatomy of small joints have made it possible to arthroscopically evaluate and treat a number of conditions involving the carpometacarpal (CMC) and metacarpophalangeal joints of the hand.[1–3] Recently, it has even been proposed that arthroscopy of the proximal interphalangeal joint may have indications. This chapter provides an overview of relevant joint anatomy, portal placement, arthroscopic techniques, and indications for those techniques.

FIRST CMC JOINT

Arthroscopy of the first carpometacarpal joint was developed and described nearly 7 years ago.[1,2] The first carpometacarpal joint was a natural starting point for small-joint arthroscopy due to its relative depth, highly curved articular surfaces, and the nearly circumferential nature of the stabilizing ligaments. Each of these factors makes complete viewing of the joint difficult with arthrotomy, unless capsulotomies are carried out through these vital ligaments. Found to be useful for diagnosis, arthroscopy of the first CMC joint was soon applied to help visualize the adequacy of reduction of fractures involving the articular surfaces of the trapezium or first metacarpal, such as a Bennett's fracture, as well as to treat established arthritis. With miniaturization of thermocouple probes, arthroscopy can now guide shrinkage of the joint capsule in conditions of joint capsule laxity as well as arthroplasty for the treatment of end-stage arthrosis.

Indications

The principal indications for arthroscopy of the first carpometacarpal joint are, in general, the same as for other joints. Included in this list are staging evalua- tion of arthrosis, identification of a ligament injury, treatment of two-part fractures of the base of the first metacarpal, retrieval of floating loose bodies or foreign objects, and the irrigation of a septic joint.

Contraindications

The contraindications for arthroscopy of the first carpometacarpal joint are the same as for other joints, including poor soft tissue coverage, active cellulitis, and joint injury that is obviously beyond the capability of the arthroscope to address (Rolando fracture).

Regional Anatomy

The skin overlying the first CMC joint is glabrous only on the palmar surface. Immediately deep to the skin and superficial to the deep fascia are numerous veins, including the principal tributaries forming the cephalic vein system. Within the periadventitial tissue of these tributaries are the S1 and S2 divisions of the superficial radial nerve, found just deep to the veins (Figure 20.1).

Several muscles and tendons cross the joint, beginning anteriorly with the abductor pollicis brevis, which originates from the anterior surface of the trapezium (Figure 20.1). Just lateral to this is the tendon of the abductor pollicis longus, which inserts into the posterior base of the first metacarpal. The tendon of the extensor pollicis brevis passes distally just posterior to the abductor pollicis longus. Just superficial to the posterior joint capsule of the first CMC joint is the deep division of the radial artery, crossing the first CMC joint deep to the extensor pollicis longus tendon before coursing anteriorly between the proximal metaphyses of the first and second metacarpals. Between the proximal epiphyses of the first and second metacarpals is the intermetacarpal ligament, which is entirely extracapsular.

Joint Anatomy

The first CMC joint is a double saddle joint formed by the distal articular surface of the trapezium and the

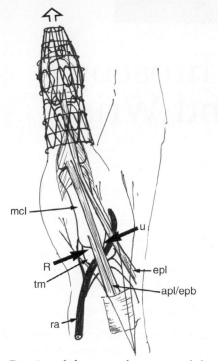

FIGURE 20.1. Drawing of the regional anatomy of the first carpometacarpal joint. mcI = first metacarpal, tm = trapezium, ra = radial artery, epl = tendon of extensor pollicis longus, apl/epb = tendons of abductor pollicis longus and extensor pollicis brevis, R and U = radial and ulnar arthroscopic portals, respectively. (Reprinted with permission, Atlas of the Hand Clinics, Sept 2001, Berger RA: Arthroscopy of the Small Joints of the Hand.)

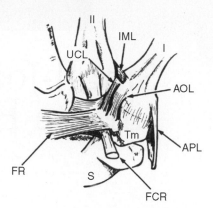

FIGURE 20.2. Drawing of the anterior surface of the first carpometacarpal joint capsule. I = first metacarpal, II = second metacarpal, Tm = trapezium, S = scaphoid, APL = tendon of abductor pollicis longus, FCR = tendon of flexor carpi radialis, FR = flexor retinaculum, AOL = anterior oblique ligament, UCL = ulnar collateral ligament, IML = intermetacarpal ligament. (Reprinted with permission, Atlas of the Hand Clinics, Sept 2001, Berger RA: Arthroscopy of the Small Joints of the Hand.)

base of the first metacarpal. The articular surface along the major axis of the trapezium is concave in the medial-lateral direction, and the articular surface along the minor axis is concave in the anteroposterior direction. The converse relationship is found with the base of the first metacarpal, where the articular surface is concave in the anteroposterior direction and convex in the medial-lateral direction. Although a joint capsule surrounds the entire joint, only three-fourths is reinforced by capsular ligaments.[4,5]

The anterior edge of the first CMC joint is reinforced by the anterior oblique ligament complex (AOL), which is composed of superficial and deep divisions (Figures 20.2, 20.3, and 20.4). The superficial division (AOLs) spans nearly the entire anterior edge of the joint and attaches to the anterior surface of the trapezium just proximal to the articular surface and just distal to the articular surface of the base of the first metacarpal. The deep division (AOLd) is a well-demarcated thickening of the superficial band found just medial to the midline of the superficial division. Often, there is a distant medial edge separating the AOLd from the AOLs (Figures 20.3 and 20.4). The deep division of the AOL is often referred to as the *beak ligament*. The orientation of the fibers of the AOLs is slightly oblique, passing proximal to distal from lateral to medial. The fiber orientation of the AOLs is

essentially proximal to distal. The extreme lateral (ulnar) surface of the joint is reinforced by the ulnar collateral ligament (UCL), which has fibers oriented in a proximal to distal direction (Figures 20.2 and 20.5). The lateral 30% of the posterior surface of the joint capsule is reinforced by the posterior oblique ligament (POL) (Figures 20.5, 20.6, and 20.7). The fiber orientation of the POL is slightly oblique, passing from proximal and medial to distal and lateral. The remaining posterior joint capsule is reinforced by the dorsoradial ligament (DRL) (Figures 20.5, 20.6, and 20.7). The fiber orientation of the DRL is generally proximal to distal. The joint capsule immediately deep to the tendon of the abductor pollicis longus is not reinforced by a ligament. Although there is a distinct border between

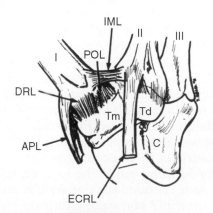

FIGURE 20.3. Drawing of the posterior surface of the first carpometacarpal joint capsule. I = first metacarpal, II = second metacarpal, III = third metacarpal, Tm = trapezium, Td = trapezoid, C = capitate, ECRL = tendon of extensor carpi radialis longus, APL = tendon of abductor pollicis longus, IML = intermetacarpal ligament, POL = posterior oblique ligament, DRL = dorsoradial ligament. (Reprinted with permission, Atlas of the Hand Clinics, Sept 2001, Berger RA: Arthroscopy of the Small Joints of the Hand.)

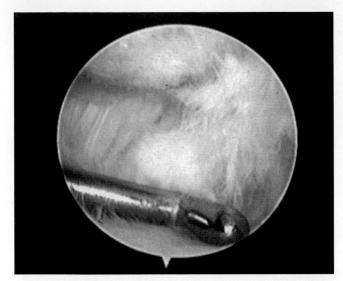

A

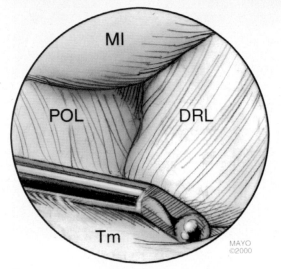

B

FIGURE 20.4. Arthroscopic photograph **(A)** and corresponding drawing **(B)** of the posterior joint capsule viewed from the 1-R portal. MI = first metacarpal, Tm = trapezium, DRL = dorsoradial ligament, POL = posterior oblique ligament. (Reprinted with permission, Atlas of the Hand Clinics, Sept 2001, Berger RA: Arthroscopy of the Small Joints of the Hand.)

the AOLs and AOLd, there are no reliable demarcations between the remaining ligaments.

Portals

The two recognized portals for arthroscopy of the first carpometacarpal joint are named according to their relationship with the extensor pollicis brevis and abductor pollicis longus tendons (Figure 20.8). The I-R portal is established at the joint line just radial to the abductor pollicis longus tendon (Figures 20.1 and 20.8). The 1-U portal is established at the joint line just ulnar to the extensor pollicis brevis tendon (Figures 20.1 and 20.8).

Surgical Technique

The patient is positioned supine on the operating table with either regional or general anesthesia. Parenteral antibiotics may be administered, and a pneumatic tourniquet is typically applied to their arm. A single finger trap is secured to the thumb, and 5 to 8 pounds of longitudinal traction is applied (Figure 20.9). Using a 22-gauge hypodermic needle, the location of either the 1-R or 1-U portal is scouted by advancing the needle directly ulnarly. The needle should be angled approximately 20 to 30 degrees distally due to the curved nature of the joint surface. If there is any difficulty in

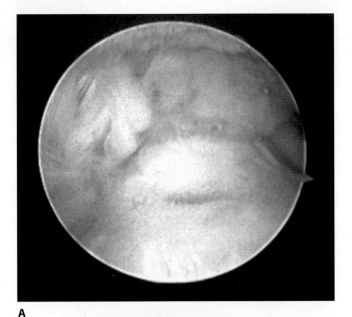

A

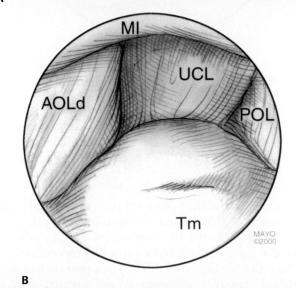

B

FIGURE 20.5. Arthroscopic photograph **(A)** and corresponding drawing **(B)** of the ulnar joint capsule viewed from the 1-R portal. MI = first metacarpal, Tm = trapezium, POL = posterior oblique ligament, UCL = ulnar collateral ligament, AOLd = deep portion of the anterior oblique ligament. (Reprinted with permission, Atlas of the Hand Clinics, Sept 2001, Berger RA: Arthroscopy of the Small Joints of the Hand.)

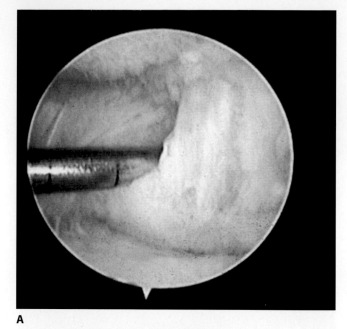

A

sected bluntly to the joint capsule level to be certain that underlying neurovascular tissues are displaced from harm's way. Depending upon the surgeon's preference, a 1.5 to 2.4 mm diameter arthroscope may be utilized (Figure 20.10). The arthroscope sheath is then introduced with a tapered trocar in one portal, and a small probe is introduced in the other portal. It is rare that an outflow device is needed, particularly with judicious control of inflow fluid volume and rate. If an outflow tract is necessary, however, a large-bore hypodermic needle may be introduced, or a shaver may be used to evacuate excess or cloudy fluid. It may also

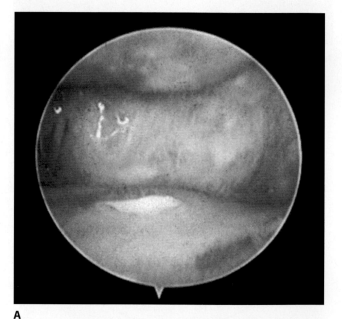

A

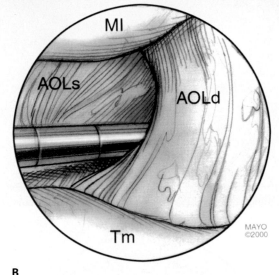

B

FIGURE 20.6. Arthroscopic photograph **(A)** and corresponding drawing **(B)** of the anterior joint capsule viewed from the 1-U portal. MI = first metacarpal, Tm = trapezium, AOLd = deep portion of the anterior oblique ligament, AOLs = superficial portion of the anterior oblique ligament. (Reprinted with permission, Atlas of the Hand Clinics, Sept 2001, Berger RA: Arthroscopy of the Small Joints of the Hand.)

passing the needle into the joint or if there is any concern about the proper identification of the joint, intraoperative radiographs or fluoroscopy may be used to verify the level of the needle prior to proceeding.

Once the proper level of the joint portals has been identified, small stab wounds are created with a scalpel, either transversely or longitudinally. I would advocate making the incisions for both portals at the beginning of the procedure. This facilitates switching portals during the operation without disturbing the cadence of the procedure. Subcutaneous tissues are dis-

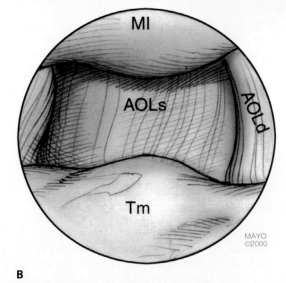

B

FIGURE 20.7. Arthroscopic photograph **(A)** and corresponding drawing **(B)** of the anterior joint capsule viewed from the 1-U portal. MI = first metacarpal, Tm = trapezium, AOLd = deep portion of the anterior oblique ligament, AOLs = superficial portion of the anterior oblique ligament. (Reprinted with permission, Atlas of the Hand Clinics, Sept 2001, Berger RA: Arthroscopy of the Small Joints of the Hand.)

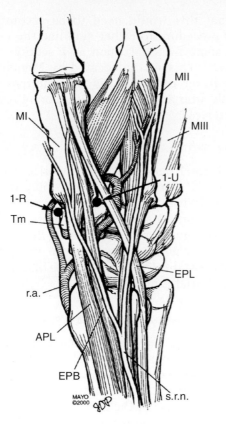

FIGURE 20.8. Landmarks used to establish the portals for the first carpometacarpal joint arthroscopy. IMC = first metacarpal, MII = second metacarpal, MIII = third metacarpal, Tm = trapezium, APL = tendon of abductor pollicis longus, EPB = tendon of extensor pollicis brevis, 1-R = radial CMC portal.

be necessary to debride excess synovial tissue in order to visualize the joint surfaces and the ligaments. This may be accomplished with either a small shaver or a suction punch.

I typically orient the camera and orient the lens of the arthroscope in a manner that places the image of the base of the first metacarpal at the top and the trapezium at the bottom. A comprehensive inspection of the articular surfaces is carried out. Next, an inspection of the intra-articular appearance of the capsular ligaments may be completed. It is best to use the probe to validate the integrity of these structures, rather than simply relying on their visual appearance.

The dorsoradial ligament, posterior oblique ligament, ulnar collateral ligament, and deep portion of the anterior oblique ligament can typically be visualized from the 1-R portal (Figures 20.3, 20.4, 20.5, and 20.7). The superficial and deep portions of the anterior oblique ligament, ulnar collateral ligament, and posterior oblique ligament can be visualized through the 1-U portal (Figures 20.3, 20.4, 20.5, and 20.7).

Procedures

The following procedures have been proposed, although this list is largely based upon personal com-

munications and anecdotal experiences and is by no means meant to be all-inclusive.

SYNOVECTOMY

A partial or radical synovectomy can be carried out arthroscopically using a shaver less than 3 mm in diameter and a thermocouple probe system or a small suction punch device. Care should be exercised when using the shaver or a punch to avoid iatrogenic compromise of the capsular ligaments themselves. Because of the small diameter of the shaver, the suction sheath frequently becomes clogged with debrided tissue. This requires frequent cleaning, which may frustrate some surgeons.

CAPSULAR SHRINKAGE

It may be advantageous in some circumstances to be able to shrink, hence stiffen, the joint capsule, such as in a substantially lax individual with early arthrosis of the first CMC joint. Commercially available thermocouple probe systems, in a diameter suitable for this joint, are available, but little experience has been gained in this specific joint at this time.

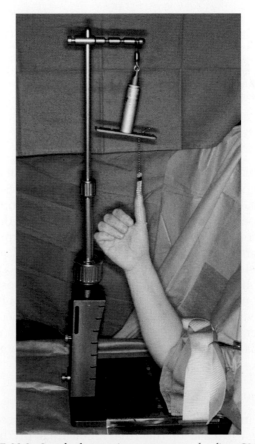

FIGURE 20.9. Standard operating room setup for first CMC joint arthroscopy. The thumb is suspended with 5 to 8 lbs. of traction. (Reprinted with permission, Atlas of the Hand Clinics, Sept 2001, Berger RA: Arthroscopy of the Small Joints of the Hand.)

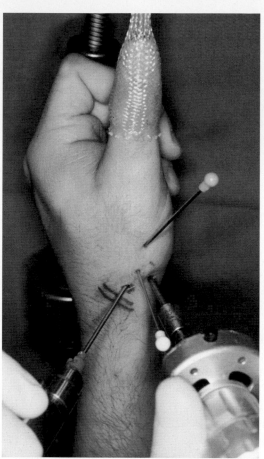

FIGURE 20.10. Arthroscopy of the first CMC joint. The arthroscope is in the 1-U portal and a shaver is in the 1-R portal. Provisional K-wires have been placed for fixation of a Bennett fracture reduced arthroscopically. (Reprinted with permission, Atlas of the Hand Clinics, Sept 2001, Berger RA: Arthroscopy of the Small Joints of the Hand.)

Staging Arthritis

The precise staging of arthritic involvement of the articular surfaces of the first CMC joint is easily accomplished with the arthroscope.[6] This is important in those patients with painful instability of the first CMC joint on whom one is considering performing an extra-articular ligament reconstruction.[7] If substantial arthrosis is present, but not radiographically evident yet, a ligament reconstruction would be considered contraindicated. The most common locations for initial involvement of articular cartilage destruction in degenerative arthritis are the central aspect of the trapezial surface and the ulnar third of the metacarpal surface.

Resection/Interposition Arthroplasty

There may some indication for partially resecting wither the base of the first metacarpal or the distal surface of the trapezium, although one would

think that this would need to be accompanied by another procedure to either stabilize the joint or interpose some material, such as a section of tendon or fascia.[6,8] This was advocated by Menon, where a strip of flexor carpi radialis was interposed arthroscopically after arthroscopic resection of the arthritic joint surfaces.[2]

Septic Arthritis

Although rarely encountered, the irrigation and debridement of a septic first CMC joint is easily accomplished with the arthroscope and a shaver. A large volume of normal saline can be passed through the joint by simply running the shaver in the middle of the joint space while connecting the inflow to a wide-open source of fluid. Cultures can be obtained by sampling the initial aspirate.

Reduction of Intra-Articular Fracture

The arthroscope may be a valuable adjunct to the treatment of simple intra-articular fractures involving the base of the first metacarpal. Bennett's fractures involve an intra-articular fracture through the ulnar condyle of the base of the first metacarpal. They may produce problems due to intra-articular stepoff or instability. The instability is generated by the uncompromised pull of the abductor pollicis longus on the large fragment with loss of contact with the ulnar collateral ligament. Since the first CMC joint is nearly circumferentially covered with stabilizing ligaments, any attempt to visualize the fracture line in a Bennett's fracture will necessarily compromise these ligaments. Accurate visualization of the adequacy of reduction by closed means using radiographic imaging is difficult due to the highly curved nature of the articular surfaces of the joint.

When contemplating an arthroscopically assisted fixation of a Bennett's fracture, it must first be determined that the fracture is mobile. It is important to remember that the arthroscope is not a reduction device per se. It is merely a means of visualizing the reduction carried out by other means. Regional or general anesthesia is required, and the patient should be prepared for the possibility that the procedure may be converted to an open reduction or aborted altogether if the arthroscopic procedure is not possible. The easiest way to assess whether the fracture is mobile, and potentially amenable to closed reduction under arthroscopic assessment, is to distract the thumb on the operating table. Under fluoroscopy, the distal fragment is manipulated while observing the fracture. Typical manipulation maneuvers include axial rotation, with the goal of reducing the large fragment (in the surgeon's grasp) to the small fragment (the ulnar condyle of the first metacarpal base). If the fracture moves close to what is considered an adequate reduction, one may proceed with arthroscopy.

Next, a 0.045 K-wire is advanced into the base of the first metacarpal under fluoroscopic guidance in a line that will either skewer the small fragment upon reduction or will penetrate an adjacent bone to stabilize the reduction (Figure 20.10). The arthroscope is introduced in the standard fashion, as is a small shaver. The shaver is used to evacuate the intra-articular hematoma universally present. A careful assessment of the articular surfaces and the capsular ligaments is made. Once clear visualization is possible, the fracture is manipulated into an acceptable reduction under arthroscopic guidance. Once an acceptable reduction is achieved, the assistant advances the previously placed K-wire for secure fixation of the fracture. Final radiographs are obtained, and external dressings with reinforcement are applied, just as in an open reduction procedure.

Because of the severe comminution and soft tissue disruption in a Rolando fracture, this fracture pattern should be viewed as a relative contraindication for arthroscopic reduction. Logically, there is no advantage to using an arthroscope for an extraarticular fracture pattern. It should be possible to use the arthroscope for intra-articular fractures of the trapezium, but the author has had no experience with this approach.

METACARPOPHALANGEAL JOINTS

Arthroscopy of the metacarpophalangeal (MCP) joints of the hand is rarely performed, but may have limited applications.[2,9] One must remember the advantages versus limitations of open versus arthroscopic procedures before deciding which technique to use. The advantage of open procedures is typically in the access to regions for procedural tasks, while the disadvantages are surgical scars, potential soft tissue destabilization, and limitation of visualization in deep recesses. Arthroscopy offers the advantages of superior visualization of most regions of a joint otherwise difficult to access in an open procedure through very small incisions with minimal impact on the status of contiguous tissues. The major disadvantages of arthroscopic procedures lie in the limits of procedural maneuvers allowed through the very small incisions. This dilemma is most evident in the MCP joint. Although a lengthy skin incision may be needed for an open exposure of the MCP joint, leaving largely a cosmetic effect, the disturbance of the soft tissues (extensor mechanism and joint capsule) probably has a

minimal effect, especially with the proper postoperative rehabilitation protocol. However, there may be an occasion when arthroscopy of the MCP joint may be an attractive option.

Indications

Indications for arthroscopy of the MCP joints are poorly worked out at this time, but may include assessment of arthritis,[10,11] synovectomy,[10,12,13] irrigation of a septic joint, retrieval of foreign bodies, and the identification and possible reapproximation of collateral ligaments avulsed from either the proximal phalanx or the metacarpal.[2]

Contraindications

The contraindications for arthroscopy of the MCP joints are the same as for other joints, including poor soft tissue coverage, active cellulitis, and joint injury that is obviously beyond the capability of the arthroscope to address. To date, the techniques of arthroscopic reduction and fixation of intra-articular fractures of the metacarpal head or proximal phalanx base have not been determined for general application.

Regional Anatomy

The skin over the dorsal surfaces of the MCP joints is typically held loosely to subcutaneous incisions, so care must be exercised when marking palpated landmarks so that stretching the skin prior to committing to an incision location does not displace the marks. Immediately deep to the skin are cutaneous sensory nerves (superficial radial and lateral antebrachial cutaneous nerves for the thumb, index and long fingers, and the dorsal sensory branches of the ulnar nerve for the ring and small fingers). The major veins draining the fingers are typically found in the intermetacarpal valleys, well away from most arthroscopic approaches.

The tendons on the dorsal surfaces of the MCP joints share a common feature: the extensor hood (Figure 20.11). At the level of the joint, the extensor hood is composed of the extrinsic extensor tendon(s) and the sagittal fibers passing toward the volar plate. The extensor tendons for the thumb include the extensor pollicis brevis (radially) and longus (ulnarly). For the index through small fingers, the extensor digitorum communis tendon passes across the MCP joint as the radial-most tendon. Each finger also has an independent proprius tendon, although the extensor indicis proprius and extensor digiti minimi (quinti) tendons are the most widely

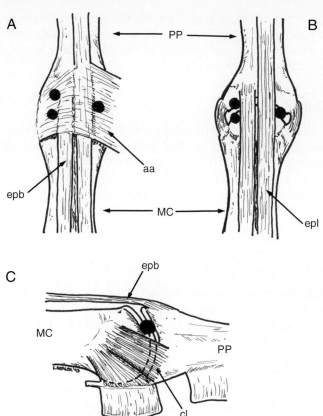

FIGURE 20.11. Drawings of the relevant anatomy for metacar-pophalangeal (MP) joint arthroscopy. **A.** Thumb MP joint showing the extensor hood formed in part by the adductor aponeurosis (aa) and the extrinsic extensor tendons (epb = extensor pollicis brevis). **B.** Thumb MP anatomy after removal of the extensor hood, revealing the tendon of extensor pollicis longus (epl). **C.** Lateral view of the MP joint demonstrating the relationships between the metacarpal (MC), proximal phalanx (PP), tendon of extensor pollicis brevis (epb), and the collateral ligament system (cl). The black dots represent the location of recommended arthroscopic portals. (Reprinted with permission, Atlas of the Hand Clinics, Sept 2001, Berger RA: Arthroscopy of the Small Joints of the Hand.)

recognized. These tendons do not insert directly into the proximal phalanx, but are connected to the dorsal joint capsule and, hence, indirectly insert into the phalanx.

Intra-Articular Anatomy

The intra-articular anatomy of the first through fifth MCP joints is similar. The joint is described as a shallow glenoid-type joint. The articular surface of the second through fifth metacarpal heads is largely spherical, but widens palmarly in the transverse plane. The first metacarpal has little medial-lateral variance. The bases of the proximal phalanges have a shallow glenoid shape for articulation with the metacarpal head.

The lateral joint capsule is reinforced by the collateral ligament system. The true collateral ligaments span the distance from a depression on the lateral and medial surfaces of the head of the metacarpal to the palmar half of the proximal rim of the proximal phalanx. The accessory collateral ligaments are fan-shaped extensions of the true collateral ligaments that attach to the lateral edges of the volar plate.

The volar plate forms the palmar surface of the MCP joint capsule. It has a poorly defined proximal attachment to the metacarpal, but has a definite attachment along the palmar rim of the base of the proximal phalanx. Often, there is a meniscal rim of the volar plate protruding into the joint space, biased toward the distal end of the volar plate.

The dorsal joint capsule is thick and redundant, extending proximally to a line that is proximal to the level of collateral ligament attachment to the metacarpal head.

Portals

The two recognized portals for arthroscopy of the metacarpophalangeal joints (Figure 20.11) are named according to their relationships with the extensor tendons. The radial portal is established at the joint line just radial to the extrinsic extensor tendons. The ulnar portal is established at the joint line just ulnar to the extrinsic extensor tendons.

Surgical Technique

The patient is positioned supine on the operating table; either regional or general anesthesia is administered. Parenteral antibiotics may be administered, and a pneumatic tourniquet is typically applied to the arm. A single finger trap is secured to the thumb or finger to be evaluated, and 5 to 8 pounds of longitudinal traction is applied (Figure 20.12). Using a 22-gauge hypodermic needle, the location of either the I-R or I-U portal is scouted by advancing the needle directly palmarly. If there is any difficulty in passing the needle into the joint or if there is any concern about the proper identification of the joint, intraoperative radiographs or fluoroscopy may be used to verify the level of the needle prior to proceeding.

Once the proper level of the joint portals has been identified, small stab wounds are created with a scalpel, either transversely or longitudinally. I would advocate making the incisions for both portals at the beginning of the procedure. This facilitates switching portals during the operation without disturbing the cadence of the procedure. Subcutaneous tissues are dissected bluntly to the joint capsule level to be certain that underlying neurovascular tissues are displaced from harm's way. The arthroscope sheath is then introduced with a tapered trocar in one portal; a small probe is introduced in the other portal. It is rare that

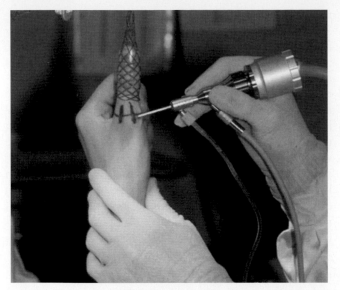

FIGURE 20.12. Standard operating room setup for thumb MCP joint arthroscopy. Longitudinal traction of 5 lbs. is applied through a finger trap. The arthroscope is in the radial portal. Note the definition of the extensor tendons defining the landmarks used to establish the portals. Arthroscopy of the first CMC joint. The arthroscope is in the 1-U portal and a shaver is in the 1-R portal. Provisional K-wires have been placed for fixation of a Bennett fracture reduced arthroscopically. (Reprinted with permission, Atlas of the Hand Clinics, Sept 2001, Berger RA: Arthroscopy of the Small Joints of the Hand.)

an outflow device is needed, particularly with judicious control of inflow fluid volume and rate. If an outflow tract is necessary, however, a large-bore hypodermic needle may be introduced, or a shaver may be used to evacuate excess or cloudy fluid. It may also be necessary to debride excess synovial tissue in order to visualize the joint surfaces and the ligaments. This may be accomplished with either a small shaver or a suction punch.

A comprehensive inspection of the articular surfaces is carried out. Next, an inspection of the intra-articular appearance of the collateral ligaments and volar plate may be completed. It is best to use the probe to validate the integrity of these structures, rather than simply relying on their visual appearance.

Procedures

The following procedures have been proposed, although largely based upon personal communications and anecdotal experiences. This is by no means meant to be an all-inclusive list.

Synovitis

Synovial biopsy is easily performed through standard portals with a 2-mm shaver or arthroscopic grabber. Similarly, a radical synovectomy can be carried out with a shaver in all joint regions.

Septic Arthritis

Irrigation and debridement of a septic MCP joint are easily accomplished with the arthroscope and a shaver. This may be considered particularly useful in so-called "fight bites" in which an open intrusion of the joint has occurred during an altercation where contact with an opponent's teeth creates a septic hazard for the joint. A large volume of normal saline can be passed through the joint simply by running the shaver in the middle of the joint space while connecting the inflow to a wide-open source of fluid. Cultures can be obtained by sampling the initial aspirate.

Diagnosis of Collateral Ligament Injury

Most ligament injuries about the MCP joints are treated well with closed means. However, the Stener-type lesion creates a situation that is less likely to result in successful closed management. In the Stener lesion, the distally avulsed collateral ligament is displaced and trapped under the free proximal edge of the extensor hood.[14] Although injury to the ulnar collateral ligament of the thumb is the most common avulsion injury associated with a Stener lesion, it is possible in the fingers.[3,8,14] This is particularly so with the ulnar collateral ligament of the index finger MCP joint and the radial collateral ligament of the small finger MCP joint. The arthroscope provides a minimally invasive means of readily identifying the presence of a Stener-type lesion in any of the digits.

Additionally, in a subacute setting of instability following injury, it may prove to be a difficult task to know if the injury has occurred from the proximal or distal attachment of a finger MCP collateral ligament. Because scar tissue has likely developed, the surgeon will have a difficult time knowing where the injury occurred, leading to potential complications of elevating the wrong end of the ligament during open repair. Again, the arthroscope offers a ready means of identifying the level of the injury prior to converting to an open procedure.

Reapproximation of Collateral Ligament Avulsion Injury

Ryu has advocated the use of the arthroscope as the definitive treatment for thumb Stener lesion injuries of the ulnar collateral ligament.[3] After verifying the presence of the Stener lesion, the ligament is "hooked" by the probe and drawn back deep to the adductor aponeurosis, where it comes to rest adjacent to the normal attachment point on the ulnar rim of the base of the proximal phalanx. From here, it is treated as a nondisplaced collateral ligament injury.

Depending upon its size, type, and location, it may be possible to retrieve a foreign body in the PIP joint arthroscopically through standard portals using an arthroscopic grabber.

PROXIMAL INTERPHALANGEAL JOINT

Arthroscopy of the proximal interphalangeal (PIP) joint has not been widely accepted as a useful technique at this time. This is no doubt due in large part to the relatively restricted number of indications due to the technical limitations.

Indications

The indications for PIP joint arthroscopy are essentially the same as those for metacarpophalangeal joint arthroscopy, and would include assessment or staging of arthritis,[11] synovial biopsy,[11] irrigation of a septic joint, and retrieval of foreign bodies.[15]

Contraindications

The contraindications for arthroscopy of the PIP joints are the same as for other joints, including poor soft tissue coverage, active cellulitis, and joint injury which is obviously beyond the capability of the arthroscope. To this date, the techniques of arthroscopic reduction and fixation of intra-articular fractures of the proximal phalangeal head or middle phalanx base have not been reported.

Regional Anatomy

The proximal interphalangeal joint is formed by the articulation of the head of the proximal phalanx and the base of the middle phalanx. The skin overlying the joint is a distal reflection of the skin over the main part of the hand, with relatively thin, mobile skin dorsally and thick, glabrous palmar skin. The palmar skin displays several colinear transverse creases at the level of the joint, while the dorsal skin is redundant and displays concentric elliptical creases. The dorsal skin is separated from the extensor mechanism by a layer of loose aponeurotic tissue. The extensor mechanism at the level of the PIP joint undergoes a transition from the discrete intrinsic and extrinsic systems proximally to the combined extensor mechanism distally. Identifiable elements at this level include the central slip, radial and ulnar lateral bands, the transverse retinacular ligament, and, although difficult to define discretely, the proximal

fibers of the oblique retinacular ligament (Figure 20.13). The radial and ulnar proper neurovascular bundles are seen coursing distally just anterior to the midlateral plane of the finger, channeled by Grayson's and Cleland's ligaments. The flexor digitorum superficialis and profundus tendons are encased within the flexor tendon sheath system. At the level of the PIP joint, this system is composed of the PIP joint volar plate, the A3 pulley, and the tenosynovial sheath. The volar plate stabilizes the PIP joint from excessive hyperextension due to stout insertions of the check rein ligaments into the neck of the proximal phalanx and distal attachments to the medial and lateral ridges of the base of the middle phalanx. The volar plate is further stabilized through the accessory collateral liga-

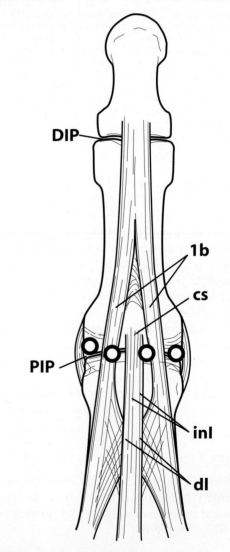

FIGURE 20.13. Drawings of the relevant anatomy for proximal interphalangeal (PIP) joint arthroscopy. Left: dorsal view of a finger. Right: lateral view of a finger. DIP = distal interphalangeal joint, PIP = proximal interphalangeal joint, lb = lateral band, cs = central slip, dl = dorsolateral portal, between a lateral band and the central slip.

ments that attach to the lateral recesses of the head of the proximal phalanx, confluent with the proximal attachments of the proper collateral ligaments. From these recesses, the proper collateral ligaments course distally to attach to the lateral ridges of the base of the middle phalanx. Finally, the palmar skin is richly invested with a venous network. The dorsal skin is innervated by terminal fibers of either the superficial radial nerve for the radial digits or the dorsal sensory branch of the ulnar nerve for the ulnar digits. The palmar and lateral skin are innervated by the underlying proper digital nerve.

Intra-Articular Anatomy

The PIP joint is a bicondylar joint. As such, a medial and lateral condyle form the head of the proximal phalanx, and corresponding medial and lateral fossae form the base of the middle phalanx. The condyles are separated by a sagittal groove called the intercondylar groove, while the fossae on the base of the middle phalanx are separated by a corresponding interfossal ridge. All of these regions are covered in articular cartilage. The dorsal aspect of the middle phalanx base forms a rim where the central slip of the extensor mechanism inserts. The volar plate often has a mensicuslike, wedge-shaped prominence intruding into the palmar aspect of the joint.

Portals

Several portals have been described for arthroscopy of the PIP joint. On either the radial or ulnar surface of the digit (or both surfaces), portals have been described in the intervals between the central slip and the lateral bands,[15] or between the lateral bands and the collateral ligaments (Figure 20.13).[11,15] Although a dorsal portal has been described, it has not been recommended for general use because of difficulty in obtaining useful imaging and the possibility of damage to the central slip.[15] Similarly, a volar portal has been described and abandoned, due to the difficulty of traversing the flexor tendons, volar plate, and neurovascular bundles.[15]

Surgical Technique

Most authors have advocated using a horizontal position of the extremity to maximize mobility of the arthroscope and equipment in multiple planes about the finger. Regional or general anesthesia has been reported most often, although there does not seem to be a strong reason not to do this procedure with a digital block and finger tourniquet. The

use of parenteral antibiotics is at the surgeon's discretion. The finger is supported in slight flexion with a towel, and manual distraction is applied if necessary.

The joint is distended by inserting a 25-gauge needle into the joint either dorsally or transversely deep to the extensor mechanism and introducing 2 cc of normal saline. Small longitudinal incisions are made in the skin over the designated portal sites, and subcutaneous tissues are bluntly separated to the level of the extensor mechanism.

A 1.5-mm arthroscopic needle system is advocated, and 2-mm shavers may be used. A tapered trocar for the arthroscopic sheath is advanced into the distended joint through the desired portal interval, and the sheath is then advanced over the trocar. A probe or shaver may be introduced into the remaining portal. Inflow is maintained through an indwelling needle through the dorsal capsule while an assistant intermittently infuses the joint with normal saline. It is best to exchange the arthroscope between portals in order to ensure maximum joint visualization.

Once the procedure is completed, the skin is closed with simple sutures, and a soft sterile dressing is applied after removal of the tourniquet and confirmation of reperfusion has been made. The use of a splint is at the surgeon's discretion, dependent upon what condition is present and what procedure was performed. Sutures are removed 10 to 14 days postoperatively.

Procedures

The following procedures may have applications similar to the metacarpophalangeal joint. As for the MCP joint, this is by no means meant to be an all-inclusive list.

SYNOVITIS

Synovial biopsy is easily performed through standard portals with a 2-mm shaver or arthroscopic grabber. Similarly, a radical synovectomy can be carried out with a shaver in all joint regions except the volar 50%.

SEPTIC ARTHRITIS

Irrigation and debridement of a septic PIP joint are easily accomplished with the arthroscope and a shaver. A large volume of normal saline can be passed through the joint simply by running the shaver in the middle of the joint space while connecting the inflow to a wide-open source of fluid. Cultures can be obtained by sampling the initial aspirate.

FOREIGN BODY RETRIEVAL

Depending upon the size, type, and location of the foreign body in the PIP joint, it may be possible to retrieve such a structure arthroscopically through standard portals using an arthroscopic grabber.

Complications

Few complications should be encountered with careful application of standard arthroscopic principles. The most serious complications are potential injury to cutaneous nerves, which can be avoided with careful dissection techniques based upon a sound understanding of the underlying anatomy. Iatrogenic injury to the articular surfaces is easily encountered unless a very gentle approach to the use of instruments is maintained. It is important to remember that the arthroscope typically moves only a few millimeters in a telescoping fashion to cover the entire joint. Do not force the arthroscope where it doesn't want to go. Infection remains a risk, regardless of surgical procedure. Many surgeons prefer to administer a prophylactic dose of parenteral antibiotics prior to initiating a joint-related procedure.

CONCLUSION

Arthroscopy of the small joints of the hand has become a reliable clinical tool, although somewhat limited in diagnostic applications. Therapeutic options are becoming increasingly available but must be balanced against the efficacy of open procedures. The arthroscopy of these joints is safe, but only if the relevant anatomy is thoroughly understood by the surgeon.

References

1. Berger RA. A technique for arthroscopic evaluation of the first carpometacarpal joint. *J Hand Surg* 1997;22(A):1077–1080.
2. Menon J. Arthroscopic management of trapeziometacarpal arthritis of the thumb. *Arthroscopy* 1996;12:581–587.
3. Ryu J, Fegan R. Arthroscopic treatment of acute complete thumb metacarpophalangeal ulnar collateral ligament tears. *J Hand Surg* 1995;20(A):1037–1042.
4. Bettinger PC, Linscheid RL, Berger RA, et al. An anatomic study of the stabilizing ligaments of the trapezium and trapeziometacarpal joint. *J Hand Surg* 1999;24(A):786–798.
5. Bettinger PC, Berger RA. Functional ligamentous anatomy of the trapezium and trapeziometacarpal joint. *Hand Clin* 2001; 17:151–168.
6. Culp RW, Rekant MS. The role of arthroscopy in evaluating and treating trapeziometacarpal disease. *Hand Clin* 2001;17: 315–319.
7. Eaton RG, Littler JW. Ligament reconstruction for the painful thumb carpometacarpal joint. *J Bone Joint Surg* 1973;55A: 1655–1666.
8. Ishizuki M. Injury to collateral ligament of the metacarpophalangeal ligament of a finger. *J Hand Surg* 1988;13A:444–448.
9. Slade JF 3rd, Gutow AP. Arthroscopy of the metacarpophalangeal joint. *Hand Clin* 1999;15:501–527.
10. Ostendorf B, Dann P, Wedekind F, et al. Miniarthroscopy of metacarpophalangeal joints in rheumatoid arthritis. Rating of diagnostic value in synovitis staging and efficiency of synovial biopsy. *J Rheumatol* 1999;26:1901–1908.
11. Sekiya I, Kobayashi M, Taneda Y, et al. Arthroscopy of the proximal interphalangeal and metacarpophalangeal joints in rheumatoid hands. *Arthroscopy* 2002;18:292–297.
12. Debrecq G, Schmitgen G, Verstreken J. Arthroscopic treatment of metacarpophalangeal arthropathy in haemochromotosis. *J Hand Surg Br* 1994;19:212–214.
13. Wei N, Delauter SK, Erlichman MS, et al. Arthroscopic synovectomy of the metacarpophalangeal joint in refractory rheumatoid arthritis: a technique. *Arthroscopy* 1999;15:265–268.
14. Stener B. Displacement of the ruptured ulnar collateral ligament of the metacarpo-phalangeal joint of the thumb. A clinical and anatomical study. *J Bone Joint Surg* 1962;44B:869–879.
15. Thomsen NO, Nielsen NS, Jorgensen U, et al. Arthroscopy of the proximal interphalangeal joints of the fingers. *J Hand Surg Br* 2002;27:253–255.

21

Proximal Row Carpectomy

Matthew A. Bernstein and Randall W. Culp

HISTORICAL PERSPECTIVE

Proximal row carpectomy is a recognized treatment option for arthritic disease of the proximal carpal row. Since its original description in 1944, proximal row carpectomy has been a controversial surgical alternative and has had an intermittently questionable reputation in the literature.[1] The complex link joint biomechanics of the wrist are converted to a sloppy ball-and-socket joint by removal of the proximal carpal row.[1] Criticism has included: loss of motion and strength, progressive radiocapitate arthritis, and unpredictability of outcome; however, much of this criticism has been anecdotal.[2] Recent investigations have reported successful results that appear to be similar to those reported for more complex reconstructions or other salvage procedures.[3–10]

Patient satisfaction and pain relief are noted in a high percentage of patients. Wrist motion has been shown to be equal to, or slightly less than, that noted preoperatively. Grip strength has been shown to range between 64% and 100% of the contralateral normal wrist.[4,7,11–15] Normal longitudinal compressive loads across the radiolunate articulation have been reported as 40% and those across the radioscaphoid articulation as 60%. Following proximal row carpectomy, the initial load across the lunate fossa to capitate articulation is 100%, however, as dead space diminishes and is replaced by scar formation, this new tissue more evenly distributes the compressive load across a broader area. The radius of curvature of the capitate is about two-thirds that of the lunate fossa, motion between the capitate and the radius is translational, and the onset and progression of radiocapitate arthrosis have been demonstrated radiographically by Imbriglia; progression of arthrosis has not been of clinical consequence, however.[15]

Arthroscopy has developed into an established tool in orthopaedic surgery. Over the last several years, with the advent of smaller-diameter arthroscopes and instruments, wrist arthroscopy has resulted in significant improvement in the care and treatment of wrist pathology. In addition to using arthroscopy in diagnosis and treatment of triangular fibrocartilage complex (TFCC) tears, radiocarpal fractures, cartilage damage, loose bodies, and debridement and synovectomies, bony resections—including radial styloidectomy and proximal row carpectomy—can be performed. The latter technique involves removal of the scaphoid, lunate, and triquetrum, thus allowing the capitate to migrate proximally and articulate with the lunate fossa of the radius.

Literature pertaining to the results of arthroscopic proximal row carpectomy is sparse; the majority of the literature mentions arthroscopy as a technique for proximal row carpectomy without discussing clinical results.[5,16–19]

INDICATIONS AND CONTRAINDICATIONS

The same indications hold for arthroscopic proximal row carpectomy as for the standard open technique. Proximal row carpectomy is an option for patients with symptomatic arthritic disease secondary to a number of diseases, including scaphoid nonunion, scapholunate dissociation, and osteonecrosis of the lunate. It has also been described in the treatment of failed carpal implants, cerebral palsy, spasticity, acute and chronic fractures and dislocations, and replantation. We do not currently recommend arthroscopic proximal row carpectomy in this latter subset of patients. Relative contraindications to the procedure include preexisting arthritis of the proposed radiocapitate articulation, multicystic carpal disease, and preexisting ulnar translocation of the carpus.[20] Due to the overwhelming majority of poor results of open proximal row carpectomy in their patients with rheumatoid arthritis, both Culp et al and Ferlic et al do not recommend its use in rheumatoid patients.[4,21]

SURGICAL TECHNIQUE

Arthroscopic proximal row carpectomy can be carried out under general or regional anesthesia, as bone grafting is not necessary and operative times are generally under 120 minutes. In the operating room, the video monitor, light source, power source, and inflow pump are positioned contralateral to the limb on which surgery is being performed. The patient is positioned supine on the operating table with a radiolucent hand table in place.

After prophylactic antibiotics, routine skin preparation, and sterile draping around a well-padded arm tourniquet, the arm is placed into a sterile traction tower. The forearm is suspended in finger traps and, via the traction tower, distraction is accomplished by a strap placed above the elbow, securing the arm to the tower base. This tower allows the surgeon to "dial in" the amount of distraction, most commonly 10 to 15 pounds. After distraction is obtained, landmarks are outlined on the dorsum of the wrist, and the portals are made. The tourniquet is routinely inflated without additional exsanguination.

Routinely the 3-4 portal is the first viewing portal. Longitudinal incisions, breaching only the skin, are used. To avoid tendon and nerve injuries, a hemostat is used to spread through the subcutaneous tissue down to and, with the tips of the hemostat closed, through the capsule. Then, using the blunt trocar, the arthroscopy cannula is introduced into the joint, directed along the sagittal plane, at an angle of approximately 11 degrees proximal to the perpendicular of the long axis of the radius. This angle approximates the normal volar inclination of the distal radius articular surface.

After the 2.7-mm arthroscope is placed into the joint, outflow is established through the 6-R portal, identified by triangulation and direct visualization upon entering the joint at the prestyloid recess. A mechanical pump is used to maintain a constant intra-articular pressure and flow rate. First, a routine evaluation of the joint is carried out; particular attention is given to the lunate fossa of the distal radius. The radial volar extrinsic ligaments, particularly the radioscaphocapitate ligament, are identified and will be preserved during the procedure.

The arthroscope is then directed ulnarly, and the TFCC and extrinsic ulnar ligaments are identified. Next, the midcarpal joint must be well visualized to ensure an adequate proximal capitate cartilaginous surface. If the status of the capitate joint is questionable, then an alternative procedure is performed: 4-corner fusion, capitolunate arthrodesis, proximal row carpectomy with interposition arthroplasty, or wrist arthrodesis. Assessment of the midcarpal articular surfaces is accomplished through the radial midcarpal portal, which is approximately 1 cm distal to the 3-4 portal. Arthroscopic instruments that will be needed to perform the proximal row carpectomy include: a hook probe, a 2.9 shaver or radiofrequency device, a 4.0 bur, small sharp osteotomes, pituitary rongeurs, and an image intensifier.

The first step in performing the proximal row carpectomy, after one is satisfied with the cartilage status of the proximal pole of the capitate and the lunate fossa, is to remove the scapholunate and luna-

totriquetral ligaments with a shaver or radiofrequency device. This is performed through the 4-5 and/or 6-R portals. Next, the core of the lunate is removed with a bur; care is taken to avoid damaging the lunate fossa and proximal capitate by leaving an "eggshell" rim of lunate, which is morcellized with a pituitary rongeur under direct vision and/or with image intensification. Next, using the 3-5 or 4-5 portal as a working portal, the scaphoid and triquetrum are fragmented with an osteotome and bur under image intensification and removed by piecemeal with a pituitary rongeur. Coring out and fragmenting the carpal bones allows for easy removal, as well as protection of the articular cartilage. Great care is taken to avoid damaging the articular cartilage. Great care is taken to avoid damaging the volar extrinsic ligaments, especially the radioscaphocapitate, which will be responsible for maintaining the stability of the capitate in the lunate fossa.

After the entire proximal row is removed, the wrist is examined under radiographic image intensification. Care is taken to ensure that there is no impingement of the trapezium against the radial styloid. Some authors advocate a modest styloidectomy; while we rarely perform this procedure, it can be done arthroscopically with the aid of image intensification, if needed.

Posterior interosseous neurectomy may be performed through a separate 1.5-cm longitudinal incision just ulnar to Lister's tubercle. The fourth compartment is partially opened on the radial side. One centimeter of the nerve is resected with bipolar electrocautery. The fourth compartment is then repaired with absorbable suture. All wounds are closed with 4-0 nylon monofilament suture.

Patients are placed in a short-arm plaster splint for approximately 3.5 to 4 weeks. Sutures from the portals are removed at 10 days. Gentle range of motion exercises are begun after splint removal at 4 weeks, and strengthening is begun at approximately 8 weeks postoperatively.

COMPLICATIONS

There are several potential complications associated with proximal row carpectomy. When the procedure is done arthroscopically, the cartilaginous surfaces of the proximal capitate and lunate fossa must be protected from instrument damage. Also, care must be taken not to disrupt the volar extrinsic carpal ligaments, as they are later necessary for long-term radiocarpal stability (Figure 21.1). Visualization is often greater arthroscopically than open; we sometimes leave behind a shell of cortical bone attached to the ligaments to avoid ligamentous injury. There is also the potential complication of irritation of the nerves, especially the dorsal ulnar sensory branch, and po-

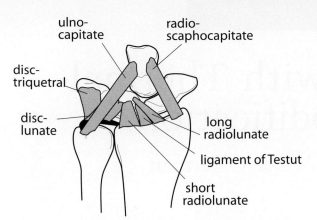

FIGURE 21.1. Diagram of the important stabilizing volar extrinsic radiocarpal and ulnocarpal ligaments. (1) Radioscaphocapitate. (2) Ulnocapitate ligament, important due to its position and contribution to the ulnar limb of the arcuate ligament and its attachment to the capitate.

tential for damage to the median and ulnar nerves, especially the ulnar nerve, while using the osteotomes. The dorsal capsuloligamentous structures are not significantly disrupted when the arthroscopic technique is utilized. Thus, there is less dorsal scar formation, and dorsal instability may occur, though we have not seen this clinically. While we have not had to do this, should dorsal capsular laxity present as a problem, concurrent or later electrothermal capsulorrhaphy may be performed.

ADVANTAGES

As with any arthroscopic procedure, the surgery is less invasive than an open procedure. Also, there is little damage to the dorsal ligaments, which are left essentially intact, in contrast to standard open proximal row carpectomy. Better visualization of the volar extrinsic ligaments increases the likelihood of preservation. Finally, there is a more acceptable scar and less stiffness, secondary to minimal capsular dissection.

CONCLUSION

Overall patient satisfaction with this procedure has been excellent. Immediate postoperative pain seems to be less than that experienced by those who have undergone open proximal row carpectomy. In our experience, all patients reported satisfactory pain relief, functional wrist motion, and effective grip strength.

References

1. Stamm TT. Excision of the proximal row of carpus. *Proc Roy Soc Med* 1944;38:74–75.
2. Lee RW, Hassan DM. Proximal row carpectomy: In Watson HK, Weinzweig J, (ed.) *The Wrist.* Philadelphia, PA: Lippincott Williams & Wilkins, 2001, pp. 545–554.
3. Culp RW. Proximal row carpectomy. *Operat Tech Orthop* 1996;2:69–71.
4. Culp RW, McGuigan FX, Turner MA, et al. Proximal row carpectomy: a multicenter study. *J Hand Surg* 1993;18A:19–25.
5. Roth JH, Poehling GG. Arthroscopic "-ectomy" surgery of the wrist. *Arthroscopy J Arthroscop Relat Surg* 1990;6(2):141–147.
6. Siegel JM, Ruby LK. A critical look at intercarpal arthrodesis: review of the literature. *J Hand Surg* 1996;21A:717–723.
7. Tomaino MM, Delsignore J, Burton RI. Long-term results following proximal row carpectomy. *J Hand Surg* 1994;19A:694–703.
8. Wyrick JD, Stern PJ, Kiefhaber TR. Motion-preserving procedures in the treatment of scapholunate advance collapse wrist: proximal row carpectomy versus four-corner arthrodesis. *J Hand Surg* 1995;20A:965–970.
9. Cohen MS, Kozin SH. Degenerative arthritis of the wrist: proximal row carpectomy versus four corner arthrodesis. *J Hand Surg* 2001;26A:94–104.
10. Culp RW, Williams CS. Proximal row carpectomy for the treatment of scaphoid nonunion. *Hand Clin* 2001;17(4):663–669, x.
11. Begley BW, Engber WD. Proximal row carpectomy in advanced Kienbock's disease. *J Hand Surg* 1994;19A:1016–1018.
12. Nevaiser RJ. On resection of the proximal carpal row. *Clin Orthop* 1986;202:12–15.
13. Nevaiser RJ. Proximal row carpectomy for posttraumatic disorders of the carpus. *J Hand Surg* 1983;8A:301–305.
14. Clendenin MB, Green DP. Arthrodesis of the wrist—complications and their management. *J Hand Surg* 1981;6A:253–257.
15. Imbriglia JE, Broudy AS, Hagberg WC, et al. Proximal row carpectomy: clinical evaluation. *J Hand Surg* 1990;15A:462–430.
16. Culp RW, Osterman AL, Talsania JS. Arthroscopic proximal row carpectomy. *Tech Hand and Upp Ext* 1997;2(1):116–119.
17. Gupta R, Bozentka DJ, Osterman AL. Wrist arthroscopy: principles and clinical applications. *J Am Acad Orthop Surg* 2001;9(3):200–209.
18. Nagle DJ. Laser-assisted wrist arthroscopy. *Hand Clin* 1999;15(3):495–499, ix. Review.
19. Atik TL, Baratz ME. The role of arthroscopy in wrist arthritis. *Hand Clin* 1999;15(3):489–494. Review.
20. Calandruccio JH. Proximal row carpectomy. *J Am Soc Surg Hand* 2001;2(1):112–122.
21. Ferlic DC, Clayton ML, Mills MF. Proximal row carpectomy: review of rheumatoid and non-rheumatoid wrists. *J Hand Surg* 1991;16A:420–424.

22

Trapeziectomy with Thermal Capsular Modification

Scott G. Edwards and A. Lee Osterman

As recently as 10 years ago, the thumb carpometacarpal (CMC) joint, or basal joint, was inherently difficult to evaluate intraarticularly. Its curved articular surfaces required an extensive arthrotomy through much of its nearly circumferential stabilizing ligaments. The introduction of a small arthroscope allowed the thumb CMC articulation to be completely visualized without destabilizing the joint.[1,2] Diagnostic thumb CMC arthroscopy eventually led to therapeutic arthroscopy, including the treatment of basal thumb arthritis, the most common hand arthrosis. With advancing technology, end-stage and intermediate-stage arthrosis may now be treated by arthroscopically-guided arthroplasty of the thumb basal joint. The development of miniaturized thermocouple probes allowed conditions of joint capsule laxity to be treated by thermal capsular shrinkage. Although early results are promising and the advantages over traditional open procedures are obvious, these techniques are still evolving and the long-term benefits and complications require further study. The purpose of this chapter is to present the current knowledge of arthroscopic treatment for thumb CMC arthrosis and joint hyperlaxity.

GROSS AND ARTHROSCOPIC ANATOMY

Several superficial structures cross the thumb CMC joint, beginning volarly with the abductor pollicis brevis (APB), which originates from the anterior surface of the trapezium. Lateral to the APB are the tendon of the abductor pollicis longus (APL) and the tendon of the extensor pollicis brevis (EPB), which lies posterior to the APL. The deep division of the radial artery crosses the posterior capsule of the thumb CMC joint and travels deep to the extensor pollicis longus (EPL) tendon before coursing anteriorly between the proximal metaphyses of the first and second metacarpals. The extracapsular intermetacarpal ligament resides at the most posterior and ulnar aspect of the thumb CMC joint, between the first and second metacarpal bases. Immediately deep to the skin overlying the joint are

numerous veins, including the principal tributaries forming the cephalic venous system. Intermingled with these veins are the S1 and S2 branches of the superficial radial nerve.[3]

The basal joint of the thumb consists of four trapezial articulations: the trapeziometacarpal (TM), trapeziotrapezoid, scaphotrapezial (ST), and trapezium-index metacarpal articulations. Of these joints, only the TM and ST lie along the longitudinal compression axis of the thumb. The TM articulation may be thought of as a double saddle joint. The articular surface of the trapezium is concave in the mediolateral direction and convex in the anteroposterior direction. The converse relationship is found at the base of the first metacarpal, where the articular surface is concave in the anteroposterior direction and convex in the mediolateral direction. These surfaces form a shallow double saddle that offers little intrinsic osseous stability and must rely on static ligamentous constraints to restrict translation (Figure 22.1). Since a strong association has been observed between excessive basal joint laxity and premature degenerative changes, careful consideration must be given to these ligamentous stabilizers when preparing for any surgical intervention.

Although a capsule surrounds the entire thumb CMC joint, capsular ligaments reinforce only three-fourths of the circumference. Sixteen ligaments have been identified about the trapezium,[4–6] of which seven are directly responsible for stabilizing the thumb CMC joint. These are the superficial anterior oblique ligament (AOLs), deep anterior oblique ligament (AOLd), dorsoradial ligament (DRL), posterior oblique ligament (POL), ulnar collateral ligament (UCL), intermetacarpal ligament, and dorsal intermetacarpal ligament. The remaining eight ligaments stabilizing the trapezium are the dorsal trapeziotrapezoid ligament, ventral trapeziotrapezoid ligament, dorsal trapezio-second metacarpal ligament, volar trapezio-second metacarpal ligament, trapezio-third metacarpal ligament, volar scaphotrapezial ligament, radioscaphotrapezial ligament, and the transverse carpal ligament.

The bulk of the ligamentous structures about the thumb CMC joint cannot be visualized from outside the joint. In fact, several structures attached to the tra-

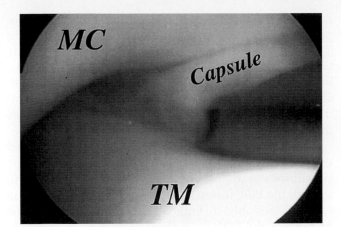

FIGURE 22.1. Arthroscopic view of the trapeziometacarpal joint. Note the double saddle articulation formed by the metacarpal (MC) and trapezium (TZ).

pezium may only be appreciated after violating the more superficial ligaments or tendons. The arthroscopic perspective of the CMC stabilizers is substantially less complicated than the same anatomy viewed externally, because a number of structures can be easily viewed from within the joint. Our understanding of the anatomy and biomechanics of the thumb basal joint has been greatly enhanced through arthroscopic assistance.

Due to the limitations of safe portal placement, the arthroscopic view is limited to the anterior, ulnar, and posterior surfaces of the joint. This does not prove to be a significant handicap, however, as the volar and radial portions of the joint capsule lack ligamentous reinforcements. The capsuloligamentous structures readily visible with standard arthroscopic portals are the AOLs, AOLd, DRL, POL, and the UCL (Figure 22.2A,B).

Superficial Anterior Oblique Ligament (sAOL)

The AOLs is a capsular ligament that originates from the volar tubercle of the trapezium 0.5 mm proximal to the articular surface and inserts broadly across the volar ulnar tubercle of the first metacarpal 2 mm distal to the articular margin of the volar styloid process. This creates a capsular recess between the AOLs and the first metacarpal that appears lax and redundant. This may represent normal and appropriate laxity to allow pronation of the thumb to occur. However, in extremes of rotation and in extension, the AOLs becomes taut.

The AOLs may be viewed through the 1-R, but is more readily inspected through the 1-U portal. It spans almost the entire anterior surface of the joint, with fibers oriented slightly oblique distally and ulnarly. When viewed from within the joint, the AOLs may be partially obscured by the deep anterior oblique ligament (AOLd), which lies in the arthroscopic foreground. While the AOLs and AOLd are virtually indistinguishable from an external approach, a probe from within the joint can easily separate the AOLs and the AOLd (Figure 22.3).

Deep Anterior Oblique Ligament (AOLd)

The AOLd or "beak ligament" is an intra-articular ligament that originates from the volar central apex of the trapezium at the ulnar edge of the trapezial ridge and inserts just ulnar to the volar styloid process at the base of the first metacarpal (beak). The orientation of its fibers is slightly oblique, and it passes proximal to distal from lateral to medial. The AOLd is shorter than the AOLs and consequently becomes taut before the AOLs in wide palmar and radial abduction and extension. This allows the AOLd to function as a pivot

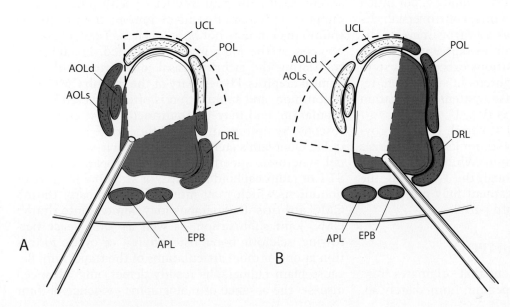

FIGURE 22.2. Schematic view of the ligaments within the trapeziometacarpal (TM) joint from two portals (in axial cross-section). By using both 1-R and 1-U portals, nearly the entire intra-articular anatomy is visualized. **A.** View of the TM joint from a distal perspective showing the arthroscope in the 1-R portal. **B.** View of the TM joint from a distal perspective showing the arthroscope in the 1-U portal. (Adapted from PC Bettinger and RA Berger: *Hand Clinics* 17(2) Functional ligamentous anatomy of the trapezium and trapeziometacarpal joint, pp. 151–168, © 2001, with permission from Elsevier Science.

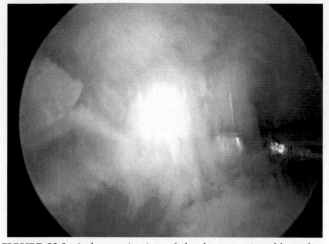

FIGURE 22.3. Arthroscopic view of the deep anterior oblique ligament (foreground) and the superficial anterior oblique ligament (background). The probe separates the two layers of ligamentous tissue.

point for rotation. By becoming taut with continued abduction, the AOLd stabilizes the metacarpal on the trapezium and prevents ulnar subluxation. Because the other thumb basal joint ligaments are still lax in wide palmar abduction, there can be further rotation, especially pronation, about the axis of the AOLd.

The AOLd can be best visualized through the 1-U portal. The orientation of its fibers runs obliquely from proximal-radial to distal-ulnar. A free edge on the radial side of the ligament can be easily probed and separated from the AOLs, which lies in the arthroscopic background.

Dorsoradial Ligament (DRL)

The DRL is a wide, capsular, fan-shaped ligament that originates from the dorsoradial tubercle of the trapezium and broadly inserts into the dorsal edge of the base of the metacarpal. This large, strong ligament is clearly important to thumb CMC stability, but much about its biomechanics remains controversial. Its function may be thought of as a mirror image of the AOL complex. The DRL becomes taut with a dorsal or dorsoradial force in all positions except full extension. In addition, the DRL tightens in supination, regardless of joint position. It also tightens in pronation when the thumb CMC joint is flexed.

Best viewed through the 1-R portal, the DRL covers a large percentage of the posterior joint and merges with the POL at its ulnar margin. While the ligament may be seen tangentially through the 1-U portal, the most radial portion of the ligament may not be visible using either of the standard portals.

Posterior Oblique Ligament (POL)

The POL is a capsular ligament that originates from the dorsoulnar side of the trapezium immediately ad-

jacent to the DRL and inserts into the dorsoulnar aspect of the metacarpal and the volar-ulnar tubercle. The POL merges with the intermetacarpal ligament, which resides outside the capsule and is not readily visualized arthroscopically. The POL is taut in wide abduction, opposition, and supination. It also resists ulnar translation of the metacarpal base during abduction and opposition.

Under arthroscopic observation, the POL fibers are oriented from proximal-radial to distal-ulnar, and are continuous with the DRL at its ulnar margin. Although the POL is best visualized through the 1-R portal, it is possible to tangentially examine the entire breadth of the POL from the 1-U portal.

Ulnar Collateral Ligament (UCL)

The UCL is an extracapsular ligament that originates from the trapezial ridge ulnar to the origin of the transverse carpal ligament and inserts into the volar-ulnar tubercle of the metacarpal superficially and ulnarly to the AOLs. Like the AOLs and AOLd, the UCL is taut in extension, abduction, and pronation and restricts volar subluxation of the metacarpal.

Through either the 1-R or 1-U portals, fibers of the UCL run nearly vertically across the ulnar aspect of the joint. It typically overlaps the AOLs by 2 to 3 mm, and in most areas, the fibers of the UCL appear to merge with those of the AOLs.

CLINICAL PRESENTATION

Although the conditions are most commonly associated with women in their fifth decade and older, virtually every skeletally mature patient is susceptible to thumb CMC joint arthrosis and hyperlaxity, regardless of activity level. Patients will present with severe basal joint pain interfering with pinching and gripping activities. Recent or remote trauma to the thumb may or may not be associated. Tenderness and effusion at the joint may be palpated. Loading and translating the arthritic basal joint often will elicit painful crepitus. Hyperlaxity of the thumb CMC joint is common, and subluxation is often detected by manipulation, and may be confirmed by dynamic fluoroscopy. Symptoms must be differentiated from those of De Quervain's stenosing tenosynovitis, carpal tunnel syndrome, superficial radial neuropathy, isolated STT or radioscaphoid arthritis, or scaphoid fracture or nonunion, which may mimic or accompany thumb CMC arthritis. Radiographs may demonstrate thumb CMC joint subluxation, as well as joint space narrowing, sclerotic bone, osteophytes, or cystic formation at one or more articulations of the trapezium. Because plain radiographs readily detect only advanced disease, the absence of radiographic evidence of joint degeneration does not preclude the diagnosis of arthritis. Currently, the only method of definitively evaluating the extent of arthritis is direct inspection through the arthroscope.

DIAGNOSTIC ARTHROSCOPY

Indications

Diagnostic arthroscopy of the thumb CMC joint is indicated in patients where standard clinical and radiographic images do not provide sufficient diagnostic information. The technique may be helpful in quantifying and staging the degree of thumb basal joint arthrosis. In our experience, arthroscopic evaluation often reveals active synovitis and significant chondromalacia when plain radiographs show no abnormalities. Therapeutically, loose body removal, septic joint irrigation, and synovectomy are easily accomplished. Thumb CMC arthroscopy is useful in the evaluation and reduction of intra-articular fractures, such as the Bennett or Rolando type, as well as in ligamentous injuries. Finally, we have been applying it to the arthritic basal joint where trapezial resection and thermal capsular modification provide an alternative treatment for thumb CMC arthrosis. Contraindications include poor soft tissue coverage or active cellulitis over the thumb CMC joint.

Preparation

The patient lies supine on the operating table with the involved arm at a right angle to the body on a hand table. General or regional anesthesia is similar to that for other upper extremity arthroscopic procedures. A single sterile finger trap on the thumb suspends the extremity vertically. In order for the axis of the thumb metacarpal to remain aligned with the axis of the radius, the wrist must be positioned in neutral and ulnar deviation. Once the metacarpal-radius axis is aligned, 5 to 10 pounds of longitudinal traction is applied to the thumb (see Figure 22.4). A pneumatic tourniquet is placed prior to draping; this can be inflated to 250 mmHg intraoperatively at the surgeon's discretion.

Landmarks and Portals

By following the contour of the metacarpal proximally, the thumb CMC joint is palpated and the joint line is marked. The abductor pollicis longus (APL), extensor pollicis brevis (EPB), and extensor pollicis longus (EPL) are also identified and marked. At the level of the thumb basal joint, one cadaveric study demonstrated that the radial artery lies ulnar to the EPB at an average distance of 11 mm and a range of 4

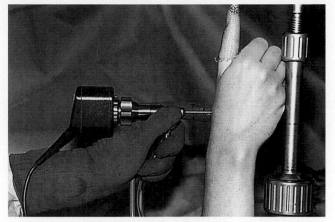

FIGURE 22.4. Traction tower arrangement for thumb carpometacarpal joint arthroscopy.

to 17 mm. The artery lies within 1 mm of the EPL, however, in 7 of 11 cadaveric specimens.[7]

In order to avoid injury to the radial artery but achieve appropriate triangulation of instrumentation within the joint, 2 portals are planned and marked accordingly along the basal joint line: one immediately radial to the APL (volar), 1-R portal, and the other immediately ulnar to the EPB (dorsal), or 1-U portal (Figure 22.5). The distance between each portal is approximately 1 cm. In order to estimate the angle of entry, a 20-gauge needle is advanced into the joint just proximal to the line drawn demonstrating the level of the base of the first metacarpal through the planned portal site. This confirms the appropriate entry angle for the arthroscope and allows insufflation of the joint with 1 to 2 milliliters of normal saline. An incision is made with a number 11 scalpel over each portal mark, cutting only the dermis. Subcutaneous tissues are bluntly dissected using a small hemostat to avoid branches of the superficial radial nerve and deep and superficial branches of the radial artery. Steinberg et al identified 2 branches of the superficial radial nerve, namely the SR2 and SR3, that surround the arthroscopic field.[3] Gonzalez et al studied the distribution of the superficial radial nerve in the area of CMC arthroscopic portals in cadaveric thumbs.[7] Of the 11 specimens examined, 7 specimens demonstrated at least one branch of the superficial radial nerve lying dorsal to the EPB tendon; 6 specimens demonstrated at least one branch over the APL tendon; and all 11 specimens demonstrated at least one branch over the EPL tendon. Careful blunt dissection is imperative to reduce the risk of injury to these branches.

Once the blunt dissection reaches the thumb CMC joint capsule, a 1.9-mm tapered trocar and its sheath are introduced through each portal site, generally with a slightly distal inclination. The joint capsule immediately deep to the APL and 1-R portal is not reinforced by a ligament. Through the 1-U portal, how-

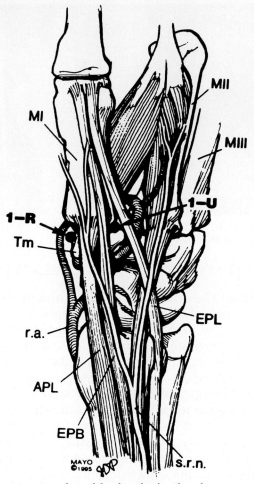

FIGURE 22.5. Portals and landmarks for thumb carpometacarpal joint arthroscopy. (Reprinted from RA Berger. A technique for arthroscopic evaluation of the first carpometacarpal joint. *J Hand Surg* 22:1022–1080, © 1997, with permission of Elsevier Science).

ever, the trocar attempts to pierce between the DRL (volarly) and the POL (dorsally). It is sometimes helpful to sweep the trocar gently in order to find the natural division between the ligaments and fibers of the joint capsule, particularly through the 1-U portal. Fluoroscopic confirmation of trocar placement within the thumb CMC joint can be reassuring if the surgeon is unfamiliar with the technique or initial visualization of intra-articular landmarks is poor. It is sometimes easy to inadvertently fall into the STT joint. The 1-U portal commonly is established first and serves as the primary viewing portal. Under direct visualization, the 1-R portal is established and serves as the primary working portal. Viewing and working portals are frequently interchanged during the procedure to ensure complete visualization and treatment of the entire CMC joint.

Surgical Technique

Initially, visualization may be difficult because of the arthritic changes in the joint. Hypertrophic synovium

may be removed with mechanical debridement or thermal ablation. Mechanical debridement is most often performed using a 2.0-mm shaver or 2.0-mm synovial suction resector. Thermal ablation may be performed using either laser or radiofrequency technology. Radiofrequency energy can be either monopolar (Oratec, Menlo Park, CA) or bipolar (Arthrocare, Sunnyvale, CA; Mitek VAPR, Westwood, MA). Each form of energy has its own advantages and disadvantages, and the choice is dependent largely on surgeon preference. Because of the small diameter of shavers necessary to debride the thumb CMC joint, the suction sheath often becomes obstructed with tissue and requires frequent cleaning. Of the many brands of thermal ablators commercially available, the authors prefer the monopolar variety rather than the bipolar. While the bipolar ablator is very aggressive and efficient in removing intra-articular soft tissues, the authors have encountered elevated temperatures within the joint that have led to thermal injury. The monopolar devices seem to control intra-articular temperatures more effectively. Regardless of the type of thermal ablator used, the joint must be continuously irrigated through the arthroscope using normal saline and a small joint pump. Continuous irrigation not only helps to clear debris and enhance visualization, but also dissipates heat produced within the joint.

The thumb basal joint is systematically inspected. Moving the thumb identifies the base of the first metacarpal. Following this, the trapezium is inspected from the ulnar to the radial side. Chondral defects and osteophytic formation are noted. The greatest chondral degeneration typically is found on the volar aspect of the trapezium. Through the 1-U portal, the AOLs and AOLd are identified on the volar aspect of the joint, and their integrity is inspected using a probe. Moving more ulnarly, the UCL is inspected through the same portal. Switching the arthroscopic camera to the 1-R portal, the POL may be inspected radial to the UCL. Continuing to the dorsoradial aspect of the joint, the DRL can be visualized using the same portal, and its inspection completes the thumb CMC ligamentous examination through the arthroscope (Figure 22.2A, B). It is important to remember that the arthritic thumb basal joint is usually tight and may not allow for easy arthroscopic maneuvering initially. Care must be taken to preserve the remaining articular cartilage. Arthroscopic examination of the STT joint through standard midcarpal portals may provide the surgeon with more information regarding the entire trapezium and help to guide therapeutic interventions.

Postoperative Care

Following diagnostic arthroscopy of the thumb CMC joint, patients are placed in a thumb spica splint for comfort and instructed to elevate the hand as much as possible to decrease swelling and allow for rapid clearing of irrigation fluid that has extravasated into the subcutaneous tissues. Immediate motion of the uninvolved digits is encouraged. Splint and sutures are removed in 7 to 10 days, and the patient is released to activities as tolerated.

PARTIAL OR COMPLETE RESECTION OF THE TRAPEZIUM

Arthroscopic partial or complete trapeziectomy has several attractive aspects. The technique is less invasive compared to conventional open procedures, it offers an opportunity to detect articular damage long before radiographic changes become apparent, there is less chance of injury to the sensory branches of the radial nerve, and it is easily converted to a standard reconstruction. Partial trapeziectomy, although effective in relieving pain in many cases, should be considered a provisional treatment for patients who are otherwise not candidates for complete trapeziectomy. Culp and Rekant[8] reported 88% excellent or good outcomes following arthroscopic partial or complete trapeziectomy without interposition in 24 thumbs. Thermal capsular modification was included in all patients. They noted that subsidence of the first metacarpal was between 2 and 4 mm, pinch strength improved 22%, and patients had no complications. Although they reported short-term follow-up (14 to 48 months) at the time of this publication, no patients have required revision surgery.

Indications

Surgery is considered when all nonoperative modalities, such as splinting, physiotherapy, and oral and injectable medications have failed to provide satisfactory relief for thumb CMC arthritis. Partial trapeziectomy is indicated in a young or high-demand older patient with thumb CMC degeneration, but without involvement of the STT joint. While infrequently a permanent solution, the procedure has the advantage of preserving the mechanical thumb height and is easily revised to a more complex reconstruction if needed. Complete trapeziectomy is mandated if there is degenerative involvement of the STT joint. Arthroscopic complete trapeziectomy has emerged as an attractive option in response to recent reports that trapeziectomy with ligament reconstruction offers little clinical advantage over trapeziectomy alone.[9,10] Routing of tendon graft through the vacant space may be performed arthroscopically as well, should interposition arthroplasty be preferred. Thumb CMC joint laxity may be addressed with arthroscopic thermal capsular modification as an adjuvant to partial or complete trapeziectomy, and is not considered a contraindication.

Surgical Technique

The patient is prepared and portals are made as described previously. Once all hypertrophic synovium has been removed, a 2.9-mm bur is introduced through one of the portals, and the articular surface of the trapezium is removed in a systematic fashion from ulnar to radial. The resection continues until 3 to 4 mm of bone are removed. The bur is used as a measurement guide to estimate the amount of bone that has been resected. Buring must continue until all hard subchondral bone is removed and only cancellous bone is visualized (Figure 22.6). Every attempt is made to maintain smooth and level surfaces and avoid creating troughs with the bur. All loose fragments are removed by continuous irrigation and suction. Larger loose bodies may require removal by a 2.0-mm arthroscopic grasper. Once 3 to 4 mm of bone have been removed from the most ulnar to the most radial aspect of the trapezium, the bur is switched to the other portal. This additional perspective ensures that the resection is complete and spans all aspects of the trapezium. Once fluoroscopic examination confirms osteophyte removal and ample joint space is created, traction is released from the thumb, and thermal capsular shrinkage is performed. Mild traction is reapplied to the thumb metacarpal so that the basal joint assumes its anatomic position. Under fluoroscopic guidance, the thumb CMC joint is pinned with a 0.045-inch Kirschner wire from the radial aspect of the metacarpal into the remainder of the trapezium (Figure 22.7). Once this is fixed in place, final tensioning of the joint may be performed by shrinking the surrounding ligaments and capsule.

As mentioned previously, the authors recommend visualizing the STT joint through standard midcarpal portals to assess the status of the entire trapezium more completely. If the degenerative process also involves the STT joint, a complete resection of the trapezium must be performed. Complete trapezial resec-

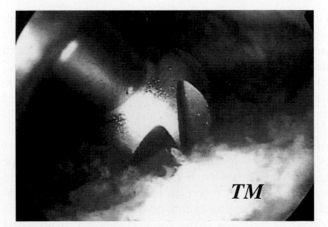

FIGURE 22.6. Trapezial resection with 2.9 bur. Note the exposure of cancellous bone during the partial trapeziectomy pictured.

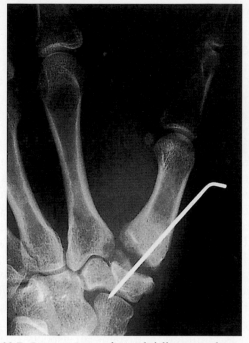

FIGURE 22.7. Postoperative radiograph following arthroscopic partial trapeziectomy. Note that the thumb column height is maintained with a 0.045-inch Kirschner wire.

tion is accomplished primarily through the 1-R and 1-U portals, but may be assisted using standard midcarpal portals. Care must be taken when resecting the volar aspect of the proximal trapezium, as the FCR tendon passes through a narrow bony groove. Once complete trapezium excision is arthroscopically and fluoroscopically confirmed, thermal capsular shrinkage with or without joint pinning is performed, advancing the Kirschner wire into the body of the scaphoid. Achieving reduction of the joint after complete trapeziectomy, however, may be somewhat more difficult, and careful fluoroscopic attention may be required.

Postoperative Care

Following arthroscopic partial or complete trapeziectomy, patients are placed in a thumb spica splint and instructed to elevate the hand as much as possible to decrease swelling and allow for rapid clearing of irrigation fluid that has extravasated into the subcutaneous tissues. Immediate motion of the uninvolved digits is encouraged. Sutures are removed in 7 to 10 days, and the patient is placed in a thumb spica cast. After 3 to 4 weeks, the pin is removed, and the cast is replaced by a removable thumb spica splint to be worn at all times with the exception of bathing and hand therapy. At 6 weeks, therapy is advanced to include strengthening exercises. During the third month following surgery, patients are weaned from their splints and resume activities of daily living. After 3

months, patients return to their previous lifestyles with minimal restrictions.

THERMAL CAPSULAR MODIFICATION

Since a strong association has been observed between excessive basal joint laxity and premature degenerative changes,[11,12] the diagnosis and treatment of such laxity have become more aggressive. Thermal modification of capsular and ligamentous tissues has broadened the role of arthroscopy in the thumb CMC joint. Under thermal modification, capsular shrinkage occurs initially at the time of surgery and, some believe, continues several months postoperatively as the capsule inevitably thickens.[13] Not only does the technique offer a less invasive alternative to other open capsular tightening procedures, but thermal modification, by nature of the process, disrupts afferent sensory fibers in the capsular tissue, which consequently decreases pain in the joint.

Much of our understanding of thermal capsular shrinkage in the thumb CMC joint has been derived and extrapolated from other larger joints, such as the shoulder, knee, and wrist, as well as from animal studies.[13–16] Capsular and ligamentous tissues are comprised primarily of type I collagen molecules, each tightly wound to form triple helical peptide chains. Each collagen molecule is bound to the next by intermolecular bonds that are resistant to heat (heat stable). Intramolecular bonds that are susceptible to separating under heat (heat labile) connect the tight triple helical structure of peptides. By applying high temperatures to the collagen, thermal modification denatures the protein, causing the triple helix to unwind; but tension is maintained and shrinkage occurs by preserving the intermolecular bonds.

Currently, thermal shrinkage may be performed with either laser or radiofrequency technology. Laser technology provides an obvious and immediate discoloration of the modified tissue and consequently allows the surgeon to visually appreciate the amount and depth of shrinkage more precisely. Only one laser probe is required for tissue ablation, coagulation, and shrinkage; it is directed by varying the distance between the probe and the tissue. Inconvenient and inefficient probe changing is not necessary with laser technology. It has been postulated that laser energy enhances healing by stimulating collagen synthesis; however, as of yet, no study has compared the nonthermal effects of the various heating modalities. On the other hand, laser heating causes local dehydration of the tissues due to evaporation, a problem not encountered with hydrothermal heating.

Radiofrequency is a form of electromagnetic energy. When applied to tissues, a rapidly oscillating electromagnetic field causes movement of charged particles within the tissue, and the resultant molecular motion generates heat. Radiofrequency is less expensive than laser, has fewer safety concerns, and allows the surgeon to manipulate the malleable probe to reach awkward areas. The energy is available in two forms: monopolar or bipolar. Monopolar radiofrequency energy (Oratec, Menlo Park, CA) heats tissue by ionic agitation current that flows between a probe tip and a grounding pad placed in a remote location on the patient's body. This form of energy is less effective in ablating floating debris, unless it is trapped between the probe tip and healthy tissue, but is quite effective for the purposes of tissue shrinkage since joint capsules and ligaments are usually well grounded in structure and ionic potential. Since monopolar energy conducts through tissue to a grounding pad, there has been some question regarding the depth of thermal modification. This concern is amplified in the thumb CMC joint, where nerves and vessels are located within 1 to 2 mm of the tissues being modified. Bipolar radiofrequency energy (Mitek VAPR, Westwood, MA; Arthrocare, Sunnyvale, CA) follows the path of least resistance through conductive irrigating solution between the tips of the probe. This method is aggressive and does not require trapping loose bodies between the probe and healthy tissue. Depth of heating is not as much of a concern as with monopolar energy; however, bipolar probes have been noted to reach extremely high intra-articular temperatures and have caused inadvertent thermal injury to the joint directly and indirectly by heating the irrigating fluid. Continuous irrigation of normal saline through the thumb CMC joint is required for any thermal shrinkage technique, but is particularly necessary when using bipolar radiofrequency.

Regardless of the source of thermal energy, studies have shown that histologic, ultrastructural, and biomaterial alterations induced by laser or radiofrequency energy have been similar.[16] The amount of shrinkage depends upon several factors including the age of the tissue, the degree of tissue temperature achieved, the duration of heat exposure, and the irrigation solution used during the procedure. As tissue ages, there is an increase in the ratio of intermolecular bonds (heat stable) to intramolecular bonds (heat labile). As a result, higher temperatures are required to cause the same degree of shrinkage in an older individual as opposed to a younger one. Higher temperatures not only may increase the extent of shrinking, but also increase the stiffness of the tissues and may make the capsule more vulnerable to mechanical loading. For individuals of all ages, the optimal temperature that induces the greatest degree of shrinkage without untoward effects on the tissue appears to be between 60 and 67.5 degrees C. Heating at higher

temperatures may result in hyalinization, extensive thermal damage, and necrosis of the tissue. Newer models of thermal modifier systems feature sensors on their probes that monitor and automatically regulate tissue temperatures to ensure optimal capsulodesis effects. Although these devices are thought to provide the highest margin of safety and efficiency, no data have been published to support this claim. Within the optimal range, however, shrinkage increases with increased exposure until it reaches a plateau beyond which no additional shrinkage is observed. Clinically, it is futile to pass the thermal probe over an area repeatedly with the desire to achieve a greater degree of shrinkage. As the tissue is cooled to room temperature, some collagen molecules regain their former triple-helical structure and undergo renaturation. This may be accompanied by relaxation of up to 10% of the total amount of initial shrinkage achieved.[13]

While the collagen is denatured at these temperatures, it is not permanently damaged, because residual populations of fibroblasts are allowed to migrate into the affected areas and repair the damaged tissue with new collagen. The reparative process begins one week after insult to the tissue and continues for 3 months. Currently, there is no consensus regarding the time required for thermally modified tissues to regain their normal material and biomechanical properties. Although hypothesized, the role and extent of further capsular contraction during the reparatory phase has not been established.

Although the effect of heat energy on collagen molecules has been well documented in the literature, the actual factors responsible for the reported benefits of thermal capsular modification are not completely understood. It is reasonable to assume that some combination of factors contributes to the success of the technique: the initial connective tissue shrinkage, which appears to tighten and stabilize the joint; the fibroplasia, capsular thickening, and secondary cicatrix formation that occur in response to the traumatic insult; and the loss of afferent sensory stimulation due to the destruction of sensory receptors.

As with many new techniques, questions sometimes arise more rapidly than they can be definitively answered. Although numerous in vitro and in vivo experimental studies have investigated the biology and biomechanics of thermally modified tissues, there is still no consensus regarding the optimal degree of shrinkage, the most appropriate postoperative regimen, the ultimate mechanism of reported clinical improvements, or the long-term fate of the modified tissues. Regardless of these unanswered questions, thermal capsular modification presents an attractive, minimally invasive option for patients with pathologies that are difficult to manage by other means.

Indications

Excessive capsular laxity has been attributed to several thumb basal joint problems. Arthroscopic thermal capsular modification is indicated as a primary procedure in patients with painful subluxation of the thumb CMC joint. Combined with joint debridement, the technique may also address mild degenerative arthritis (stage I or II, Eaton[17] or Burton[18] classification). Finally, it may act as an adjuvant treatment to partial or complete trapeziectomy for severe arthritic conditions (stage III or IV) about the basal joint. Regardless of whether the trapezium is resected, the goal of thermal capsular modification is the same: to tighten the capsule and ligaments of the thumb CMC joint in a minimally invasive manner. Relative contraindications to thermal capsular modification include excessive thumb metacarpophalangeal joint hyperextension and connective tissue disorders, such as Ehlers-Danlos.

Surgical Technique

Patient preparation and portals are achieved as previously described, and a complete diagnostic arthroscopy of the thumb CMC is performed. Traction on the thumb is reduced to relax the joint but still allow adequate visualization. All intracapsular ligamentous structures are identified and probed to assess their laxity. Careful attention is given to the degree of joint distraction prior to shrinking.

Using the 1-U portal to visualize the joint, the thermal modification probe is placed through the 1-R portal. The probe is passed over the capsule and ligaments in a smooth and systematic manner. To move too quickly over the tissue may not allow the probe to reach optimal temperature; to move too slowly may risk thermal injury, particularly if using laser or bipolar energy. Damage to the tendons of the flexor carpi radialis (FCR) and flexor pollicis longus have been recognized as complications of this procedure.[19] Reducing the wattage output to the probe may be prudent around these structures. Progressing systematically allows the tissue to be modified in the most efficient manner while avoiding needless passes over maximally affected tissue. The authors prefer to begin at the AOLd and AOLs, continuing volarly and ulnarly to the UCL and as much of the POL as can be visualized from the 1-U portal. At this point, the visualizing and working portals are switched so that the arthroscope is inserted through the 1-R portal and the probe is in the 1-U portal. With this vantage point, the remainder of the POL, as well as the DRL may be addressed.

As the probe comes in contact with the tissue, some degree of immediate shrinkage occurs, which is accompanied by a subtle change of color and texture, or "caramelization" of the tissue (Figure 22.8). With some

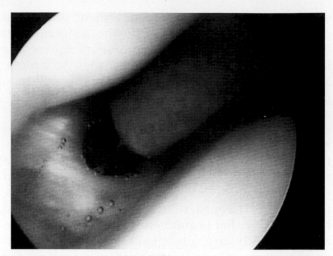

FIGURE 22.8. Monopolar radiofrequency probe shrinking the anterior oblique ligament. Note the "caramelization" and associated color change of the thermally modified tissue.

regularity, it is preferable to leave a small area of healthy tissue between areas of modified tissue to allow for fibroblasts to repair the adjacent denatured collagen. Complete caramelization of the capsule is not desirable. Despite the satisfaction of witnessing immediate shrinking of the tissue during the procedure, up to 10% of the collagen will renature and relax as it cools.[13] This phenomenon should be anticipated and tensioning should be appropriately adjusted. Furthermore, some believe that the majority of the tensioning of the collagen occurs several weeks later during the reparative process, but this is debated in the literature.[13–15]

After partial or complete trapeziectomy is performed, the thumb CMC joint is reduced under arthroscopic and fluoroscopic visualization in order to restore anatomic thumb column height. Under this distraction, one 0.045-inch Kirschner wire is inserted through the radial side of the metacarpal and advanced proximally through the thumb CMC joint and into the remains of the trapezium in cases of partial resection, or into the body of the scaphoid in cases of complete resection. Although the majority of thermal capsular modification is performed prior to anatomic reduction and pinning, final tensioning of the joint may be performed by shrinking once the pin is in place. Although the origins of the capsule and intracapsular ligaments have been variably elevated or detached from the trapezium, the soft-tissue envelope remains intact through the periosteal continuum and contains collagen susceptible to thermal modification. If tendon interposition is considered, it must follow thermal modification, as the graft would obstruct any accessibility to the capsule.

Postoperative Care

Patients undergoing thermal capsular modification, when performed alone or accompanying minor debridement or trapeziectomy, are placed in a thumb spica splint postoperatively and instructed to elevate the hand as much as possible to decrease swelling and allow for rapid clearing of irrigation fluid that has extravasated into the subcutaneous tissues. Immediate motion of the uninvolved digits is encouraged. Sutures are removed in 7 to 10 days, and the patient is placed in a thumb spica cast. After 3 to 4 weeks, the pin is removed, and the cast is replaced by a removable thumb spica splint to be worn at all times with the exception of bathing and hand therapy. At 6 weeks, therapy is advanced to include strengthening exercises. During the third month following surgery, the patients are weaned from the splint and resume activities of daily living. After 3 months, patients return to their previous lifestyles with minimal restrictions.

TENDON INTERPOSITION

Following arthroscopic partial trapeziectomy, Menon[20] described a technique that interposes autologous FCR tendon, fascia lata allograft, or a Gore-Tex cardiovascular patch between the partially resected trapezium and first metacarpal. Thermal capsular modification was not performed. With an average follow-up of 37 months, complete pain relief was achieved in 25 of 33 patients. Four patients had persistent pain and required a second operation. All patients maintained their preoperative range of motion, and the average pinch strength nearly doubled. Although 18 of 19 patients receiving Gore-Tex interposition had good clinical outcomes, recent studies have demonstrated that Gore-Tex can cause particulate disease, and it largely has been abandoned. Autologous tendon has emerged as the standard material for interposition.

Menon believed that his technique was contraindicated in patients with metacarpal base subluxation greater than one-third the diameter of the joint surface, metacarpophalangeal hyperextension of greater than 10 degrees, or fixed metacarpal adduction contractures.[20] In the advent of thermal capsular shrinkage, significant subluxation of the thumb CMC joint may no longer be considered an absolute contraindication. Although not originally described by Menon, it would be reasonable to apply the technique to conditions requiring complete trapeziectomy.

Indications

Arthroscopic tendon interposition is indicated for patients undergoing concomitant partial or complete trapeziectomy. Though no data support the clinical advantages of interposition arthroplasty over trapeziectomy alone, many believe the tendon anchor acts as a collagen scaffolding that supports the first metacarpal and facilitates scar formation and resulting joint stabilization.

Surgical Technique

Partial or complete arthroscopic trapeziectomy is performed as previously described. Although it was not originally described by Menon, the authors recommend thermal capsular shrinkage prior to introduction of the tendon graft. At least 10 cm of palmaris longus tendon or three-quarters width of the FCR tendon is harvested using multiple transverse incisions. A large curved needle is attached to one end of the graft by absorbable suture. While the 1-U serves as the viewing portal with the arthroscope, the 1-R portal is enlarged to about 1 cm, and the skin edges are retracted using skin hooks. It is helpful to illuminate the 1-R capsular opening with the arthroscope. The large curved needle is passed through the opening in the 1-R portal and is brought through the joint. The needle exits through the volar capsule and thenar musculature and is pulled out through the skin over the thenar eminence. By pulling the suture, the end of the tendon graft is introduced into the joint and can be visualized through the arthroscope. The end of the tendon is advanced until it abuts the volar capsule and is unable to advance further. The remaining tendon is packed into the joint using a forceps. The arthroscope is withdrawn and the joint capsule closed. A 0.045-inch Kirschner wire is passed through the base of the first metacarpal into the remaining trapezium in cases of partial resection, or into the body of the scaphoid in cases of complete resection.

Postoperative Care

Postoperative care following arthroscopic partial or complete trapeziectomy with tendon interposition is identical to that of arthroscopic partial or complete trapeziectomy alone.

COMPLICATIONS

There are few complications associated with thumb CMC joint arthroscopy, and they are comparable to arthroscopy of other joints in regard to infection and iatrogenic articular damage. Specific to the thumb CMC joint, the creation of portals may damage one or more of the many sensory branches of the radial nerve that typically surround the arthroscopic field. Injury to these branches, namely the SR2 and SR3, potentially may result in sensory loss or neuroma formation. The radial artery passes within a few millimeters of the EPB at the level of the thumb CMC joint and may also be injured while creating the portals. Blunt dissection to the joint capsule should help to reduce both of these potential complications. Unintentional insertion of the arthroscopic instruments into the radioscaphoid or scaphotrapezial joints, due to their close proximity to the thumb CMC joint, may occur and should be recognized quickly. Careful attention to bony and soft tissue landmarks, and even fluoroscopy confirmation prior to portal placement, will help to minimize this risk. The authors recommend using fluoroscopy liberally to confirm the placement of the arthroscope if the surgeon is unfamiliar with the intra-articular anatomy of the involved carpal joints.

Complications due to thermal capsular modification within the thumb CMC joint relate to the close proximity of the structures that lie just exterior to the capsule being heated. Injury to the FCR and FPL tendons has been reported.[19] Reduction in wattage output is advised when performing shrinkage around these structures, particularly when using monopolar radiofrequency or laser energy. Heat may accumulate within the joint, causing thermal necrosis to intra-articular tissues, particularly if using bipolar radiofrequency. Continuous irrigation of normal saline through the joint will help to dissipate the heat and reduce the risk of thermal injury. Currently, known complications of thermal capsular modification are short-term complications. Like the long-term benefits of capsular shrinkage, the long-term complications of the procedure are speculative at this time and require further investigation. The extent of relaxation of thermally modified tissue has not been established. In addition, the disruption of the afferent sensory fibers in the capsular tissue offers the short-term benefit of providing anesthesia to the joint, but the long-term effects are unclear. Some have suggested that the loss of neurosensory input could cause the joint to become more susceptible to future injury due to loss of reflex-protective muscle activity.[13] There are no scientific data, however, to support this theory.

CONCLUSION

Arthroscopic trapeziectomy and thermal capsular modification have demonstrated favorable early results in the treatment of thumb CMC arthritis. The various indications and options for arthroscopic intervention are summarized in Table 22.1. However, these are evolving techniques and have yet to withstand the test of time and critical review, particularly in regard to thermal capsular modification. We must approach these techniques cautiously and conscientiously and recognize that excellent outcomes may be achieved using traditional open procedures. On the other hand, arthroscopy offers a minimally invasive

TABLE 22.1. Indications and Options for Arthroscopic Treatment of the Arthritic Thumb Carpometacarpal Joint.

Eaton or Burton stage	Options for arthroscopic treatment
I	Thermal shrinkage, possible pinning
II	Thermal shrinkage, debridement, possible hemitrapeziectomy, possible pinning
III	Thermal shrinkage, debridement, hemi- or complete trapeziectomy, pinning
IV	Thermal shrinkage, complete trapeziectomy, pinning

alternative to traditional techniques to treat basal joint arthrosis and hypermobility. As with all exciting new techniques, science and time will eventually resolve whether arthroscopic treatments of the thumb CMC joint should be included in the armamentarium of every hand surgeon.

References

1. Berger RA. Arthroscopy of the small joints of the hand. In: Osterman AL, Geissler WB (eds), *Atlas of Hand Clinics: New Techniques in Wrist Arthroscopy.* Philadelphia, PA: W.B. Saunders, 2001, pp. 389–408.
2. Berger RA. A technique for arthroscopic evaluation of the first carpometacarpal joint. *J Hand Surg* 1997;22:1077–1080.
3. Steinberg BD, Plancher KD, Idler RS. Percutaneous Kirschner wire fixation through the snuff box: an anatomic study. *J Hand Surg* 1995;20A:50–62.
4. Bettinger PC, Berger RA. Functional ligamentous anatomy of the trapezium and trapeziometacarpal joint (gross and arthroscopic). *Hand Clin* 2001;12(2):151–168.
5. Bettinger PC, Linscheid RL, Berger RA, et al. An anatomic study of the stabilizing ligaments of the trapezium and trapeziometacarpal joint. *J Hand Surg* 1999;24A(4):786–789.
6. Bettinger PC, Smutz WP, Linscheid RL, et al. Material properties of the trapezoid and trapeziometacarpal ligaments. *J Hand Surg* 2000;25A(6):1085–1095.
7. Gonzalez MH, Kemmler J, Weinzweig N, et al. Portals for arthroscopy of the trapeziometacarpal joint. *J Hand Surg* 1997;22B(5):574–575.
8. Culp RW, Rekant MS. The role of arthroscopy in evaluating and treating trapeziometacarpal disease. *Hand Clin* 2001;17(2):315–319.
9. Davis TR, Brady O, Barton NJ, et al. Trapeziectomy alone, with tendon interposition or with ligament reconstruction? A randomized prospective study. *J Hand Surg* 1997;22B(6):689–694.
10. Lins RE, Gelberman RH, McKeown L, et al. Basal joint arthritis: trapeziectomy with ligament reconstruction and tendon interposition arthroplasty. *J Hand Surg* 1996;21A:202–209.
11. Eaton RG, Lane LB, Littler JW, et al. Ligament reconstruction for the painful thumb carpometacarpal joint: A long-term assessment. *J Hand Surg* 1984;9A:692–699.
12. Pellegrini VD. The basal articulations of the thumb: pain, instability, and osteoarthritis. In: Peimer CA, (ed). *Surgery of the Hand and Upper Extremity,* vol 1. New York: McGraw-Hill, 1996:1019–1039.

13. Arnoczky SP, Aksan A. Thermal modification of connective tissues: basic science considerations and clinical importance. *J Am Acad Orthop Surg* 2000;8:305–313.

14. Hayashi K, Markel M. Thermal modification of joint capsule and ligamentous tissues. *Tech Sports Med* 1998;6:120–125.

15. Hayashi K, Peters D, Thabit G, et al. The mechanism of joint capsule thermal modification in an in vito sheep model. *Clin Orthop Rel Res* 2000;370:236–249.

16. Osmond C, Hecht P, Hayashi K, et al. Comparative effects of laser and radiofrequency on joint capsule. *Clin Orthop Rel Res* 2000;375:286–294.

17. Eaton RG, Littler JW. Ligament reconstruction for the painful thumb carpometacarpal joint. *J Bone Joint Surg* 1973;55A:1655–1666.

18. Burton RI. Basal joint arthrosis of the thumb. *Orthop Clin North Am* 1973;4:331–348.

19. Sweet S, Weiss LE. Applications of electrothermal shrinkage in wrist arthroscopy. In: Osterman AL, Geissler WB (eds), *Atlas of Hand Clinics: New Techniques in Wrist Arthroscopy*. Philadelphia: WB Saunders, 2001;6(2):203–210.

20. Menon J. Arthroscopic management of trapeziometacarpal arthritis of the thumb. *Arthroscopy* 1996;12:581–587.

23

Resection of Volar Ganglia

Christophe Mathoulin

Dorsal wrist ganglia are usually caused by a capsular abnormality. More often than not, degenerative pseudocysts develop within the dorsal capsule of the wrist and involve the scapholunate ligament. Their arthroscopic resection is well-documented.[1-6] Cysts of the volar face of the wrist account for 20% of all synovial cysts of the hand. They usually appear between the flexor carpi radialis tendon and the abductor pollicis longus tendon. Their origin is usually radiocarpal and the cyst may be at some distance from its origin (Figure 23.1). There are also volar capsular abnormalities in the region of the scapholunate interosseus ligament.

Various treatments have been suggested ranging from complete abstention of therapy to open surgery. Surgical treatment is the most curative, but it can be responsible for numerous problems such as an unsightly scar, neuromas on the terminal branches of the radial nerve, or joint stiffness. In addition, the proximity of the radial nerve and artery make this surgery riskier. Arthroscopic resection of palmar synovial cysts of the wrist has several advantages. The postoperative follow-up is very simple, and this technique avoids the majority of the complications described above.

SURGICAL TECHNIQUE

All patients in our series were operated on as outpatients under local regional anesthetic using a pneumatic tourniquet. We use a 2.4-mm arthroscope with a 30-degree visual angle, a shaver, and miniaturized instruments. The arm is fixed to an arm table and the elbow flexed to 90 degrees with the wrist in vertical traction using a "Japanese" hand. First, the position of the cyst is located and the outline is drawn. The arthroscope is positioned using the 3-4 radiocarpal opening. In our experience, most cysts develop inside the radiocarpal joint.

The first step is to locate the origin of the cyst. Pressure is applied to the cyst, which enables its origin to be seen clearly. It is usually situated between the radioscaphocapitate and the radiolunotriquetral ligaments (Figure 23.2A,B). It is easy to find the ganglion stalk inside the joint.

A 1-2 radiocarpal surgical approach is performed. To avoid damaging any vital structures, a transverse 3-mm incision of the skin is performed in line with the cutaneous folds. Then, using mosquito forceps, we enter directly through the capsule, retracting the adjacent structures. With the help of a shaver introduced through this lateral surgical approach, the ganglion stalk is resected and then the fine anterior capsule between the two ligaments is resected. (It makes it easier if you press on, or ask an assistant to press on, the cyst.) When the cyst wall opens in the joint, the mucus from the cyst clouds the arthroscopic vision. The shaver vacuums up this mucous liquid. Then, under arthroscopic control, the joint capsule, the tendon synovitis, and the ganglion sac are resected using a shaver (Figure 23.3A,B). The limits of the palmar capsulectomy are difficult to define, but our experience has shown that when the capsular resection becomes more difficult the capsule is healthy again. The general rule is a resection of about 1 cm. The flexor pollicis longus tendon and flexor carpi radialis tendon can be seen perfectly at the end of the operation, and care must be taken not to damage these tendons with the shaver.

We do not close the incisions, thus allowing evacuation of any surplus water inside the joint. The patient is discharged the same day with the hand and wrist free. The wrist and hand can be used normally as soon as the anesthetic has worn off.

RESULTS

We have operated on 12 patients using this technique, 27 women and 5 men. The average age was 46 years old (18 to 76). The average length of time between the apparition of the cyst and surgical resection was 13 months (between 3 and 52). Mobility was normal in all cases. Muscular strength was diminished in all cases, but only moderately, and was about 75% compared to the opposite side. The wrists were more often than not painless. The reason for the operation was usually aesthetic.

Our average follow-up is 26 months (between 12 and 39 months). At the longest follow-up none of the patients had complained of pain. Mobility was normal in all cases and strength identical to the opposite side.

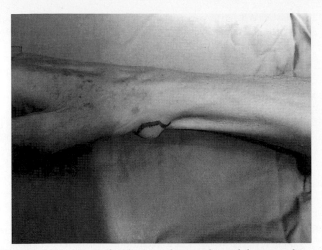

FIGURE 23.1. View of a classic volar ganglion of the wrist, located in front of radiocarpal joint, lateral to the FCR tendon.

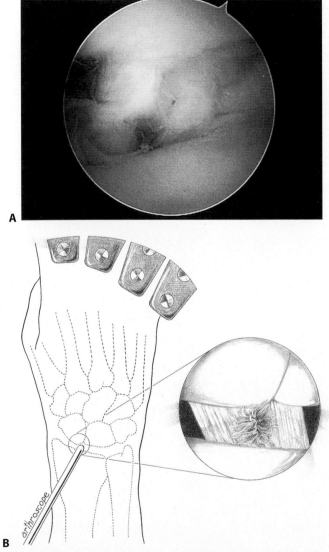

FIGURE 23.2. A. Operating view showing the location of the radiocarpal palmar ganglion. The ganglion stalk is located between the radioscaphocapitate ligament and radiolunotriquetral ligament. **B.** Diagram showing the location of the radiocarpal palmar ganglion between the radioscaphocapitate ligament and radiolunotriquetral ligament.

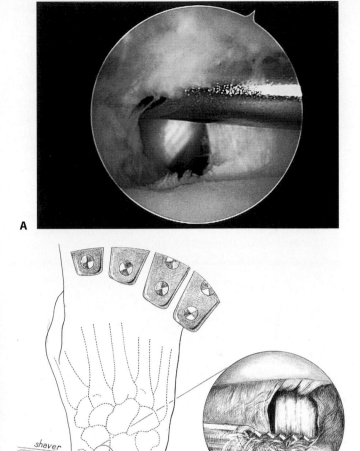

FIGURE 23.3. A. Operating view showing the capsular and cyst resection with a shaver placed through a 1-2 radiocarpal lateral approach. We can see the flexor pollicis longus tendon after cyst resection. **B.** Diagram showing the capsular and cyst resection with a shaver.

The small 3-mm horizontal incisions, which we performed to position the arthroscope, meant that the scars became totally invisible.

We had no radial artery lesions. One patient, the eldest, presented a moderate hematoma, which spontaneously resolved in three days. To date there have been no recurrences.

CONCLUSION

If the excision of the dorsal synovial cyst of the wrist has become a routine practice, arthroscopic resection of palmar synovial cysts of the wrist appears to be a reliable and elegant solution, particularly as standard surgical resection is not exempt from complications.

The description of palmar cyst resection technique was described by Mathoulin in Paris[7] and Ho in Hong Kong. In 2003, Ho reported his experience of six palmar ganglions resected using arthroscopy with simple postoperative follow-up and no recurrences.[8] It is a sure and easy technique that allows a satisfactory resection of the cyst and the adjoining joint capsule, provided that the limits of the cyst are located accurately. The satisfaction level of the patients is very high, helped by the fact that there are no cutaneous sutures and no wrist immobilization.

References

1. Fontes D. Ganglia treatment by arthroscopy. In: Saffar P, Amadio PC, Foucher G. (eds). *Current Practice in Hand Surgery*. London: Martin Dunitz, 1997, pp. 283–290.

2. Geissler WB. Arthroscopic excision of dorsal wrist ganglia. *Techniques in Hand and Upper Extremity Surgery* 1998;2:196–201.

3. Luchetti R, Badia A, Alfarano M, et al. Arthroscopic resection of dorsal wrist ganglia and treatment of recurrences. *J Hand Surg* 2000;25B(1):38–40.

4. Osterman AL, Raphael J. Arthroscopic resection of dorsal ganglion of the wrist. *Hand Clin* 1995;11:7–12.

5. Pederzini L, Ghinelli L, Soragni O. Arthroscopic treatment of dorsal arthrogenic cysts of the wrist. *J Sports Traumatol Rel Res* 1995;17:210–215.

6. Whipple TL. Arthroscopic surgery. *The Wrist*. Philadelphia: J.B. Lippincott; 1992, pp. 82–84.

7. Mathoulin C. Résection arthroscopique des krystes synoviaux du poignet. In: SFA, (ed.) *Perspectives en arthroscopie*. France: Springer-Verlag, 2003;3:105–108.

8. Ho PC, Lo WN, Hung LK. Arthroscopic resection of volar ganglion of the wrist: a new technique. *Arthroscopy* 2003;19:218–221.

24

Clinical Approach to the Painful Wrist

Andrea Atzei and Riccardo Luchetti

Pain localization of the wrist is the most common cause of referral to consultation in the office of many hand and wrist surgeons. In many cases, patients' complaints are readily recognized as typical symptoms and the history pathognomonic of defined disorders. Accurate physical examination, supplemented by standard X-rays, often yields a prompt diagnosis during the first patient visit.

However, cases of chronic wrist pain, in which exact diagnosis is difficult even after several consultations, are not infrequent. This is not surprising if one considers the anatomic and biomechanical complexity of the wrist joint. Within that small area, there is a concentration of intimately related structures, including more than 20 radiocarpal, intercarpal, and carpometacarpal joints, as well as the distal radioulnar joint (DRUJ), 26 carpal ligaments and the triangular fibrocartilage complex (TFCC), each of which can be source of intra-articular pathology. In addition, the 24 tendons, 2 main vascular trunks, and 6 nerves crossing the joint are all sources of extra-articular pathology.

Thorough clinical evaluation of the painful wrist should include routine steps of taking the patient's history and performing a physical examination, followed by appropriate imaging studies. During the last decade, arthroscopy has confirmed its role as a valuable tool in helping the clinician in the diagnosis of wrist disorders.[1-4]

Direct visualization of intra-articular structures allows early diagnosis and treatment of selected cases. However, limitations of arthroscopy include the fact that only intra-articular pathology can be assessed, and not all abnormalities identified by arthroscopy are necessarily responsible for the patient's complaints. Therefore, diagnostic arthroscopy is indicated only following a thorough clinical examination, during which the anatomic structures responsible for the patient's symptoms should be located with the greatest accuracy and all extraarticular causes of pain excluded. A systematic approach is suggested for the diagnosis and management of the conditions or disorders that cause wrist pain.

CLINICAL EVALUATION

History

The steps in taking a patient's history are well-defined (Table 24.1). The patient's general history should be collected first; age and sex are important as they correlate with joint wear.[5,6] Special attention should be paid to occupational and avocational activities involving the wrist, previous injuries or surgery, and other systemic illnesses and/or rheumatologic diseases. Details of wrist complaints, whether they follow injuries considered trivial and therefore initially underestimated, or result from slow progression of nontraumatic conditions, must be obtained by specific questioning during a thorough clinical history.

The most common causes of acute or chronic wrist pain[7-9] can be divided into seven main categories (Table 24.2): traumatic injuries (including acute injuries and posttraumatic conditions), degenerative and inflammatory disorders (local or systemic conditions and repetitive trauma disorders), infections, tumors, congenital and developmental disorders, neurological disorders, and vascular disorders. Categorizing the patient's wrist complaints according to these seven general causes is an important step to identify a specific disorder or to formulate a differential diagnosis to guide physical examination and further investigation.

Physical Examination

Continuous advances in our understanding of wrist anatomy and kinematics have increased the importance of physical examination as the basic diagnostic tool over imaging techniques, whose most valuable contribution is in differential diagnosis in selected cases.[10] Examination should be extended to the entire upper extremity, including the cervical spine and all other joints or areas of symptomatology.

Evaluation of the painful wrist begins with an accurate inspection for specific areas of swelling or obvious deformities, erythema, warmth, nodules or skin lesions, and prior surgical scars. Assessment of pas-

TABLE 24.1. Steps in Taking a Patient History.

Patient's general history	Wrist complaint history
1. Age	1. Classification of chief complaint
2. Handedness	2. Onset, location, and nature of symptoms
3. Occupation	3. Symptom's relation to specific activities
4. Avocational activities	4. Factors exacerbating or improving symptoms
5. Previous wrist injuries	
6. Previous wrist surgery	5. Frequency and duration of postactivity ache
7. Other orthopedic/ rheumatologic disorders	6. Subjective loss of wrist motion
8. Other medical/ dismetabolic disorders	7. Abnormal sounds or sensations with wrist motion
	8. Efficacy of prior treatments
	9. Current work status
	10. Involvement of worker's compensation claim

sive and active range of motion of both wrists usually follows. A loss of motion is consistently associated with a disorder primarily affecting the wrist joint, either posttraumatic or degenerative. Measurement of grip strength has proved to be a reliable index of wrist

impairment,[11] especially when the rapid exchange grip technique is used to detect submaximal effort.[12]

Palpation is the next step of physical examination. Diagnostic ability depends essentially on a thorough knowledge of both soft tissue and bony topographic anatomy of the wrist: recognition of underlying soft tissue and bone structures as sources of pain is a fundamental step towards diagnosis, as it allows correlation of clinical complaints with anatomical damage.[13] A systematic approach to correlating the pain symptom to topographic anatomy of the wrist can be achieved by dividing the dorsal and palmar aspect of the wrist surface into three areas: radial, central, and ulnar (Figure 24.1). A total of six areas are defined by using prominent bony landmarks and easily palpable tendons as reference points.

Proceeding from radial to ulnar on the dorsal surface of the wrist, the following landmarks are located (Figure 24.1A): the dorsoradial border of the compartment for the abductor pollicis longus (APL) and the extensor pollicis brevis (EPB) tendons [i.e., the first extensor compartment of the wrist, a longitudinal line

TABLE 24.2. Most Common Causes of Wrist Pain.

			Chondritis/Osteochondritis/ Posttraumatic arthritis	
Traumatic Disorders	**Fracture and Malunion** Radius—ulna Scaphoid Other carpal bones	**Nonunion** Scaphoid Capitate Hamate	SNAC SLAC Piso-triquetral arthrosis Hamate-triquetral arthrosis Hyperextension radioscaphoid impingement (Gymnast's wrist) Ulno-carpal impingement	
	Ligamentous Injuries and Instability Perilunate (scapholunate, lunotriquetral) Midcarpal (intrinsic, extrinsic) Radiocarpal (ventral or dorsal subluxation, ulnar translocation) Dorsal wrist syndrome Distal radioulnar joint (luxation, subluxation, TFCC injury) Carpo-metacarpal J (1st CMC; 2nd–3rd CMC, carpal boss; 4th–5th CMC)		**Extensor Carpi Ulnaris Tendon Subluxation**	
Degenerative Inflammatory Disease	**Connective Tissue Diseases** Rheumatoid arthritis Systemic erythematous lupus	**Metabolic Diseases** Gout/pseudogout Hyperparathyroidism Chondrocalcinosis	**Tendonitis Tenosynovitis Repetitive Strain Injury**	**Chondritis/ Primary Arthrosis**
Infective Disorders	**Common Bacterial/Atypical Agent**		**Specific Granulomatous Disease**	
Neoplastic Disorders	**Ganglia** (extraosseous/ intraosseous/occult) **Tendon Cysts**	**Bone Tumors** Enchondroma, osteoid osteoma, chondromatosis, etc.	**Soft Tissue Tumors** Pigmented villonodular synovitis, Giant cell tumor, etc.	**Malignant Tumors** **Metastasis**
Congenital and Developmental Disorders	**Simple Osseous Cyst**	**Madelung's deformity**	**Muscular Anomalies** Extensor brevis manus	**Carpal Coalition** Scapholunate Scaphotrapezial Lunotriquetral
Neurological Disorders	**Traumatic** Palmar branch median n. (from section) Sens. branch radial n. (from injection) Dorsal sens. branch ulnar n. (direct contusion) Distal post. interosseous n. (recurrent ganglion)		**Compressive** Carpal tunnel syndrome (CTS) Wartemberg's syndrome Guyon's syndrome T.O.S. Radicular compression	
Vascular Disorders	Aneurysm/thrombosis of the ulnar artery Avascular necrosis of the lunate (Kienboeck's disease); of the scaphoid (Preiser's disease); of the capitate; of the triquetrum			

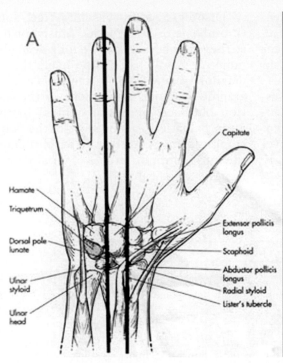
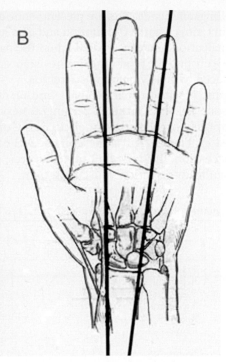

FIGURE 24.1. Topographic anatomy of the wrist. **A.** Dorsal surface of the wrist. Landmarks for reference are the dorso-radial border of the first extensor compartment, a longitudinal line passing over Lister's tubercle, a line continuing proximally from the middle axis of the ring finger and passing between the fourth and fifth extensor compartment, and the ulnar border of the sixth extensor compartment. Three areas are defined between these landmarks: radial dorsal area corresponding to the "anatomical snuffbox," central dorsal area, and ulnar dorsal area. **B.** Palmar surface of the wrist. Landmarks for reference are the dorsoradial border of the first extensor compartment, the ulnar border of the FCR, a line continuing proximally from the middle axis of the ring finger and passing just radial to the volar aspect of the distal radioulnar joint, and the ulnar border of the sixth extensor compartment. Three areas are defined between these landmarks: radial palmar area, central palmar area, and ulnar palmar area.

passing over Lister's tubercle, and a line that extends along the middle axis of the ring finger proximally—this line usually passes between the fourth and fifth extensor compartment of the wrist—and the ulnar border of the flexor carpi ulnaris (FCU) tendon.

Consequently, three dorsal areas are defined as follows: the radial dorsal area between the dorsoradial border of the first extensor compartment of the wrist and the longitudinal line passing over Lister's tubercle, including the area of the "anatomical snuffbox"; the central dorsal area between the longitudinal line passing over Lister's tubercle and the line continuing the middle axis of the ring finger; and the ulnar dorsal area between the line continuing the middle axis of the ring finger and the ulnar border of the FCU tendon.

On the palmar surface of the wrist, the following landmarks are located (Figure 24.1B): the dorsoradial border of the first extensor compartment, the ulnar border of the flexor carpi radialis (FCR) tendon, a line continuing proximally along the middle axis of the ring finger (this line usually passes just radial to the volar aspect of the DRUJ), and the ulnar border of the FCU tendon. Consequently, the palmar surface of the wrist is divided in three areas between these landmarks: the radial palmar area between the dorsoradial border of the first extensor compartment and the ulnar border of the FCR tendon; the central palmar area between the ulnar border of the FCR tendon and the

line continuing proximally along the middle axis of the ring finger; and the ulnar palmar area between the line continuing proximally along the middle axis of the ring finger and the ulnar border of the FCU tendon.

A comprehensive and careful examination of the diffusely painful wrist will enable the surgeon to elicit a patient's symptoms by palpating specific spots. Palpation of an osseous prominence may evoke pain in the case of fracture or nonunion or avulsion of the ligaments inserting on it. A joint rim is usually felt as a small depression between two bony ends. Gentle palpation may show swelling in the case of synovitis, or in the presence of small ganglia, direct pressure over the capsule may exacerbate pain. Firm palpation of the joint surface may provoke pain in the case of osteochondritis or avascular necrosis.

A series of maneuvers exerting axial load on the different joints are utilized to elicit pain and/or crepitation in degenerative joint diseases. In these cases, joint compression or, when possible, palpation of the degenerated articular surfaces increases pain, while axial distraction maneuvers usually relieve it. Pain is also present following those maneuvers that stress the joint ligaments in an attempt to sublux the joint itself, as well as following direct pressure over the torn ligament. In the presence of complete ligament disruption, malalignment of the bony ends and widening of the joint space are common findings.

Pain, swelling, and tenderness are present along a tendon's course in tenosynovitis. Crepitation and pain are reproduced by palpation and exacerbated when the patient is asked to actively pull the tendon against resistance. Pain is also reproduced by passive tendon stretching.

A complaint of painful paresthesias and/or dysesthesias is associated with either a peripheral nerve injury or compression; paresthesia elicited by digital nerve percussion (Tinel's sign) is present just at the level of nerve compression. In the case of mixed nerves, early signs of muscular dysfunction must be sought.

Disorders of the vascular tree, such as arterial thrombosis or aneurysms, must not be overlooked, as they may be responsible for a deep, dull wrist ache radiating to the palm and fingers that is difficult to diagnose except by a clinical and/or ultrasonographic vascular assessment of the hand. Information obtained from the clinical history and from joint palpation, according to the suggested topographic approach, allows the clinician to focus on the most common causes of wrist pain for the symptomatic area (Table 24.3).

TABLE 24.3. Common Causes of Wrist Pain According to Topographic Areas.

	Volar areas			Dorsal areas		
	Radial	*Central*	*Ulnar*	*Radial*	*Central*	*Ulnar*
Traumatic Disorders	**Fractures** Scaphoid* Radial styloid* Trapezium Base 1st MC* Trapezoid **Nonunion** Scaphoid **Post-trauma Arthrosis** SNAC;* SLAC*	**Fractures** Lunate hamate	**Fractures** Pisiform Hook of the hamate **Arthrosis Post-traumatic** Piso-triquetral* **Lig. Injuries** TFCC injuries (*type 1B and C*)* DRUJ.Inst.*	**Fractures** Radial Styloid* Scaphoid* Trapezium* Trapezoid* Base 1st MC* **Inst./Lig. Injury** 1 CMC **Nonunion** Scaphoid **Post-tr. Athro.** SNAC;* SLAC* R-S impingement*	**Fractures** Lunate Capitate Radius (dye punch) **Inst./Leg Injury** Scapholunate Inst.* 2nd –3rd C-MC inst. (Carpal-boss) Midcarpal inst.	**Fractures** Triquetrum Base 4th–5th MC **Nonunion** Ulnar styloid **Post-Tr. Arthrosis** Triq-hamate* Ulno-carp. imping.* **Inst./Lig. Inj.** TFCC injuries (*type 1B–D and 2*)* DRUJ. Inst.* Lunotriq. inst.* Midcarpal inst. 4th–5th CMC inst.
Degenerative Inflammatory Disorders	**Tendonitis** FCR **Prim. Arthrosis** Basal thumb* Triscaphe*	**Tendonitis** Trigger finger	**Tendonitis** FCU **Prim. arthrosis** Piso-triquetral	**Tendonitis** de Quervain Intersection s.	**Tendonitis** EPL EIP	**Tendonitis** ECU (subluxation) **Prim. Arthrosis** Triq hamate*
Infective Disorders	No specific location					
Neoplastic Disorders	**Cysts** Articular;* Tendinous	**Cysts** Articular;* Osseous		**Cysts** Articular;* Osseous	**Cysts** Articular;* Osseous	
Congenital and Developmental Disorders	**Skeletal anomalies** Scaphotrapezial synostosis	**Skeletal anomalies** Scapholunate synostosis	**Skeletal anomalies** Lunotriquetral synostosis	**Skeletal anomalies** Scaphotrapezial synostosis	**Extensor manus brevis** **Madelung's disease**	**Madelung's disease**
Neurological Disorders	**Traumatic** Cut. palm. br. Median nerve	**Compressive** CTS	**Compressive** Guyon's syndrome	**Traumatic** Sens. br. rad. n. **Compressive** Wartemberg's syndrome	**Traumatic** Post. inteross. n.	**Traumatic** Dorsal br. Ulnar nerve
Vascular Disorders	**Preiser's disease**	**Avascular necrosis of the capitate**	**Ulnar artery aneurysm-thrombosis**	**Preiser's disease**	**Kienboeck's disease**	**Avascular necrosis of pisiform**

*Indicates disorders for which diagnostic or therapeutic arthroscopy is indicated.

SNAC = scaphoid nonunion advanced collapse; SLAC = scapholunate advanced collapse; CMC = carpometacarpal joint; ECV = extensor carpi ulnaris; CTS = carpal tunnel syndrome.

Provocative Maneuvers

Differential diagnosis and/or confirmation of the suspected diagnosis is achieved by means of special provocative maneuvers and diagnostic tests. Not only ligaments and osteoarticular structures should be tested, but also the numerous tendons, vessels, and nerves crossing the wrist. Table 24.4 summarizes the tests and maneuvers most commonly used in clinical practice categorized by the six topographic areas in which the patient's major complaint is localized.

Taken by itself, information from each of these tests may not yield an exact diagnosis. To reach a presumptive diagnosis, results from each test should be compared with those from other tests, with the patient's clinical history, and with the pathomechanics of known wrist trauma.

Anesthetic Examination

As a part of the clinical evaluation of wrist pain, an injection of a small amount of local anesthetic (0.5 to 0.8 mL of lidocaine) is essential to determine whether there is a multiplicity of causes to confirm the clinical diagnosis. In addition, an anesthetic injection may be of help in demonstrating to the patient the degree of pain relief that might be obtained with surgery.

IMAGING INVESTIGATIONS

In those complicated cases in which history and clinical examination are insufficient to formulate an exact diagnosis, the clinician should plan further evaluations. The introduction of many new imaging modalities has expanded the use of diagnostic imaging to be frequently abused or overused without a clear understanding of the indications for specific pathologic conditions. As a general rule, imaging techniques should be used to confirm or exclude a clinically presumptive diagnosis or to improve definition of a treatment plan.

Unless otherwise indicated by clinical findings, the initial radiographic examination should consist of three views:[14,15] standard posteroanterior (PA), oblique (PA oblique or AP oblique), and lateral views. The conventional radiographs are examined for bony abnormalities (fractures, cortical interruption, degree and pattern of mineralization) and the width and symmetry of joint spaces. The ligamentous architecture is assessed by determining whether the three carpal arcs of the wrist and parallelism of the joints are maintained.[14] Any arc interruption usually indicates disruption of joint integrity at that site. The lateral view is extremely important for evaluation of radiolunocapitate alignment and assessment of radioscaphoid,

TABLE 24.4. Common Diagnostic Tests and Provocative Maneuvers According to Topographic Areas*.

Area	Radial	Central	Ulnar
Dorsal	1 CMC Grind Test 2–3 CMC Shear Test Palpation of Anatomic snuffbox/Articular-Nonarticular Junction of Scaphoid (ANAJ) Intersection Syndrome Tinel's sign over the sensory branch of Radial Nerve (Wartenberg's Neuralgia)	Finger Extension Test (FET) Scaphoid shift (Watson's) Maneuver SL Shear Test "Catch-up clunk" (Lichtman's) Test EPL Test EIP Test Radio-Carpal Subluxation Test Palpation of Extensor Digitorum Brevis Manus	LT Shear Test Derby's Method for LT dissociation Ballottement Test Triquetral Impingement Ligament Tear (TILT) Test Ulnar Snuff Box Compression test Piano Key Test Press Test Ulno-Carpal impaction test Ulnar styloid impaction test EDM test EUC Palpation Test EUC Subluxation Provoc Test Tinel's sign over the Dorsal Branch of Ulnar Nerve
Volar	1 CMC Grind Test Palpation of STT joint Finkelstein's Test FRC Palpation Test Tinel's sign over the Palmar Cutaneous Branch of Median Nerve	FDC Palpation Test Phalen's Test Tinel's sign over the Median Nerve	Palpation of the Hook of the Hamate Piso-Triquetral Grind Test FUC Palpation Test Tinel's sign over the Ulnar Nerve

*See Suggested Readings for literature about various tests.

scapholunate, and scaphocapitate angles. Additional views of the wrist should be dictated by the findings of the clinical examination, such as the carpal tunnel view to evaluate the bony tubercles of the carpal tunnel, "clenched-fist" radiographs for enhancing detection of scapholunate dissociations, and spot films or tangential films of the painful region for patients with pain isolated at one site.

When clinical examination suggests superficial involvement, and extraarticular pathology is suspected, an ultrasound examination should be the next step. Musculoskeletal ultrasound is a quick and easy method of excluding soft tissue abnormalities, particularly tendon damage, ganglia, and synovial cysts. Although it allows for dynamic studies and bilateral comparisons with low patient discomfort, the quality and interpretation of ultrasound findings are operator-dependent, and therefore its use is limited.

If the history and physical examination (clicking or snapping) suggest that the patient's problems arise from interosseous ligamentous or TFCC injuries, cineradiography or an arthrogram under fluoroscopic control may be done. In cineradiography, the wrist is moved through full range of motion, with specific attempts to re-create stresses and positions known by the patient in order to reproduce that altered movement between the carpal bones responsible for the painful click.[16]

Subsequent examination is arthrography, which serves to establish the integrity of the capsular structures and intrasynovial interosseous ligaments, especially the scapholunate and lunotriquetral ligaments and the triangular fibrocartilage.[17] It may also show abnormal infolding of the synovium or the corrugated appearance consistent with localized synovitis. Arthrograms are diagnostic when they show an abnormal leak of opaque material between the radiocarpal and midcarpal or distal radioulnar spaces. To confirm the diagnosis, the flow of dye across these articulations is viewed directly by fluoroscopy. This finding must be

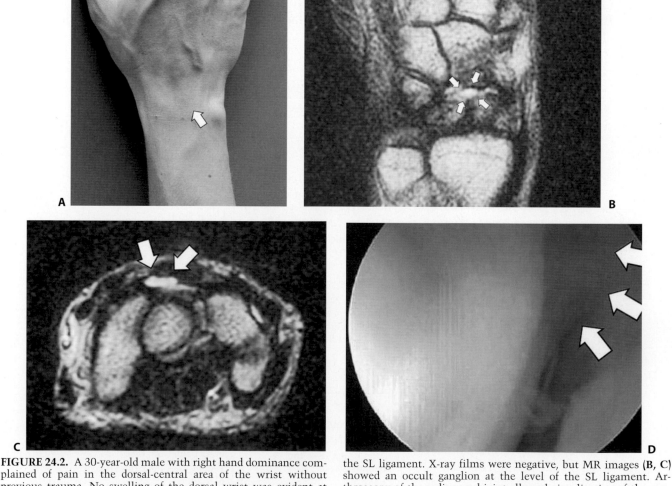

FIGURE 24.2. A 30-year-old male with right hand dominance complained of pain in the dorsal-central area of the wrist without previous trauma. No swelling of the dorsal wrist was evident at clinical evaluation **A.** Pain was exacerbated by palpation of the dorsal aspect of SL ligament. Positive a FET confirmed pathology of the SL ligament. X-ray films were negative, but MR images (**B, C**) showed an occult ganglion at the level of the SL ligament. Arthroscopy of the radiocarpal joint allowed visualization of the ganglion stalk, arising from the distal part of the dorsal aspect of the SL ligament **D.**

evaluated carefully, however, in relation to the patient's age, complaints, and clinical findings. As reported by several authors, communication between the different compartments of the wrist is not necessarily the result of trauma or disease.[15,18]

The computed axial tomography (CAT) scan has been used in the diagnosis of carpal pathology, but its only advantage is a better definition of the static alterations of the relationships between the carpal bones and the distal extremities of the radius and the ulna.

The MRI has recently been introduced for studying wrist anatomy and various other pathological conditions, such as avascular necrosis, tumors of the soft tissues, and carpal tunnel syndrome. Good-quality MRI can occasionally visualize the ligamentous and cartilaginous structures of the wrist, particularly the triangular fibrocartilage complex, and can reveal the presence or absence of occult ganglia and tendinitis.[19,20] Even though the application possibilities for studying injuries to the intercarpal ligaments are still being studied, this exam has shown a fair degree of accuracy in identifying TFCC injuries and intercarpal ligament disorders when its results are compared to arthroscopy.[21–23]

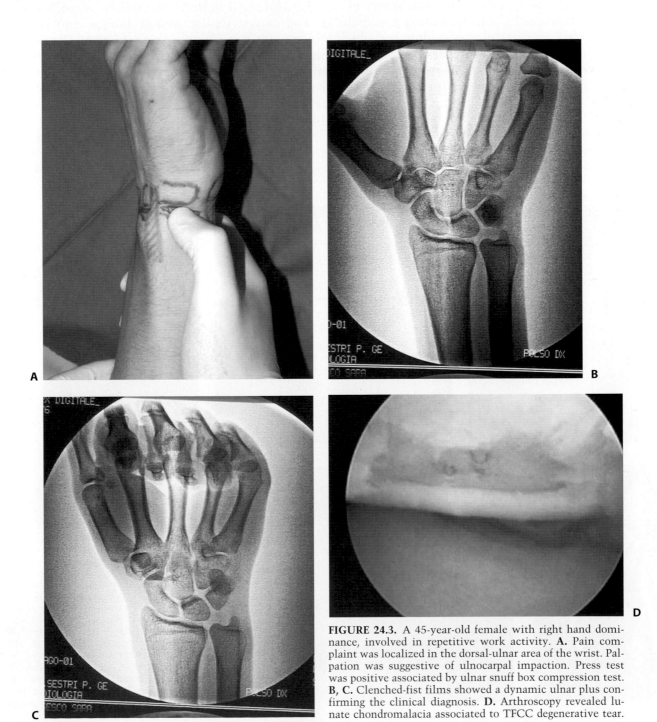

FIGURE 24.3. A 45-year-old female with right hand dominance, involved in repetitive work activity. **A.** Pain complaint was localized in the dorsal-ulnar area of the wrist. Palpation was suggestive of ulnocarpal impaction. Press test was positive associated by ulnar snuff box compression test. **B, C.** Clenched-fist films showed a dynamic ulnar plus confirming the clinical diagnosis. **D.** Arthroscopy revealed lunate chondromalacia associated to TFCC degenerative tear.

DIAGNOSTIC ARTHROSCOPY

When pathologies of extraarticular origin can be clinically excluded but physical examination does not point to a certain diagnosis of the disorder affecting the intra-articular structures, and even imaging techniques do not shed enough light on the causes of the patient's problem, arthroscopy must be performed to reach a diagnosis. Arthroscopy has increased the surgeon's knowledge about the origin of wrist pain, allowing not only a direct view of the anatomic elements involved in the pathological process, but also enabling the surgeon to appreciate the consistency of intra-articular structures by palpation using a second instrument (probe). In particular, regarding pathologies of the intra-articular soft tissues, arthroscopic examination gives precise information about the location and dimensions of ligamentous injuries (Figures 24.2 and 24.3), chondral wear (Figure 24.4), and synovitis. Partial ligamentous injuries, that at present cannot be shown even with the most sophisticated imaging equipment (Figure 24.5), are readily identifiable by arthroscopy.

Arthroscopy of the wrist is one of the more useful tools available to the physician for assessment and treatment of the intra-articular disorders of the radiocarpal, mediocarpal, and distal radioulnar joints. Arthroscopy provides an in-depth diagnostic complement to imaging examination, causes minimal invasion and allows for quick rehabilitation, usually with few complications[24,25] and with the possibility for immediate treatment.

Arthroscopy plays an important role in the diagnostic and therapeutic algorithms for the treatment of intra-articular wrist disorders (joint fractures, acute and chronic instability, osteochondrosis and intra-articular mobile bodies, and painful posttraumatic stiffness). Accurate clinical examination must precede arthroscopic evaluation. Classification of chronic wrist pain as pain of intra-articular or extraarticular origin appears to be crucial in determining when arthroscopic evaluation is indicated.

Development of the topographic approach was prompted by the need to provide the surgeon with a guide for identifying the multitude of local and

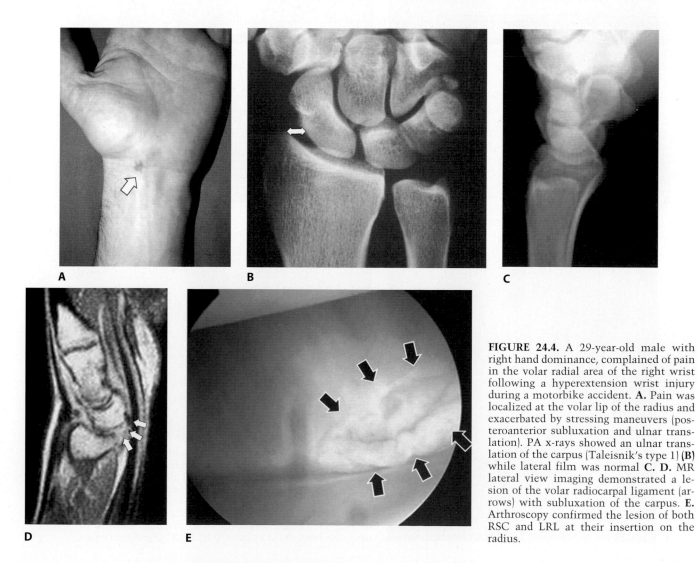

A   **B**   **C**

D   **E**

FIGURE 24.4. A 29-year-old male with right hand dominance, complained of pain in the volar radial area of the right wrist following a hyperextension wrist injury during a motorbike accident. **A.** Pain was localized at the volar lip of the radius and exacerbated by stressing maneuvers (posteroanterior subluxation and ulnar translation). PA x-rays showed an ulnar translation of the carpus (Taleisnik's type 1) **(B)** while lateral film was normal **C. D.** MR lateral view imaging demonstrated a lesion of the volar radiocarpal ligament (arrows) with subluxation of the carpus. **E.** Arthroscopy confirmed the lesion of both RSC and LRL at their insertion on the radius.

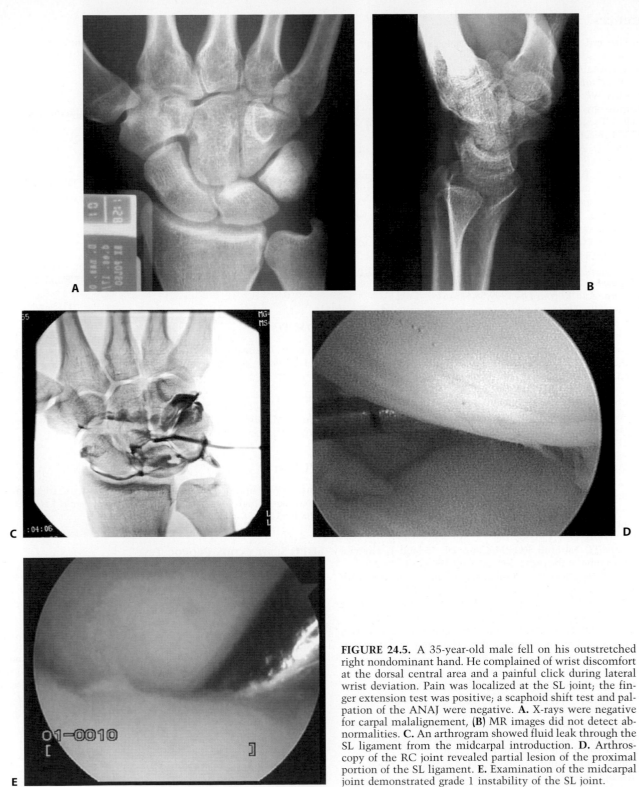

FIGURE 24.5. A 35-year-old male fell on his outstretched right nondominant hand. He complained of wrist discomfort at the dorsal central area and a painful click during lateral wrist deviation. Pain was localized at the SL joint; the finger extension test was positive; a scaphoid shift test and palpation of the ANAJ were negative. **A.** X-rays were negative for carpal malalignement, **(B)** MR images did not detect abnormalities. **C.** An arthrogram showed fluid leak through the SL ligament from the midcarpal introduction. **D.** Arthroscopy of the RC joint revealed partial lesion of the proximal portion of the SL ligament. **E.** Examination of the midcarpal joint demonstrated grade 1 instability of the SL joint.

general disorders affecting the wrist. Although it may not be exhaustive or complete, it provides a correlation between the more common disorders and the different structures forming the joint that are possible sources of intra-articular or extra-articular wrist pain. A topographic method of classification of the more commonly used clinical tests is also suggested.

Indications for both diagnostic and therapeutic arthroscopy for wrist disorders are still expanding. The asterisks in Table 24.3 mark the current best indications for arthroscopy.

References

1. Adolfsson L. Arthroscopy for the diagnosis of post-traumatic wrist pain. *J Hand Surg* 1992;17B:46–50.
2. Berger RA. Arthroscopic anatomy of the wrist and distal radioulnar joint. *Hand Clin* 1999;15:393–413.
3. Cooney WP. Evaluation of chronic wrist pain by arthrography, arthroscopy, and arthrotomy. *J Hand Surg* 1993;18A:815–822.
4. Kelly EP, Stanley JK. Arthroscopy of the wrist. *J Hand Surg* 1990;15B:236–242.
5. Mikic ZD. Age changes in the triangular fibrocartilage of the wrist joint. *J Anat* 1978;126:367–384.
6. Viegas SF, Patterson RM, Hokanson JA, et al. Wrist anatomy: incidence, distribution, and correlation of anatomic variations, tears, and arthrosis. *J Hand Surg Am* 1993;18:463–475.
7. Brown DE, Lichtman DN. The evaluation of chronic wrist pain. *Orthop Clin North Am* 1984;15:184.
8. Nagle DJ. Evaluation of chronic wrist pain. *J Am Acad Orthop Surg* 2000;8:45–55.
9. van Vugt RM, Bijlsma JWJ, van Vugt AC. Chronic wrist pain: diagnosis and management. Development and use of a new algorithm. *Ann Rheum Dis* 1999;58:665–674.
10. Nelson DL. The importance of physical examination. *Hand Clin* 1997;13(1):13–15.
11. Czitrom AA, Lister GD. Measurement of grip strength in the diagnosis of wrist pain. *J Hand Surg Am* 1988;13:16–19.
12. Hildreth DH, Breidenbach WC, Lister GD, et al. Detection of submaximal effort by use of the rapid exchange grip. *J Hand Surg Am* 1989;14:742–745.
13. Nelson DL. Additional thoughts on physical examination of the Wrist. *Hand Clin* 1997;13(1):35–37.
14. Taleisnik J. Classification of carpal instability. In: Taleisnik J, ed. *The Wrist*. New York: Churchill Livingstone, 1985, pp. 229–238.
15. Taleisnik J. Pain on the ulnar side of the wrist. *Hand Clin* 1987;3:51–68.
16. Hankin FM, White SJ, Braunstein EM. Dynamic radiographic evaluation of obscure wrist pain in the teenage patient. *J Hand Surg* 1986;11A:805–809.
17. Zinberg EM, Palmer AK. The triple-injection with arthrogram. *J Hand Surg* 1988;13A:803–809.
18. Herbert TJ, Faithfull RG, McCann DJ, Ireland J. Bilateral arthrography of the wrist. *J Hand Surg* 1990;15B:233–235.
19. Zlatkin MB, Chao PC. Chronic wrist pain: evaluation with high-resolution MR imaging. *Radiology* 1989;173:723–729.
20. Schreibman KL, Freeland A, Gilula LA, et al. Imaging of the hand and wrist. *Orthop Clin North Am* 1997;28:537–582.
21. Johnstone DJ, Thorogood S, Smith WH, Scott TD. A comparison of magnetic resonance imaging and arthroscopy in the investigation of chronic wrist pain. *J Hand Surg* 1997;22B:714–718.
22. Morley J, Bidwell J, Bransby-Zachary M. A comparison of the findings of wrist: arthroscopy and magnetic resonance imaging in the investigation of wrist pain. *J Hand Surg* 2001;26B(6):544–546.
23. Schae Del-Hoepfner M, Iwinska-Zelder J, Braus T, et al. MRI versus arthroscopy in the diagnosis of scapholunate ligament injury. *J Hand Surg* 2001;26B:17–21.
24. Whipple TL, Marotta JJ, Powell JH. Techniques of wrist arthroscopy. *Arthroscopy* 1986;2:244–252.
25. Roth JH, Haddad RG. Radiological arthroscopy and arthrography in the diagnosis of ulnar wrist pain. *Arthroscopy* 1986;2:234–243.

Suggested Readings

1CMC GRIND TEST

Swanson AB, Swanson GD. Osteoarthritis in the hand. *J Hand Surg Am* 1983;8:669–675.

2–3 CMC SHEAR TEST

Joseph RB, Linscheid RL, Dobyns JH, et al. Chronic sprains of the carpometacarpal joints, *J Hand Surg Am* 1981;6:172–180.

BALLOTTEMENT TEST

Reagan DS, Linscheid RL, Dobyns JH. Lunotriquetral sprains. *J Hand Surg Am* 1984;9:502–514.

"CATCH-UP CLUNK" (LICHTMAN'S TEST)

Lichtman DO, Schneider JR, Swafford AR, et al. Ulnar midcarpal instability of the wrist: clinical and laboratory analysis. *J Hand Surg Am* 1981;6:515–523

DERBY'S METHOD FOR LT DISSOCIATION

Burkhart SS, Wood MB, Linscheid RL. Post-traumatic recurrent subluxation of the extensor carpi ulnaris tendon. *J Hand Surg Am* 1982;7:1–3.

EDM TEST

Drury BJ. Traumatic tenosynovitis of the fifth dorsal compartment of the wrist. *Arch Surg* 1960;80:554.

EIP TEST

Spinner M, Olshansky K. The extensor indicis proprius syndrome. *Plast Reconstr Surg* 1973;51:134–138

EPL TEST

Lanzetta M, Howard M, Conolly WB. Post-traumatic triggering of extensor pollicis longus at the dorsal radial tubercle. *J Hand Surg Br* 1995;20:398–401

EUPC SUBLUXATION PROVOC TEST

Burkhart SS, Wood MB, Linscheid RL. Post-traumatic recurrent subluxation of the extensor carpi ulnaris tendon. *J Hand Surg Am* 1982;7:1–3.

FINGER EXTENSION TEST

Weinzweig J, Watson HK, Patel J, Fletcher J. The finger extension test: a reliable indicator of carpal pathology. Presentation to the 16th International Wrist Investigators' Workshop, Seattle, October 4, 2000.

FINKELSTEIN'S TEST

Finkelstein H. Stenosing tenosynovitis at the radial styloid process. *J Bone Joint Surg Am* 1930;12:509–540.

INTERSECTION SYNDROME

Wood MB, Linscheid RL. Abductor pollicis longus bursitis. *Clin Orthop* 1973;93:293–296

LT SHEAR TEST

Kleinman WB (1985): Diagnostic exams for ligamentous injuries. American Society for Surgery of the Hand, Correspondence Club Newsletter: 51

PALPATION OF ANATOMIC SNUFFBOX/ ARTICULAR-NONARTICULAR JUNCTION OF SCAPHOID (ANAJ)

Watson HK, Weinzweig J. Physical examination of the wrist. *Hand Clin* 1997;13(1):17–34

PALPATION OF EXTENSOR DIGITORUM BREVIS MANUS

Shaw JA, Manders EK. Extensor digitorum brevis manus muscle. A clinical reminder. *Orthop Res* 1988;17:867–869.

PHALEN'S TEST

Phalen GS. Spontaneous compression of the median nerve at the wrist. *JAMA* 1951;145:1128–1133

PIANO KEY TEST

Cooney WP, Bishop AT, Linscheid RL. Physical examination of the wrist. In Cooney WP, Linscheid RL, Dobyns J (eds.) *The Wrist: Diagnosis and Operative Treatment*. St. Louis: Mosby 1998, pp. 236–261.

PRESS TEST

Lester B, Halbrecht J, Levy IM, Gaudinez R. "Press test" for office diagnosis of triangular fibrocartilage complex tears of the wrist. *Ann Plast Surg* 1995;35:41–45.

RADIOCARPAL SUBLUXATION TEST

Tubiana R, Thomine JM, Mackin E. *Examination of the Hand and Wrist*. Philadelphia: Mosby, 1995, pp 185–197

SCAPHOID SHIFT (WATSON'S) MANEUVER

Watson HK, Weinzweig J. Physical examination of the wrist. *Hand Clin* 1997;13(1):17–34

SL SHEAR TEST

Dobyns J, Linscheid RL, Beabout J, et al. Traumatic instability of the wrist. AAOS Instructional Course Lectures. 1975;24:182.

TINEL'S SIGN OVER THE SENSORY BRANCH OF RADIAL NERVE (WARTENBERG'S NEURALGIA)

Lanzetta M, Foucher G. Association of Wartenberg's syndrome and De Quervain's disease: a series of 26 cases. *Plast Reconstr Surg* 1995;96(2):408–412

TRIQUETRAL IMPINGEMENT LIGAMENT TEAR (TILT) TEST

Weinzweig J, Watson HK. Triquetral impaction ligament tear [TILT] syndrome. *J Hand Surg* 1996;21B:36.

ULNOCARPAL IMPACTION TEST

Friedman SL, Palmer AK. The ulnar impaction syndrome. *Hand Clin* 1991;7:295–310.

ULNAR SNUFF BOX COMPRESSION TEST

Cooney WP, Bishop AT, Linscheid RL. Physical examination of the wrist. In Cooney WP, Linscheid RL, Dobyns J (eds.) *The Wrist: Diagnosis and Operative Treatment*. St. Louis: Mosby 1998, pp. 236–261.

Tubiana R, Thomine JM, Mackin E. *Examination of the Hand and Wrist*. Philadelphia: Mosby, 1995, pp 185–197

ULNAR STYLOID IMPACTION TEST

Topper SM, Wood MB, Ruby LK. Ulnar styloid impaction syndrome. *J Hand Surg Am* 1997;22:699–704.

Index